DIGITAL HEARING AIDS

Brad A. Stach, Ph.D.
Editor-in-Chief for Audiology

DIGITAL HEARING AIDS

JAMES M. KATES

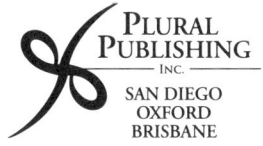

PLURAL PUBLISHING INC.
SAN DIEGO
OXFORD
BRISBANE

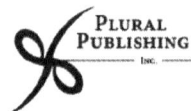

5521 Ruffin Road
San Diego, CA 92123

e-mail: info@pluralpublishing.com
Web site: http://www.pluralpublishing.com

49 Bath Street
Abingdon, Oxfordshire OX14 1EA
United Kingdom

Copyright © by Plural Publishing, Inc. 2008

Typeset in 11/13 Berkeley by John Reinhardt Book Design
Printed in the United States of America by Bang Printing

All rights, including that of translation, reserved. No part of this publication may be reproduced, stored in a retrieval system, or transmitted in any form or by any means, electronic, mechanical, recording, or otherwise, including photocopying, recording, taping, Web distribution, or information storage and retrieval systems without the prior written consent of the publisher.

For permission to use material from this text, contact us by
Telephone: (866) 758-7251
Fax: (888) 758-7255
e-mail: permissions@pluralpublishing.com

Every attempt has been made to contact the copyright holders for material originally printed in another source. If any have been inadvertently overlooked, the publishers will gladly make the necessary arrangements at the first opportunity.

ISBN-13: 978-1-59756-317-8
ISBN-10: 1-59756-317-X

Library of Congress Cataloging-in-Publication Data:
Kates, James M.
 Digital hearing aids / James M. Kates.
     p. ; cm.
  Includes bibliographical references and index.
  ISBN-13: 978-1-59756-317-8 (alk. paper)
  ISBN-10: (invalid) 1-59756-316-X (alk. paper)
  1. Hearing aids. 2. Signal processing--Digital techniques. I. Title.
 [DNLM: 1. Hearing Aids. 2. Amplifiers. 3. Analog-Digital Conversion. 4. Signal Processing, Computer-Assisted. WV 274 K19d 2008]
  RF300.K38 2008
  617.8'9—dc22

2008007416

In memory of my wife

Joanna I. Scott
(1945–2001)

Contents

Preface

1 Hearing-Aid Technology — 1

Types of Hearing Aids	1
Canal Aids	2
In-the-Ear Aids	3
Behind-the-Ear Aids	4
Open Fitting BTE Aids	4
Body-Worn Aids	4
From Analog to Digital	4
Moore's Law	6
Digital Current Drain	7
Analog and Digital Power Consumption	8
Digital Circuit Components	10
Analog-to-Digital Converter	10
Digital Signal Processor	11
Memory	12
Clock	13
Batteries	14
Concluding Remarks	15
References	16

2 Signal Processing Basics — 17

Signal and System Properties	17
Sequences	17
Linear Time Invariance	18
Convolution	19
Correlation	22
Transfer Functions	24

vii

Feedback		25
Group Delay		27
Amplitude Modulation		28
Distortion		29
Discrete Fourier Transform		30
Filters and Filter Banks		32
Filter Definitions		32
Recursive Filters		34
Nonrecursive Filters		37
Frequency Resolution and Group Delay		40
Block Processing		40
Digital System Concerns		42
Integer Arithmetic		42
Quantization Noise		43
Aliasing Distortion		46
Temporal Aliasing		46
Algorithm Complexity		47
Algorithm Interaction		48
Concluding Remarks		49
References		49
3	**The Electroacoustic System**	**51**
	Hearing Aid System	52
	Head and Ear	55
	Microphone and Receiver	61
	Vent Acoustics	62
	Acoustic Elements	63
	Vent Size	65
	Residual Ear-Canal Volume	67
	Open BTE Fitting	69
	Occlusion Effect	70
	Concluding Remarks	72
	References	72
4	**Directional Microphones**	**75**
	Hearing-Aid Microphones	76
	Microphone Construction	76
	Directional Microphones and Spatial Signal Processing	78
	Directional Response Patterns	83
	Microphone Spacing and Time Delay	83
	Microphone Mismatch	85
	Frequency Response	85

	Magnitude Frequency Response	85
	Microphone Mismatch	90
	Interaction with Vents	91
	Microphone Noise	93
	Microphones on the Head	93
	Microphone Performance Indices	98
	Front-to-Back Ratio	98
	Directivity Index	99
	Unidirectional Index	101
	The AI-DI	102
	Rooms and Reverberation	102
	Critical Distance	103
	Early Reflections	103
	Combining Noise and Reverberation	104
	Benefit in the Real World	105
	Concluding Remarks	108
	References	109
5	**Adaptive and Multimicrophone Arrays**	**113**
	Two-Microphone Adaptive Array	114
	Adaptive Delay	114
	Adaptive Gain	116
	Adaptive Filter	118
	Delay-And-Sum Beam-forming	123
	Adaptive Arrays	129
	Superdirective Arrays	133
	Widely-Spaced Arrays	136
	Array Benefits	139
	Concluding Remarks	142
	References	143
6	**Wind Noise**	**147**
	Turbulence	148
	Hearing-Aid Measurements	150
	Airflow and Turbulence	150
	Sound Pressure	155
	Signal Characteristics	158
	Spectrum	158
	Temporal Fluctuations	160
	Correlation	160
	Wind-Noise Reduction	163
	Directional Microphones	163

x   Contents

Wind Screens	164
Spectrum Algorithms	165
Correlation Algorithms	166
Adaptive Arrays	169
Concluding Remarks	171
References	172

7 Feedback Cancellation — 175

The Feedback System	176
System Equations	177
System Response	179
Gain-Reduction Solutions	185
Adaptive Feedback Cancellation	187
System Equations	188
LMS Adaptation	190
Constrained Adaptation	191
Adaptation Equations	192
Initialization	193
Simulation Results	194
Decorrelation Techniques	198
Interrupted Adaptation	199
Delay	199
Filtered-X Algorithm	199
Frequency-Domain Adaptation	203
Processing Limitations	205
Room Reflections	206
Measurement Procedure	207
Measurement Results	208
Maximum Stable Gain	212
Nonlinear Distortion	215
Concluding Remarks	216
References	217

8 Dynamic-Range Compression — 221

Does Compression Help?	222
Algorithm Design Concerns	224
Frequency Resolution	224
Processing Delay	224
Single-Channel Compression	227
Input/Output Rules	227
Volume Control	229
Envelope Detection	231

| | | Contents | xi |

	Multichannel Compression	236
	Temporal Response	236
	Swept Frequency Response	240
	Frequency-Domain Compression	242
	Ideal FFT System	242
	Practical FFT System	244
	Side-Branch Structure	246
	Frequency Warping	247
	Digital Frequency Warping	247
	Warped Compressor System	249
	System Delay Comparison	255
	Concluding Remarks	258
	References	259

9 Single-Microphone Noise Suppression 263

Properties of Speech and Noise Signals	264
Low-Level Expansion	270
Envelope Valley Tracking	272
Bandwidth Reduction	274
Adaptive High-Pass Filter	275
Adaptive Low-Pass Filter	276
"Zeta Noise Blocker"	277
Envelope Modulation Filters	278
Concluding Remarks	286
References	287

10 Spectral Subtraction 291

Noise Estimation	293
Valley Detection	293
Minima Statistics	294
Histogram	298
Wiener Filter	300
Spectral Subtraction	302
Classical Approaches	302
General Equation	304
Nonlinear Expansion	306
Ephraim-Malah Algorithm	307
Auditory Masking	309
A Fundamental Compromise	311
Algorithm Effectiveness	312
Concluding Remarks	314
References	315

xii Contents

11 Spectral Contrast Enhancement — 319

Auditory Filters in the Damaged Cochlea 320
   Physiological Measurements — 320
   Tuning Curves — 320
   Neural Firing Patterns — 321
   Perceptual Measurements — 324
Processing Strategies — 328
   Spectral Valley Suppression — 328
   Spectral Contrast Modification — 331
   Raise Spectrum to a Power — 331
   Spectral Filtering — 334
   Excess Upward Spread of Masking — 340
   F2/F1 Ratio — 341
   Processing Comparison — 342
Combining Spectral Contrast Enhancement with Compression — 345
Concluding Remarks — 348
References — 350

12 Sound Classification — 355

The Rationale for Classification — 357
Signal Features — 359
Feature Selection — 361
Mutual Information — 362
Feature Selection Using Mutual Information — 364
Classifier Algorithms — 367
Training the Classifier — 368
Types of Classifiers — 369
   Clustering — 370
   Linear Discriminant — 371
   Support Vector Machine — 372
   Neural Network — 374
   Hidden Markov Model — 377
   Bayes Classifier — 379
Personalizing the Classifier — 381
Classification Examples — 382
   Number of Features — 383
   Isolated Signals vs. Mixtures — 385
Concluding Remarks — 387
APPENDIX 12-A — 388
References — 395

13 Binaural Signal Processing — 401

The "Cocktail Party" Problem	402
Signal Transmission	404
Binaural Compression	406
Compression Using Binaural Loudness Summation	406
Auditory Efferents	409
Compression Using Auditory Efferents	410
Binaural Noise Suppression	416
Interaural Cross-Correlation	418
Binaural Wiener Filter	421
Binaural Signal Difference	423
Binaural Spectral Subtraction	425
Directional Cues	427
Localization Model	429
Dichotic Band Splitting	432
Concluding Remarks	434
References	435

Index — 441

Preface

THE HEARING AID INDUSTRY has rapidly gone from simple analog hearing aids to complex digital devices that incorporate many different signal-processing algorithms. The limited number of processing options provided in analog devices has been replaced by the ability to implement a wide variety of digital signal-processing (DSP) algorithms, and the range of adjustments has been greatly increased through sophisticated fitting software. The increase in flexibility, however, comes at a price for the audiologist or dispenser. It is now much harder to understand what is actually happening inside a hearing aid or to understand the limits on what the processing can accomplish.

My objective in writing this book is to explain the signal processing approaches used in modern digital hearing aids. I have left audiology, fitting procedures, and the design of digital hardware for other authors to cover. Although the text draws on my work for GN ReSound, my goal is to describe the principles and approaches used for different signal processing algorithms and not to dwell on any particular product or commercial implementation. I have concentrated on signal processing described in peer-reviewed articles or in the patent literature; algorithms that are described only in commercial marketing materials have been avoided because the technical explanations are generally incomplete or imprecise.

This book is intended for audiologists, hearing-aid dispensers, and graduate students in the hearing sciences. I envision the book being used in a first- or second-year graduate course in the hearing sciences or audiology. In the best of all possible worlds, this book would be used for the second semester of a two-course sequence on signal processing, with the first semester dedicated to an introductory signal processing course.

I also realize that the audience for this book may extend beyond the audiology community. For engineers conversant with digital signal processing, some of the explanations may be unnecessary or redundant, but I beg your indulgence given the intended audiology audience. I have tried to provide references to the engineering literature if more information on a particular processing approach is desired; this book is thus the starting point for exploring signal processing in hearing aids rather than the final destination.

Because this is a book about signal processing, I have assumed that the reader has some fundamental knowledge in this area and some basic mathematical skills. In Chapter 2, I review the mathematical concepts that are applied in the following chapters, and I have also provided some references to other texts that develop this basic material in more detail. In the remaining chapters, I use the minimal mathematics that I feel necessary to describe the signal processing, but in each case I have also endeavored to explain the processing in more qualitative terms so that the concepts can be grasped even if the reader is not completely comfortable with the mathematics.

The book begins in Chapter 1 with a review of the different styles of hearing aids that are available and the digital circuit components that are used to build a digital hearing aid. Basic concepts in digital signal processing are covered in Chapter 2. Chapters 3 through 7 then cover acoustics and spatial signal processing. The effects of the head, ear, and hearing-aid vent on the hearing-aid response are presented in Chapter 3. Chapter 4 describes directional microphones, and adaptive and multimicrophone arrays are treated in Chapter 5. Wind noise and algorithms designed to reduce wind noise are then presented in Chapter 6. Chapter 7 deals with acoustic feedback and feedback cancellation.

The remaining chapters deal with signal processing based on auditory physiology and perception rather than on physical acoustics. Single-channel and multichannel dynamic-range compression are covered in Chapter 8. A potpourri of single-microphone noise suppression algorithms is presented in Chapter 9, and spectral subtraction is given its own treatment in Chapter 10. Spectral modifications to improve speech intelligibility are covered in Chapter 11. Sound classification, which is used to adjust the parameters of these algorithms under different listening conditions, is presented in Chapter 12. Binaural signal processing, including dynamic-range compression and noise suppression, is described in Chapter 13, the final chapter.

This book would not have been possible without the generous support of GN ReSound. It is an enlightened company that sees the value of research and teaching, and is willing to share the knowledge of one of its people with the rest of the world. In particular, I need to thank Jos Leenen, my supervisor in Eindhoven, Laurel Christensen in Chicago, and René Mortensen in Ballerup for supporting my desire to write this book, and Henrik Schimmell for his gracious approval of this endeavor.

Many people helped with the text. Much of the material contained in this book was first presented in a graduate seminar that I taught at the University of Colorado in Boulder, and a draft of the book was subsequently used as the basis of my graduate course on digital hearing aids. I thank my students for their patience as guinea pigs in these courses. My GN ReSound colleagues Tjeerd Dijkstra, Jos Leenen, Bert de Vries, Rob de Vries, Erik van der Werf, and Alexander Ypma provided helpful comments on the chapters related to their technical expertise. My University of Colorado colleagues Kathryn Arehart and Melinda Anderson also provided useful comments. I greatly appreciate the help provided by my colleagues; those errors that remain are my own.

Hearing-Aid Technology

THE PURPOSE OF A HEARING AID is to amplify sound to overcome a hearing loss. The hearing aid is a miniature sound system that combines a microphone, amplifier, and output transducer (termed the receiver by analogy with a telephone handset). Most hearing aids available today use digital technology to process the sound, and incorporate algorithms designed to take into account the characteristics of the desired signals (e.g., speech or music) and the properties of the impaired auditory system. This chapter focuses on the physical constraints, such as size and power consumption, that are important in designing a hearing aid. The circuit components that are combined to build a digital hearing aid are also described.

Types of Hearing Aids

Hearing aids are available in several different sizes. The choice of size or style depends on factors such as the amount of amplification needed, individual vanity, and manual dexterity. The different styles commonly available for hearing aids are shown in Figure 1-1 using an illustration taken from a brochure for the ReSound Pixel™ digital product line (ReSound, 2006). Three of the hearing aids are shown worn in the ear in Figure 1-2. The illustration is, of course, designed to minimize the vis-

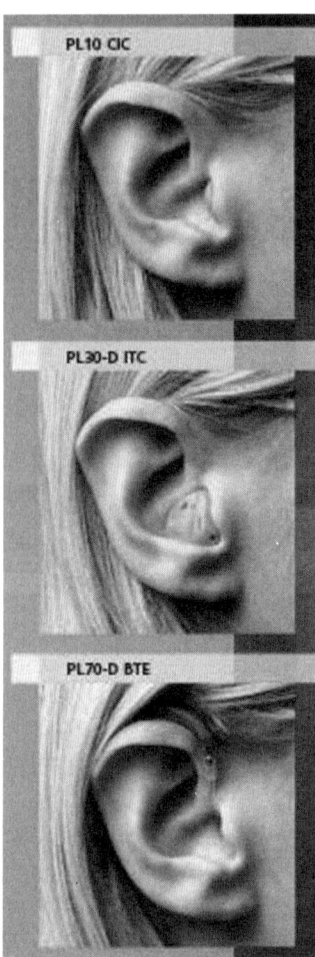

Figure 1-1. Styles of hearing aids available in the ReSound Pixel™ product line. The PL10 is a CIC instrument, the PL30 is an ITC instrument, the PL40 and PL50 are ITE instruments with small and larger shell sizes, respectively, and the PL70 is a BTE instrument.

ibility of the hearing aids, but it still gives a good sense of the differences in visibility in going from a small to a large device. The basic styles are discussed in this section in order from small to large.

CANAL AIDS

Canal aids fit entirely in the ear canal and are available in two sizes. A completely-in-the canal (CIC) hearing aid is customized to fit the size and shape of the individual ear canal. It is nearly invisible because it is seated deeply within the ear canal. However, the deep insertion can make this style of hearing aid difficult to adjust or remove. Note the cable with the ball at the end on the PL-10 devices shown in Figure 1-1; to remove the CIC hearing aid one generally grasps the ball with fingertips or fingernails and pulls on the cable as the body of the hearing aid cannot be reached.

The in-the-canal (ITC) hearing aid is somewhat larger than the CIC device. The outer surface of the ITC hearing aid generally protrudes slightly from the ear canal, which makes a CIC easier to remove than an ITC and obviates the need for the ball and pull-cable. If the target ear is small, it may not be possible to build a CIC or ITC that can hold the electronics and still fit in the ear canal. The small size of the CIC and ITC devices also makes handling them difficult, and the battery may be too small for someone with dexterity problems to be able to insert or remove. The small size of these devices also leaves only a small amount of room for the receiver, and a

Hearing Aid Technology 3

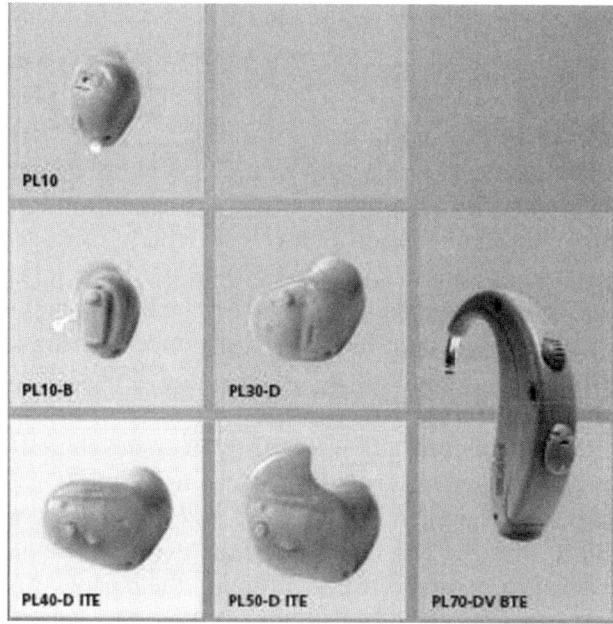

Figure 1-2. CIC, ITE, and BTE hearing aids from the ReSound Pixel™ product line shown positioned in the ear.

small receiver in turn limits the maximum power output. Thus, CIC and ITC hearing aids are most appropriate for mild to moderate-to-severe hearing losses.

IN-THE-EAR AIDS

In-the-ear (ITE) hearing aids fit completely within the outer ear. Like the CIC and ITC hearing aids, the ITE is customized to fit the individual ear. Because the ITE fills the bowl of the concha in the outer ear, it has more room for the electrical components than the CIC or ITC. Most ears that are too small for a CIC or ITC can be successfully fitted with an ITE, at the cost of the hearing aid being larger and hence more visible. The larger case, however, often leaves room for a larger receiver, so the ITE can be generally used for mild to severe hearing losses. All three types of hearing aids—CIC, ITC, and ITE—have the opening for the receiver in the ear canal, which means that the receiver can be clogged by earwax or damaged by ear drainage.

BEHIND-THE-EAR AIDS

Behind-the-ear (BTE) hearing aids house the electronics in a case that fits above and to the rear of the outer ear. A small housing can be nearly invisible when viewed from in front of the wearer, but a large housing protrudes above the ear. The output sound is generated by the receiver in the BTE case and is conducted into the ear canal through a piece of tubing. The tubing terminates in an earmold, which is a custom-molded plug that fits into the ear canal and which supports the tube. The large size of the BTE case leaves plenty of room for the battery and receiver, so BTE hearing aids can be used for mild to profound hearing losses.

OPEN FITTING BTE AIDS

A new style of BTE hearing aid has recently been developed for mild to moderate hearing losses. These new devices use a miniature BTE case that is essentially invisible from the front, and a very thin tube to conduct the sound into the ear canal. The tube diameter is small enough that the tube is also very hard to see, although the narrow tube diameter also provides some attenuation of high-frequency sounds. The tube is terminated not with an earmold, but with a soft piece of silicone that looks much like the basket at the end of a ski-pole and which is nearly transparent to sound. This open fitting provides amplification that is most appropriate for a mild to moderate hearing loss, and particularly a loss concentrated at high frequencies.

BODY-WORN AIDS

Body-worn hearing aids use a large electronics package attached to a belt or placed in a pocket. The microphone and receiver are placed in a BTE case, and the transducers are connected to the electronics package via a cable. A body aid provides the greatest possible amount of amplification, although feedback may limit the amplification achieved in practice. Body aids are typically used only for profound hearing losses.

From Analog to Digital

Hearing aids have undergone a transformation over the last decade. In 1996 a hearing aid was an analog device. It consisted of a microphone, amplifier, and receiver packaged in a case that fit behind or in the ear. The processing options available were mainly the specification of the gain-versus-frequency response built into the instrument. The same model of hearing aid would often have different internal components depending on the microphone, amplifier, and receiver chosen by the manufacturer to match the specified amplification requirement. Adjustments to the hearing-aid response were typically made with a screwdriver; potentiometers (trim-pots) were provided to give control over processing parameters such as compression threshold or output power limiting. The most advanced analog device in the marketplace provided two channels of wide dynamic-range compression.

Today hearing aids are digital devices that contain many sophisticated processing algorithms including adaptive directional microphones, feedback cancellation, multichannel dynamic-range compression, adaptive noise suppression, and spectral shaping for speech enhancement. The growth of digital hearing-aid sales is plotted in Figure 1-3. In 1996 approximately 6% of all hearing aids sold were digital (Strom, 2001). By

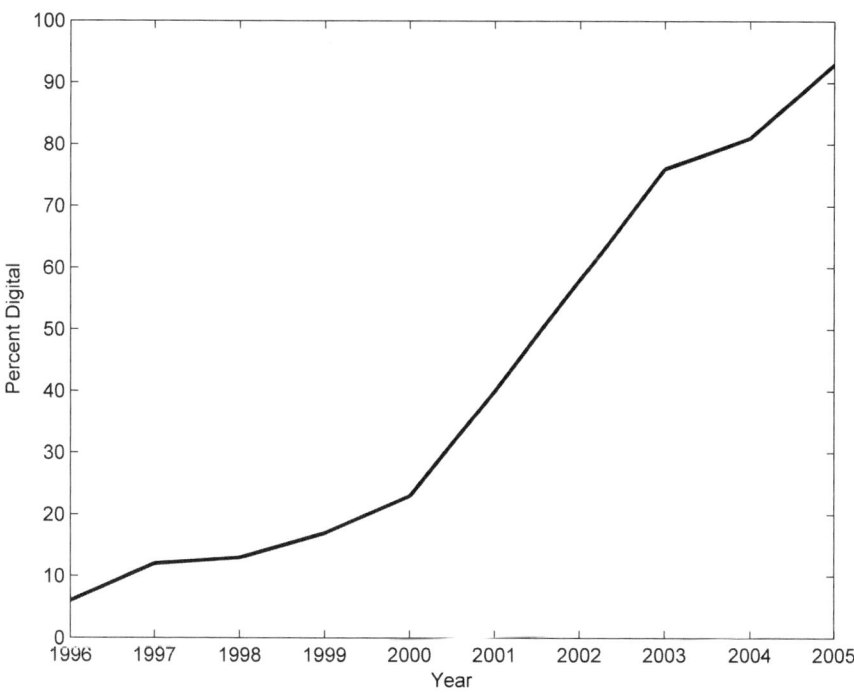

Figure 1-3. Digital hearing aids as a percent of domestic U.S. hearing-aid sales.

2005, the fraction of digital instruments had increased to 93% (Strom, 2006). Digital hearing aids were originally premium devices, but digital processing is now appearing at all price points within a manufacturer's product range. Furthermore, digital circuitry can be fitted into even very small hearing-aid shells as illustrated in Figure 1-1.

MOORE'S LAW

The advent of digital hearing aids has been fueled by the rapid advances in digital circuit manufacturing technology. Each year it is possible to put more transistors on a digital integrated circuit. Moore first observed this trend in 1965 (Moore, 1965), and predicted that the number of transistors in an integrated circuit would double every year. This observation has since come to be known as Moore's Law. In practice, circuit complexity has doubled about every 2 years, as shown on the graph of Figure 1-4. This graph shows the number of transistors used in a digital processor or computer central processing unit (CPU) over a 34-year span.

The increased integrated-circuit density comes as a result of being able to make transistors smaller. Smaller transistors require less power to operate. Thus another way of looking at Moore's Law is not in terms of increased processing complexity, but instead in terms of the reduced

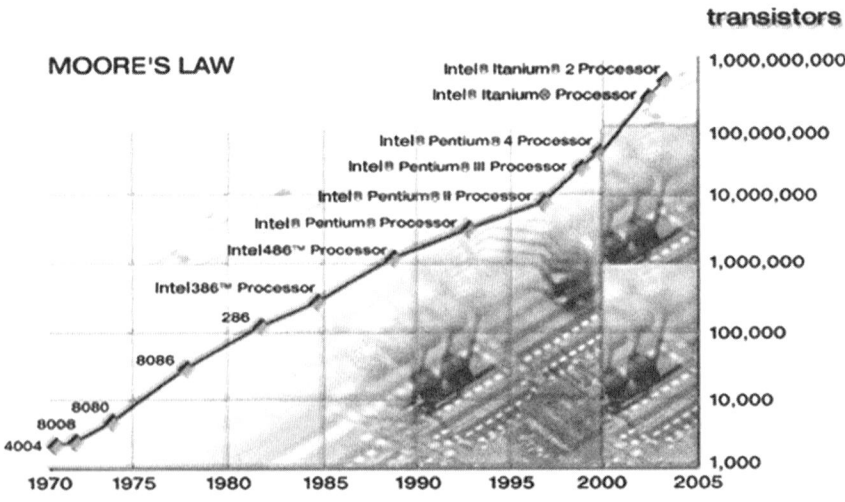

Figure 1-4. Moore's Law showing the increase in computer processor complexity over time (from Intel, 2006).

electrical power needed each year to perform a specified set of calculations (Armstrong, 2006).

Smaller transistors can be used two ways in designing a digital signal processing (DSP) circuit for a hearing aid. One can keep the integrated circuit the same size and increase the number of transistors, or one can keep the number of transistors the same and decrease the circuit size and power consumption. The basic tradeoff becomes processing complexity versus battery life, and both are important in hearing aids. Often the solution is to select a desired battery life as the target for the hearing aid, and to then design a digital processor that is consistent with that battery life.

DIGITAL CURRENT DRAIN

A battery stores a limited amount of electrical energy. The chemical reaction that occurs within the battery determines the battery voltage. The battery life then depends on the amount of power (rate of delivering energy per unit time) needed by the hearing aid. Power is the product of voltage times current. As the voltage is fixed, the power is proportional to the current needed by the hearing-aid circuit.

The current drain for a digital circuit is given by:

$$I = aC_L V_{DD} f_{clock} \quad \text{Equation (1.1)}$$

and the power consumption is given by:

$$P = IV_{DD} = aC_L V_{DD}^2 f_{clock} \quad \text{Equation (1.2)}$$

The term f_{clock} is the digital clock frequency, and V_{DD} is voltage applied to the circuit. The term C_L refers to the system load capacitance, which depends on the digital technology used to make the integrated circuit. Smaller transistors will have reduced capacitance and hence reduced power consumption. The capacitance term C_L in Eq. (1.1) is for the entire digital circuit, so it is proportional to the total number of transistors used as well as being inversely proportional to the size of the transistors. The term a refers to how often an average transistor in the circuit switches on and off, and it thus depends on the complexity of the signal-processing algorithm.

The current drain defines many of the tradeoffs in designing a digital processor for a hearing aid. A typical digital hearing aid uses 16-bit words to represent the sound samples internally. A longer word can represent a larger dynamic range with less distortion, and so would be desirable. Increasing the word size, however, will increase the number of transistors needed for fetching data from memory and for performing arithmetic. If the current consumption is to remain constant, then increasing the size of the digital words requires a reduction in the clock rate. A lower clock rate, in turn, means fewer arithmetic operations can be performed each second and would require a corresponding reduction in the algorithm complexity.

The solution to this dilemma, of course, is the continuing improvement in digital semiconductor technology. Moore's Law indicates that C_L is constantly going down, and V_{DD} is decreasing as well. Thus, each generation of digital hearing-aid circuit technology requires less power than the previous generation to perform the same operations. The continuing improvements in digital technology will lead to improvements in every aspect of digital hearing-aid circuits. Eventually, the digital circuits will be so good that it will be difficult to distinguish one hearing aid from another on the basis of the internal circuitry; the major distinction between products will be the signal-processing algorithms.

ANALOG AND DIGITAL POWER CONSUMPTION

The acceptance of digital hearing aids in the marketplace has depended on several factors, including battery life, benefit to the end user, and cost. Excessive power consumption compared to analog devices delayed the introduction of digital hearing aids compared to other types of digital electronics. The relative power consumption for analog and digital hearing aids is plotted in Figure 1-5. The power needed for analog circuits has remained relatively constant over time, whereas the power needed for digital processing has gone down over time in accordance with Moore's Law. Today power consumption no longer limits the acceptance of digital hearing aids.

The first practical digital hearing aids were released about 10 years ago. An earlier digital product was released in 1987 by Project Phoenix (Heide, 2000), but this hearing aid did not succeed in the marketplace. The digital processor was packaged in a body-worn unit that was connected to a BTE case containing the microphone and receiver. The digital processor required three batteries each the size of a quarter, and a proprietary personal computer was required to fit the hearing aid. A later version, never brought to market, fit everything into a BTE case

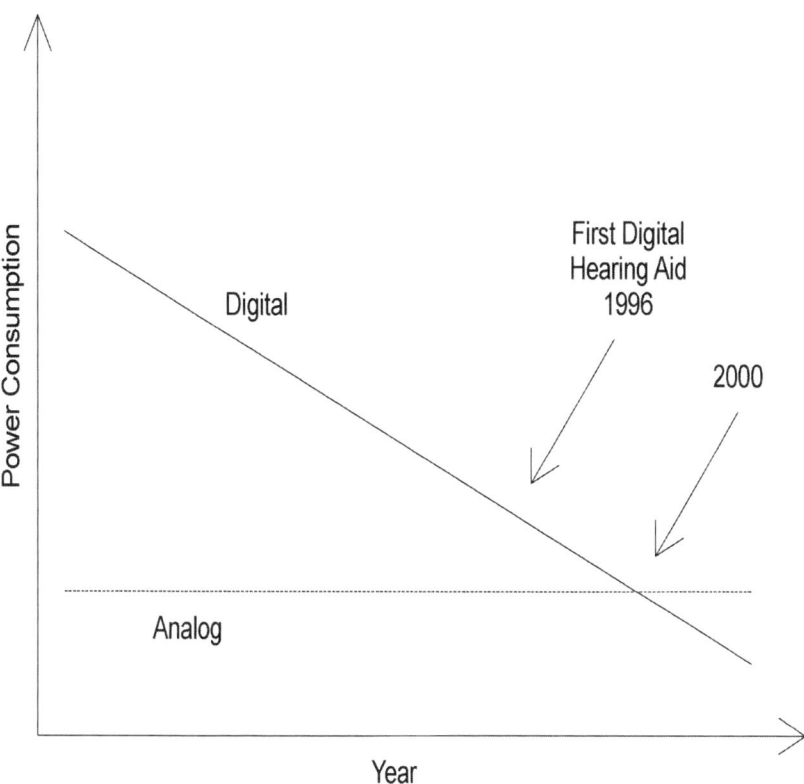

Figure 1-5. Power consumption over time for analog and digital hearing aids (after Armstrong, 2006).

and used a stack of three 675 batteries to provide the power.

The power consumption in a typical digital hearing aid is illustrated in Figure 1-6. The total current drain is about 1 mA. The microphone and analog-to-digital converter (A/D) draw about 200 µA. The digital processor, its associated memory, and the digital-to-analog converter (D/A) draw about 700 µA, and the output amplifier and receiver draw about 50 µA. Improvements in digital technology will reduce the DSP current consumption, so the limiting factor will ultimately be the current consumption of the microphone and receiver.

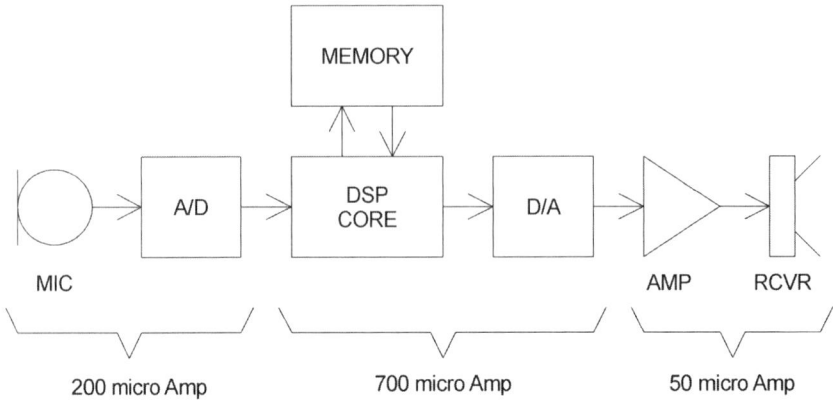

Figure 1-6. Distribution of current consumption in a programmable digital hearing aid (after Armstrong, 2006).

Digital Circuit Components

A digital hearing aid is defined more by its algorithms than by its hardware. However, the circuit components influence the performance of the overall system. In this section some of the important digital circuit components are briefly described.

ANALOG-TO-DIGITAL CONVERTER

The microphone converts the acoustic pressure fluctuations into an electrical waveform. The analog-to-digital converter converts the electrical waveform into a sequence of numbers. Two considerations are the sampling rate of the converter and the number of bits in the resulting digital sample. Many hearing aids use a sampling rate of 16 kHz and 16-bit words to represent the signal samples. The sampling rate of 16,000 samples/sec gives a bandwidth of 8 kHz, and the 16-bit word size is the same resolution as used for commercial audio CDs. These conversion parameters give good bandwidth and signal quality while minimizing the digital system power consumption.

Adding one octave, although potentially beneficial to the hearing-impaired listener (Karlsen et al., 2006), would greatly increase the hearing-aid power consumption. Increasing the sampling rate from 16 to 32 kHz, for example, would double f_{clock} in Eq. (1.2) and would approximately double the A/D converter and DSP power consumption. Thus, increased bandwidth, while desirable, will have to wait for the next generation of digital circuits to have low-enough power consumption. As explained above, increasing the digital word size would also cause a proportional increase in power consumption. In summary, current A/D and D/A characteristics are acceptable; improvements are desirable but need to be deferred to when lower power digital technology is available.

DIGITAL SIGNAL PROCESSOR

The digital processing circuit in a digital hearing aid performs all of the arithmetic operations associated with the processing algorithms. A modern computer central processing unit (CPU), such as the processor in the Microsoft Xbox 360, can operate at 6400 million instructions per second (MIPS). In contrast, the fastest processor available for a hearing aid can operate at about 8 to 16 MIPS, which is a factor 400 times slower. Thus, the signal-processing unit in a hearing aid is substantially less powerful than that found in consumer electronics devices. A personal computer can be provided with 1 to 2 Gbytes (8-bit units) of memory, whereas the processor in a hearing aid has about 4 to 8 kwords (16-bit units) available, which is a factor more than 100,000 less. The limiting factors are the size of the processor in a hearing aid, which must fit into a space much smaller than an Xbox, and the amount of power available from the small hearing-aid battery as opposed to a power supply that can be plugged into an electrical wall outlet. The processor in an Xbox draws about 20 W, whereas the processor in a hearing aid draws about 1 mW.

There are different ways to design a low-power digital signal-processing system for a hearing aid. One approach is to design the algorithm, and then design a digital processing circuit to run that algorithm and nothing else. The DSP can be optimized for the signal processing being executed, which results in the lowest possible power consumption, but it also means that the algorithm is hard wired. A new DSP circuit has to be designed whenever a change in the processing or a new algorithm is desired. The other approach is to design a general-purpose "open platform" processor, similar in concept to a computer CPU, that can be programmed to run any algorithm.

The differences in power consumption between the hardwired processor and the open platform are illustrated schematically in Figure 1-7. The vertical shift for the open platform relative to the hardwired system is approximately a factor of three in power consumption. The open plat-

12 Digital Hearing Aids

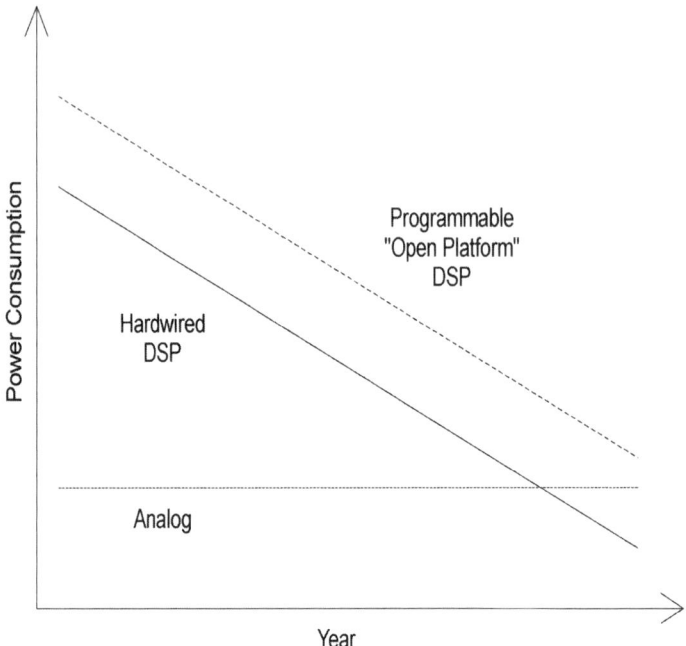

Figure 1-7. Power consumption over time for hardwired and programmable digital hearing aids (after Armstrong, 2006).

form, like a home computer, has to go through several steps in order to execute a program instruction. First it has to fetch the command from memory, then it has to decode the instruction to determine what operation should be performed, and finally it executes the instruction. The hardwired system, on the other hand, just needs to execute the instruction as everything else is predetermined. But as digital current drain continues to fall the differences in power consumption between the hardwired and open platform DSPs will become less important, and one would expect that eventually all digital hearing aids will use the open platform approach to take advantage of its processing flexibility.

MEMORY

Any digital processor needs memory to store program parameters, signal and algorithm data, and the program instructions. Several different types of memory are available that differ in their power consumption and data permanence. In a personal computer, the programs are stored on a hard disk. A program to be executed is read into memory, from which the CPU fetches the instructions to actually perform the numeric operations. A hearing aid doesn't have a hard-disk drive, so the program is stored in permanent memory called erasable programmable read-only memory (EPROM). This is the same kind of memory used in a solid-state MP3 player. The individual processing parameters are also stored in EPROM. During a fitting session for a digital hearing aid, the parameters determined for the user by the fitting software are transferred from the host computer to the EPROM in the hearing aid.

Writing data to EPROM requires a large amount of power. The battery life when recording to a portable MP3 unit is much lower than the battery life for playback. One therefore wants to use EPROM for as little data storage as possible. The incoming signal and the intermediate outputs from the various stages of signal processing do not need to be permanently stored. Once a sample is read in and processed, it is no longer needed and the memory space it used can be devoted to the next sample. These temporary values don't need to be store in EPROM, and instead are stored in random access memory (RAM). RAM requires much less power than EPROM, and is used for all temporary data storage.

A third form of memory, read-only memory (ROM), requires even less power than RAM. The problem is that one can read from ROM but cannot write to it. ROM is useless for the signal samples as these are constantly changing. However, portions of the DSP program can be stored in ROM and accessed as needed. The processing parameters are determined for each hearing-aid user and the signal samples are constantly changing, but there are program sections that are used over and over again and which are needed no matter what algorithm is being executed. For example, many algorithms want amplitude in dB rather than the linear amplitude of the input samples. A program segment that converts from linear to dB can therefore be written in advance and stored in ROM, where it can be accessed whenever it is needed. Using ROM reduces the power relative to RAM, and results in no loss of programming flexibility as the program in ROM can just be ignored if it is not needed.

CLOCK

Nearly every digital system contains a clock. The clock provides a high-frequency digital signal that controls the movement of data from one location to the next and provides the timing for the arithmetic operations and data conversion operations. As the clock frequency is not perfect, it has a small variation, termed jitter. The clock jitter means that the samples returned by the A/D converter, for example, will not be exactly uniformly spaced but instead will have some variation in the sample spacing. This variation in the sample timing is equivalent to an internal noise source, and degrades the effective signal-to-noise ratio (SNR) of the system. Thus, an ideal 16-bit A/D converter has a SNR of 107 dB, but a real A/D converter in a hearing aid will have a SNR less than 107 dB due to the clock jitter.

Batteries

The complexity of the DSP circuit is limited by the amount of power that can be supplied by the battery in the hearing aid. Hearing-aid batteries come in several different sizes, and Zinc-Air is the dominant battery technology. Batteries are compared to some common sources of energy in Table 1-1. A battery does not produce energy; rather, it stores energy produced by another source and then releases that energy in a controlled chemical reaction. The nature of the reaction determines the output voltage of the battery.

The Zinc-Air battery has the highest energy density of the technologies shown, but it still lags far behind common fuels such as Diesel fuel or gasoline. Rechargeable batteries, such as NiMH, have a much lower energy density than Zinc-Air. A NiMH battery, for example, would have

TABLE 1-1. Energy Density of Some Common Fuels and Batteries

Energy Source	Energy Density, Watt-Hours/mL
Diesel Fuel	10.7
Gasoline	9.7
Ethanol	6.1
Zinc-Air Battery	1.3
Silver Oxide Battery	0.5
NiMH Battery (AA)	0.3
NiCD Battery (AA)	0.1

TABLE 1-2. Comparison of Zinc-Air Hearing-Aid Batteries /TFN/(Data from Energizer)

Battery Size	Diameter, mm	Height, mm	Weight, g	Capacity, mAh
10	5.8	3.6	0.3	90
312	7.9	3.6	0.5	160
13	7.9	5.4	0.8	280
675	11.6	5.4	1.9	640

to be about three to four times larger than a Zinc-Air cell to provide the same amount of energy, assuming that the battery technology optimized for AA cells can be adapted to the smaller battery sizes used in hearing aids.

The common sizes of Zinc-Air hearing-aid batteries are compared in Table 1-2 compiled from the Energizer web site. Zinc-Air batteries provide a 1.4-V output. The battery capacity is measured in milli-Ampere hours (mAh). A size-10 battery, for example, can provide a current of 1 mA for a total of 90 hours, or a current of 1.5 mA for 60 hours. A typical goal in designing a hearing aid is to get at least 50 hours of operation before the battery needs to be replaced, so even the tiny size 10 Zinc-Air cell has sufficient energy to power a CIC or open-fitting BTE device.

The battery can be modeled as an ideal voltage source in series with a resistor that limits the maximum amount of current that can be delivered. If a high output level is demanded by the processing, the battery may not be able to supply the current needed to drive the receiver and the battery voltage will drop. The reduction in the battery voltage can affect all of the other circuits in the hearing aid, including the A/D and D/A converters and the DSP unit. As a result, high current demands may cause momentary bursts of distortion. This distortion can be reduced by incorporating protection circuits in the hearing aid.

Concluding Remarks

Ten years ago digital hearing aids were just beginning to penetrate the marketplace. The dominant technology was analog instruments adjusted with a screwdriver. Today the vast majority of hearing aids sold are digital. Hearing-aid manufacturers now produce systems with digital signal processing in the hearing aid adjusted through fitting software in a host computer. This chapter provided a brief review of the size, power, and circuit concerns that impact the design of digital signal processing for hearing aids. The remaining chapters focus on the signal processing and algorithms that have been proposed or implemented in digital hearing aids.

The challenge in designing a hearing aid is to fit the largest possible amount of signal processing into the smallest possible package. Hearing aids are a specialized product. The computer circuits designed for mainstream consumer electronics applications are, in general, too large and draw too much power to be used in hearing aids. However, the same technology advances that drive the progress in consumer electronics are also applicable to hearing aids. But the small size and low power requirements of hearing aids mean that the processing capability available in hearing aids will always lag several years behind what is available in mainstream consumer applications. Nonetheless, there has been a tremendous increase in the kinds of signal processing available in hearing aids and in the ability to fit the processing parameters to the individual user.

References

Armstrong, S. (2006). *Hearing aid algorithms*. American Audiology Society 2006 meeting, Scottsdale, AZ, March 7, 2006.

Heide, V. (2000). Historical perspective on digital hearing aids: The Nicolet Phoenix. *Audible Difference*. http://www.audible-difference.com/Articles/ProjectPhoenix.htm.

Intel. (2006). http://www.intel.com/technology/silicon/mooreslaw/

Karlsen, B. L., Flynn, M. C., & Eneroth, K. (2006). *The benefit of high-frequency bandwidth for hearing-impaired people under speech-in-noise conditions*. International Hearing Aid Conference, Lake Tahoe, CA, Aug. 16 to 20, 2006.

Moore, G. E. (1965). Cramming more components onto integrated circuits. *Electronics, 38*(8), 114–117.

ReSound. (2006). *ReSound Pixel™ Product Brochure*. No. MK600315 Rev. A. GN ReSound North America.

Strom, K. E. (2001). Hearing instrument dispensing in 2000: The HR dispenser survey. *Hearing Reviews, 8*(6), 20–42.

Strom, K. E. (2006). The HR 2006 dispenser survey. *Hearing Reviews 13*(6), 16–38.

2
Signal Processing Basics

THIS CHAPTER PRESENTS some basic signal processing principles that will be used in subsequent chapters. This chapter is not meant to be a replacement for a course in signal processing, but rather provides a brief review of some basic concepts that will be used throughout the book. Most of the algorithms described in this book are digital, and so this chapter emphasizes digital signal-processing concepts.

Many textbooks are available on signal processing. For an introduction to signal processing intended for the speech and hearing sciences, the reader is referred to Hartmann (2004) and Dillon (2001). More mathematical detail on digital signal processing is provided by Lyons (1996) and McClellen et al. (1997), and comprehensive engineering treatments can be found in Oppenheim et al. (1999) and Lathi (2004).

Signal and System Properties

SEQUENCES

In an analog system, a continuous-time input signal is processed to produce a continuous-time output signal. In a digital system, signal samples are processed. The signal is sampled at discrete time intervals, with each sample represented by a number. In a digital hearing aid having a 16-kHz sampling frequency, for example, the incoming signal is sampled at a rate of 16,000 times a second, or 16 times each msec. The digital signal is thus a sequence of numbers, denoted by x(n) where n is the sample index. The numbers used for the digital sequence may be continuously valued, or they may be quantized to a limited set of allowable values.

There are several sequences that are often used in digital signal processing. One is the unit impulse, or unit-sample sequence, denoted by δ(n), where

$$\delta(n) = \begin{cases} 1, & n = 0 \\ 0, & n \neq 0 \end{cases} \quad \text{Equation (2.1)}$$

The unit impulse is therefore 1 for n = 0, and all other samples are set to 0. The unit impulse has a flat frequency response (equal power at all frequencies) and zero phase shift.

Another useful sequence is the sinusoid, given by

$$x(n) = \cos(\omega n + \varphi) \quad \text{Equation (2.2)}$$

where ω is the frequency of the sinusoid in radians/sec and φ is the phase angle in radians. For a signal sampled at f_s samples/sec, the digital frequency is given by:

$$\omega = 2\pi f / f_s \quad \text{Equation (2.3)}$$

where f is the frequency of the equivalent continuous-time sinusoid. For example, if the digital system has a sampling frequency of 16 kHz, a sinusoid at a analog frequency of 1.6 kHz would have a digital frequency of ω = 2π(1.6/16) = 0.2π. From the Nyquist sampling theorem, the highest frequency that can be represented in a digital system is $f_{max} = f_s/2$, which results in ω ≤ π.

LINEAR TIME INVARIANCE

Linear time invariance in an analog system and linear shift invariance in a digital system are closely related concepts. Let $y_1(n)$ be the digital system output for the input $x_1(n)$, and let $y_2(n)$ be the system output for the input $x_2(n)$. For a linear system, the input sequence $ax_1(n) + bx_2(n)$ will yield the output $ay_1(n) + by_2(n)$. That is, the output of a linear system excited by a weighted sum of input signals is the weighted sum of the outputs due to each signal separately. If the input is doubled in amplitude, for example, the output will be doubled as well. If a linear system is excited by a sinusoid, it will have an output only at the frequency of the input. The amplitude and phase of the sinusoid will typically be changed by the linear system, but there will be no outputs at any other frequencies (including 0 Hz).

Linearity is particularly important for a system excited by a combination of sinusoids. Assume that the system output to a sinusoid at a given frequency is known. Adding a sinusoid at a second frequency to the system input will produce an additional output at this second frequency, but will not affect the amplitude or phase of the output at the frequency of the first sinusoid. The output at each frequency can be determined separately and the outputs added together. Thus, the output for a complicated signal is the sum of outputs for each individual frequency component. If the input is a combination of sinusoids at several different frequencies, only those frequencies will be present in the output as a linear system cannot have any output at a frequency that is not present in the input.

Shift invariance means that the same output is obtained whenever an identical input is applied to the system. If $y(n)$ is the system output for the input $x(n)$, then $y(n-m)$ will be the output for the input $x(n-m)$ which has been delayed by m samples. A delay of m samples in the input results in a delay of m samples in the output, and the output is not changed in any other way. Furthermore, the system does not change over time. A hearing aid that has the same frequency response no matter what the input signal level or when the signal is applied to the system is a linear shift-invariant system. A hearing aid with dynamic-range compression, however, has a gain that changes over time depending on the incoming signal characteristics and the past input samples; the compression hearing aid is therefore neither linear nor shift invariant. If the gain changes slowly over time, however, then the system can modeled as a linear system over those periods of time where the gain-versus-frequency characteristic remains essentially constant.

CONVOLUTION

A linear system can be characterized in the time domain by its impulse response. The impulse response $h(n) = \exp(-0.25n)$, $0 \leq n \leq 9$ for a filter is plotted sample-by-sample in Figure 2-1A. The response starts at

20 Digital Hearing Aids

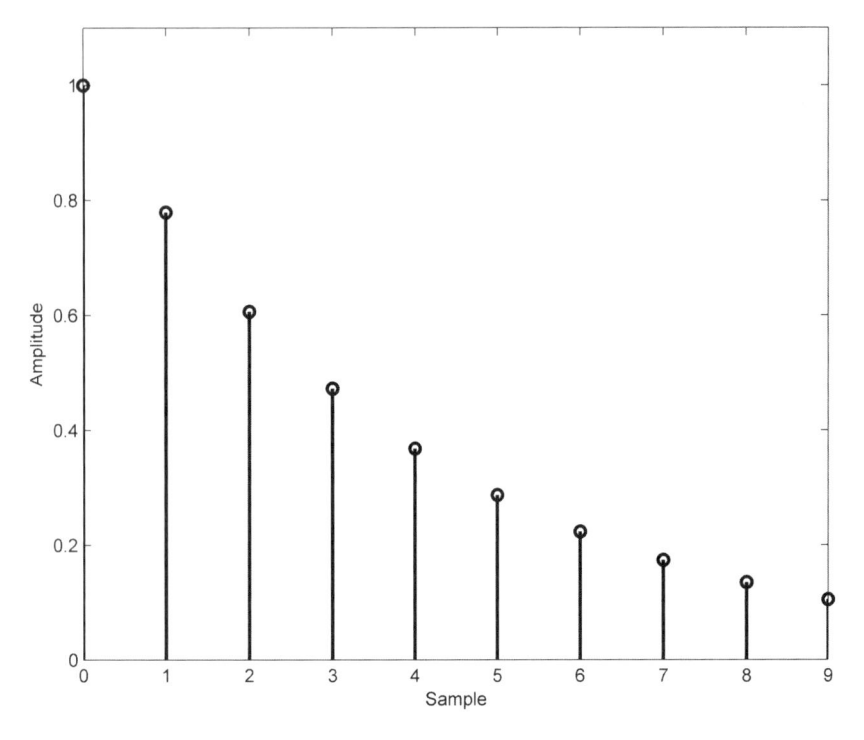

Figure 2-1A. Impulse response of a filter.

sample $n = 0$, and is zero for all earlier samples. Let $x(n)$ be the sequence input to this filter, and let $y(n)$ be the output sequence. If $x(n)$ is the unit impulse $\delta(n)$, then the output $y(n) = h(n)$. Exciting a system with a unit impulse reproduces the system impulse response by definition.

Now let $x(n)$ be a sequence consisting of many samples, each having an amplitude a_n. The sequence $x(n)$ can be written in terms of unit impulses as:

$$x(n) = a_0 \delta(n) + a_1 \delta(n-1) + a_2 \delta(n-2) + \ldots \quad \text{Equation (2.4)}$$

Each term in the sequence represents a weighted unit impulse at delays of 0, 1, 2,... samples and so on for the length of the sequence $x(n)$. A shorthand way to write the sequence $x(n)$ is:

$$x(n) = \sum_{l=0}^{L-1} a_m \delta(n-l) \quad \text{Equation (2.5)}$$

The capital Greek sigma denotes the summation over the terms that follow, and the sequence $x(n)$ is assumed to consist of L samples numbered from $l = 0$ to $l = L-1$.

The system response to the first sample of $x(n)$ is:

$$y_0(n) = a_0 h(n) \quad \text{Equation (2.6)}$$

the system response to the second sample of $x(n)$ is:

$$y_1(n) = a_1 h(n-1) \quad \text{Equation (2.7)}$$

and the response to the third sample of $x(n)$ is:

$$y_2(n) = a_2 h(n-2) \quad \text{Equation (2.8)}$$

The complete system output is the summation of the outputs for each sample of $x(n)$:

$$y(n) = \sum_{l=0}^{L-1} y_l(n) \quad \text{Equation (2.9)}$$

Substituting the terms given in Eqs. (2.6–2.8) into Eq. (2.9) leads to:

$$y(n) = \sum_{l=0}^{L-1} x(l) h(n-l) \quad \text{Equation (2.10)}$$

The mathematical operation indicated by the summation of Eq. (2.10) is termed convolution. Convolution gives the output sequence that results when an input sequence is passed through a linear system. If the input sequence comprises L samples, and the filter impulse response is M samples, then the length of the convolution output is $L+M-1$ samples.

For example, consider the filter impulse response $h(n)$ plotted in Figure 2-1A. The filter impulse response comprises $M = 10$ samples. Let the input to the filter be the sequence $x(n) = [1, 1, 1]$, so the input sequence length $L = 3$. This input sequence is plotted in Figure 2-1B. The convolution of $x(n)$ with $h(n)$ is the sequence $y(n)$ plotted in Figure 2-1C. The length of the filtered output is $10 + 3 - 1 = 12$ samples.

22 Digital Hearing Aids

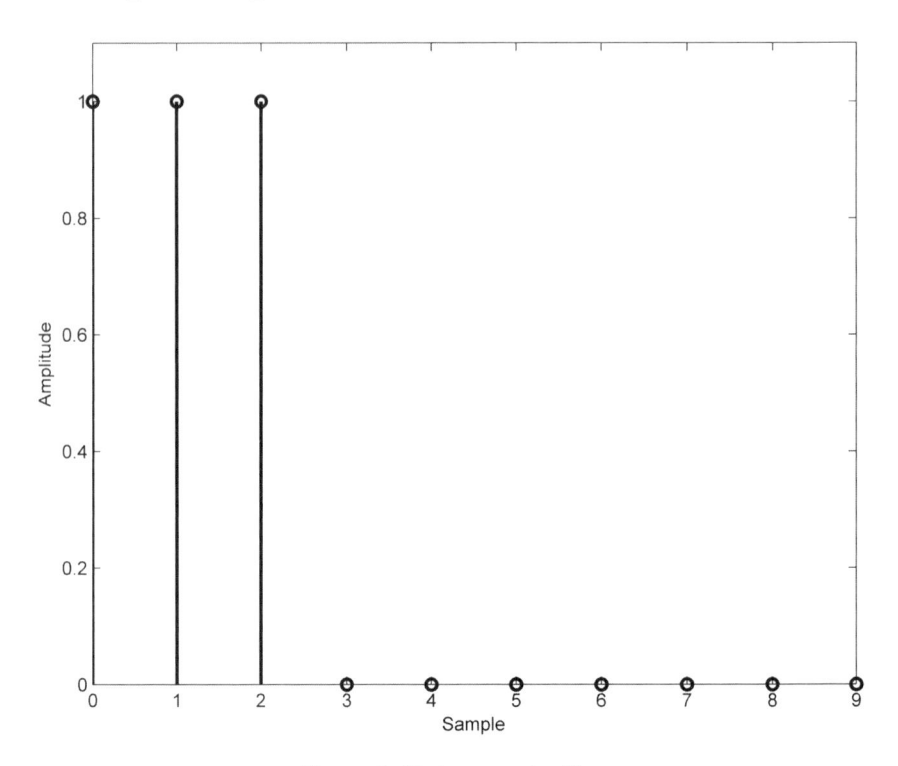

Figure 2-1B. Input to the filter.

CORRELATION

Correlation is the operation of multiplying two signals together to form their product, and then summing the samples in the resulting sequence. Correlation compares a signal with itself or with another signal. If the signal $x(n)$ is compared with itself, the result is its autocorrelation function. If $x(n)$ is compared with a different signal $y(n)$, the result is the cross-correlation function.

For the autocorrelation function, the sequence $x(n)$ is multiplied by shifted versions of itself. The autocorrelation operation is given by (Rabiner & Gold, 1975):

$$R_{xx}(n) = \frac{1}{M} \sum_{m=0}^{M-1} x(m)x(m+n) \quad \text{Equation (2.11)}$$

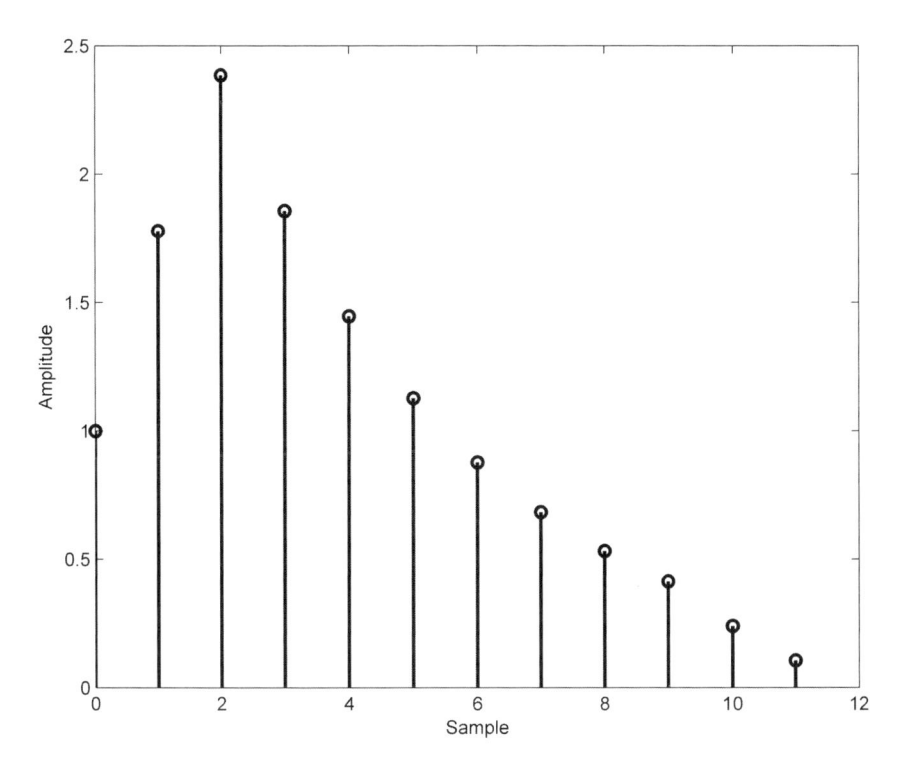

Figure 2-1C. The filter output sequence is the convolution of the input with the filter impulse response.

The autocorrelation term at zero delay, $R_{xx}(0)$, gives the mean-square value of the sequence $x(n)$. The zero-delay term is always the largest term of the autocorrelation function. If $x(n)$ is a periodic signal, then the autocorrelation function will have the same period as $x(n)$ and the value at the periodic peaks will be the same as at zero delay. In the special case of $x(n) = cos(\omega n + \varphi)$, the autocorrelation function is $R_{xx}(n) = cos(\omega n)$. If $x(n)$ is white noise, then $R_{xx}(0)$ gives the mean-square energy in the noise sequence and the remaining samples are all zero. The autocorrelation function also has even symmetry, that is, $R_{xx}(-n) = R_{xx}(n)$.

For the cross-correlation function, the sequence $x(n)$ is compared with shifted versions of the sequence $y(n)$. The cross-correlation operation is given by:

$$R_{xx}(n) = \frac{1}{M} \sum_{m=0}^{M-1} x(m) y(m+n) \quad \text{Equation (2.12)}$$

24 Digital Hearing Aids

If x(n) and y(n) are periodic and have the same period, then $R_{xy}(n)$ will also be periodic with that period. If x(n) and y(n) are periodic but have different periods, then $R_{xy}(n) = 0$. If x(n) and y(n) are statistically independent, for example, separate white noise sequences, then $R_{xy}(n) = 0$ as well.

TRANSFER FUNCTIONS

A linear system has output only at those frequencies present in the input. The output for a sinusoid will be a sinusoid at the same frequency, but which may have amplitude and phase shifts. For an input signal $x(n) = a_1 cos(\omega n + \varphi_1)$, the output will be $y(n) = a_2 cos(\omega n + \varphi_2)$. The signal has undergone an amplitude change a_2/a_1 and a phase shift $\varphi_2 - \varphi_1$. These amplitude and phase shifts will occur for each frequency present in the input signal, and may be different at each frequency. The net effect at all frequencies can be represented in the frequency domain as $Y(f) = H(f)X(f)$, where $X(f)$ is the input signal described as its amplitude and phase at each frequency f, $Y(f)$ is the output signal, and $H(f)$ is the transfer function that represents the system amplitude and phase shift as a function of frequency. The magnitude and phase angle of $Y(f)$ are given by:

$$|Y(f)| = |H(f)||X(f)| \quad \text{Magnitude}$$
$$\angle Y(f) = \angle H(f) + \angle X(f) \quad \text{Phase angle}$$

Equation (2.13)

The effects of transfer functions in series are cumulative. Figure 2-2 shows two systems in series (also termed in cascade). $Y_1(f)$ is the output of system 1 for the input $X(f)$, and is given by:

$$Y_1(f) = H_1(f)X(f) \quad \text{Equation (2.14)}$$

$Y_2(f)$ is the output of system 2 for the input $Y_1(f)$, and is given by:

$$Y_2(f) = H_2(f)Y_1(f) \quad \text{Equation (2.15)}$$

Eq. (2.14) can then be substituted for $Y_1(f)$ in Eq. (2.15), giving the output for the two systems in cascade:

$$Y_2(f) = H_1(f)H_2(f)X(f) \quad \text{Equation (2.16)}$$

```
X(f) ──→ │ H₁(f) │ ──Y₁(f)──→ │ H₂(f) │ ──→ Y₂(f)
```

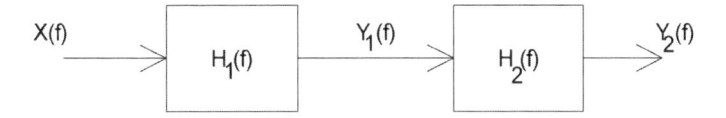

Figure 2-2. Block diagram showing two transfer functions in series.

The transfer function for two or more systems in cascade is therefore the product of the separate transfer functions for each system. The magnitudes are multiplied together, and the phase angles are summed.

Figure 2-3 shows several transfer functions in parallel. The output for the kth transfer function is given by:

$$V_k(f) = X(f)H_k(f) \quad \text{Equation (2.17)}$$

The total system output is then:

$$Y(f) = \sum_{k=1}^{K} V_k(f) = X(f)\sum_{k=1}^{K} H_k(f) \quad \text{Equation (2.18)}$$

The transfer function for two or more systems in parallel is therefore the sum of the separate transfer functions for each system. Note that the sum of the transfer functions is not simply the sum of their magnitudes but is also affected by their phase angles. Consider a parallel combination of two transfer functions. If one transfer function has a magnitude of 1 and a phase angle of 0 degrees, and the second transfer function has a magnitude of 1 but a phase angle of 180 degrees, then the two outputs will cancel each other to produce an output of zero.

FEEDBACK

Feedback is an important aspect of the hearing aid system. In acoustic feedback, for example, the sound generated by the receiver in the ear canal leaks back to the microphone and is combined with the input signal. Figure 2-4 shows a feedback system, in which the output signal $Y(f)$ is filtered by the feedback path function $G(f)$ and recombined with the input signal $X(f)$. The system can be described by the pair of equations:

$$Y(f) = S(f)H(f) \quad \text{Equation (2.19)}$$

26 Digital Hearing Aids

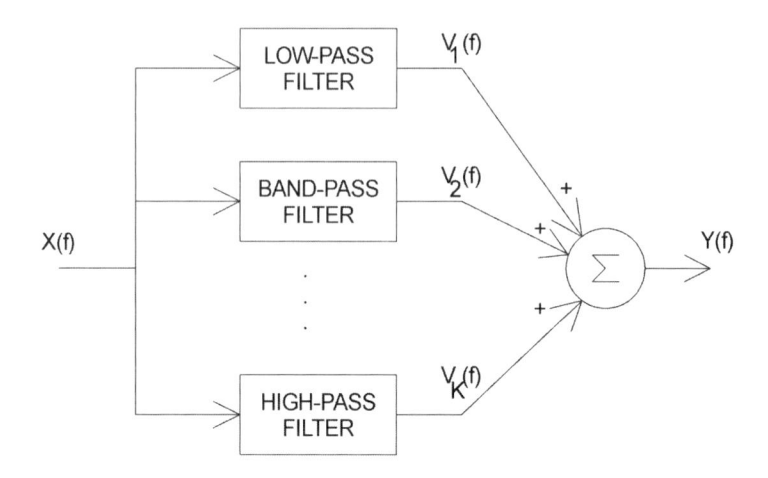

Figure 2-3. Block diagram of a multichannel filter bank showing the input signal X(f), the set of filters, and the filter outputs combined to form the system output Y(f).

and

$$S(f) = X(f) + Y(f)G(f) \quad \text{Equation (2.20)}$$

Substituting Eq. (2.19) for S(f) in Eq. (2.20) leads to:

$$\frac{Y(f)}{H(f)} = X(f) + Y(f)G(f) \quad \text{Equation (2.21)}$$

Solving Eq. (2.21) for Y(f) then gives:

$$Y(f) = X(f)\frac{H(f)}{1 - H(f)G(f)} \quad \text{Equation (2.22)}$$

If the feedback path is blocked off, that is $G(f) = 0$, then Eq. (2.22) reduces to the system $Y(f) = X(f)H(f)$. However, if at some frequency $H(f)G(f) = 1$, then the denominator of Eq. (2.22) becomes zero and the system response will become infinite. The feedback system becomes unstable. If $H(f)$ is the desired frequency response of the hearing aid, then

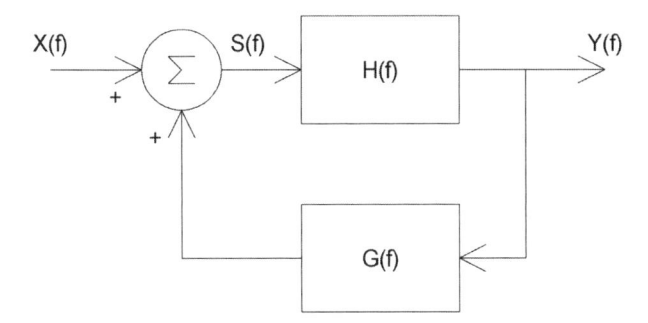

Figure 2-4. Block diagram of system with feedback. A filtered version of the output Y(f) is added back to the input X(f).

the denominator of Eq. (2.22) modifies that response and can produce undesired frequency-response peaks when $H(f)G(f) \approx 1$. Note that for the system to become unstable, the magnitude of the product $H(f)G(f)$ must equal 1 and the summed phase response of the two transfer functions in series must be zero.

GROUP DELAY

Group delay is related to the phase response of a linear system. The group delay is defined as the negative of the first derivative with respect to frequency of the transfer-function phase response. Group delay corresponds to the amount of time it takes a tone burst to propagate through a system. An example of the system group delay is shown in Figure 2-5.

A minimum-phase system is one that has the shortest possible group delay for a given magnitude frequency response. In a minimum-phase system, the group delay is related to the slope of the magnitude frequency response; the steeper the slope, the greater the delay. Analog systems tend to be minimum-phase, so response peaks in an analog hearing aid will be associated with large amounts of group delay because of the steep slopes of the response on either side of the peak. Similarly, a low-pass or high-pass filter with a steep slope will have a greater group delay, especially in the region surrounding the cutoff frequency, than a filter having a shallow slope. Group delay also influences other aspects of signal processing, and an example for feedback cancellation described in Chapter 7.

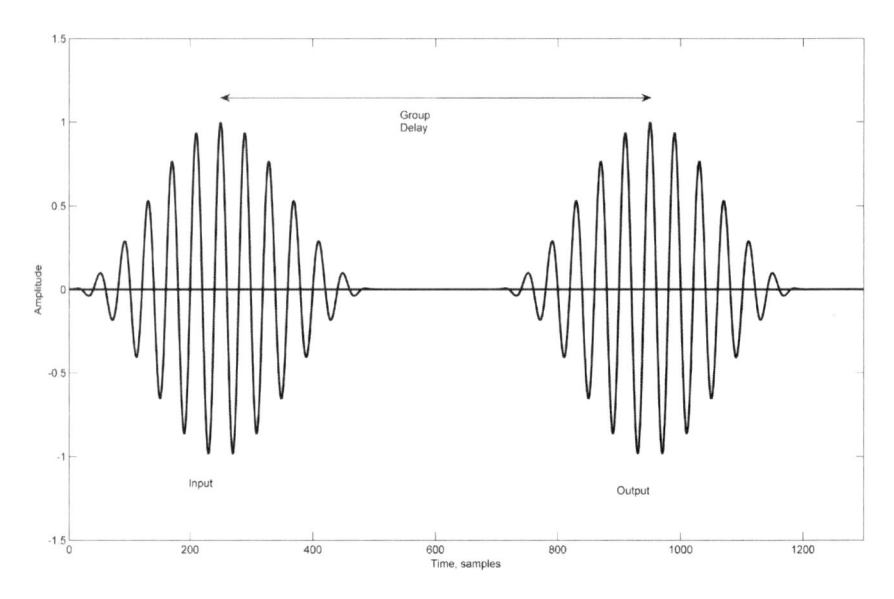

Figure 2-5. Group delay relationship for system output and input.

The basic principle of greater group delay associated with steeper filter slopes also applies to minimum-phase digital systems. However, in a digital system it is also possible to compensate for the variation of group delay with frequency and create a system with the same time delay at all frequencies. Such a system is called a linear-phase system. But nothing comes for free in signal processing, and a linear-phase system will always have a longer delay than a minimum-phase system realizing the same magnitude frequency response.

AMPLITUDE MODULATION

Speech can be modeled as the output of a bank of band-pass filters, where the signal in each frequency band is represented as a tone at a carrier frequency modulated by the speech envelope. The carrier is given by the sinusoid:

$$c(n) = cos(\omega_c n) \quad \text{Equation (2.23)}$$

at the digital carrier frequency ω_x. The modulated signal is then given by

$$x(n) = [1 + a(n)]\cos(\omega_c n) \quad \text{Equation (2.24)}$$

where $a(n)$ is the amplitude modulation waveform (Peebles, 1976).

A useful case to consider is when the modulation $a(n)$ is a sinusoid at a lower frequency than the carrier. For this case, the modulated signal is

$$x(n) = [1 + m\cos(\omega_m n)]\cos(\omega_c n) \quad \text{Equation (2.25)}$$

where ω_m is the modulation frequency and m is the modulation depth, $m \leq 1$. Expanding the trigonometric identity for the product of the cosines yields

$$x(n) = \cos(\omega_c n) + \frac{1}{2}m\{\cos[(\omega_c + \omega_m)n] + \cos[(\omega_c - \omega_m)n]\}$$

Equation (2.26)

The result of the amplitude modulation is therefore a spectrum that consists of a component at the carrier frequency having an amplitude of 1, plus two sidebands at the sum and difference frequencies each having an amplitude of $m/2$. For example, if the carrier were at 1 kHz and the modulation frequency were 50 Hz, then the sidebands would be at 950 and 1050 Hz.

DISTORTION

The term distortion has been used in different ways by different authors. One use is for distortion to mean any deviation from a flat system frequency response. A high-frequency boost, given this usage, would represent distortion (sometimes termed linear distortion). In this book, however, distortion will never be used to describe the output of a linear transformation. Distortion will be used only to mean the results of a nonlinear operation. In a linear system there can be output only at the frequencies of the input signal; in a system with nonlinear distortion, there will be output at other frequencies as well. For example, consider a system having as an input a sinusoid at 100 Hz. If the system is purely linear, there will be output at only 100 Hz. A nonlinear system will have outputs at other frequencies as well, most often at multiples of the input frequency (e.g., harmonic distortion). If the input to a nonlinear system is two sinusoids, then there may also be distortion components at the sum and difference frequencies (e.g., intermodulation distortion).

The transfer function specifies the output amplitude and phase at each frequency of the input. The amplitude and phase of the distortion products cannot be specified as a linear transformation of the input signal as the distortion product frequencies were not present in the input. Therefore, the concept of the transfer function cannot be applied to systems that have nonlinear distortion. In practice, every system tends to have small amounts of nonlinear distortion, but these small amounts of distortion are typically ignored in calculating the transfer function if the system behavior is predominantly linear.

Discrete Fourier Transform

The frequency content of a data segment is often analyzed using a Fourier transform. The fast Fourier transform (FFT) is an algorithm for the efficient computation of the discrete Fourier transform (DFT). Many different procedures can be used to calculate the DFT, all of which yield the same frequency analysis of the digital signal. The DFT is computed for a signal segment. If the segment consists of N samples, then the DFT will consist of N values. These N values comprise the component at 0 Hz (termed the DC—direct current—component), the component at the Nyquist frequency, and pairs of components at each of ($N/2-1$) uniformly spaced intermediate frequencies. For example, assume that the digital signal is sampled at 16 kHz, and the segment of the signal being analyzed is 64 samples long. There will be DFT components at 0 Hz and the Nyquist frequency of 8 kHz. The remaining DFT components will be spaced at multiples of 8000/32 = 250 Hz, which gives the frequency spacing of the FFT. Whereas a frequency analysis would be represented by $X(f)$, where f is the continuous frequency variable, the DFT is denoted by $X(k)$, where k is the analysis bin index from 0 through $N/2$.

The pairs of intermediate frequency DFT values each comprise a cosine term and a sine term. The cosine term is the real value, and the sine term is the imaginary value, based on calculus that is beyond the scope of this book. The real and imaginary values are given by

Signal Processing Basics

$$X_{real}(k) = \sum_{n=0}^{N-1} x(n)\cos\left(\frac{2\pi nk}{N}\right)$$

$$X_{imag}(k) = -\sum_{n=0}^{N-1} x(n)\sin\left(\frac{2\pi nk}{N}\right)$$

Equation (2.27)

The DFT calculation is thus equivalent to computing the correlation of the signal segment with a set of sinusoids. The frequency of each sinusoid is a multiple of the fundamental frequency determined by the inverse of the segment size. The energy in the signal segment at any given frequency is:

$$|X(k)|^2 = X_{real}^2(k) + X_{imag}^2(k) \quad \text{Equation (2.28)}$$

and the phase is:

$$\varphi(k) = a\,tan\left[\frac{X_{imag}(k)}{X_{real}(k)}\right] \quad \text{Equation (2.29)}$$

For the class of signals considered in this book, the original signal segment can be recovered from the discrete Fourier transform by computing the inverse transform:

$$x(n) = \frac{1}{N}\sum_{k=0}^{N-1}\left[X_{real}(k)\cos\left(\frac{2\pi nk}{N}\right) - X_{imag}(k)\sin\left(\frac{2\pi nk}{N}\right)\right]$$

Equation (2.30)

The function $X_{real}(k)$ was computed by cross-correlating the segment $x(n)$ with cosine functions at multiples of the period of the segment length. Cross-correlating $X_{real}(k)$ with another set of cosines recovers that part of $x(n)$ that can be represented by cosines. Similarly, the function $X_{imag}(k)$ was computed by correlating the segment $x(n)$ with sine functions, and correlating $X_{imag}(k)$ with another set of sines recovers that part of $x(n)$ that can be represented by sines. The combination of the cosine and the sine terms completely describes $x(n)$. The inverse transform of *Eq. (2.30)* is closely related to the forward transform of *Eq. (2.27)*, and the same FFT algorithm can be used to compute the inverse as for the forward transform.

The FFT is usually computed for a segment length given by a power of 2 (e.g., 32, 64, 128,...) because the earliest form of the algorithm was derived for this family of transform sizes. However, efficient algorithms now exist for any composite number, by which is meant a segment size N that can be represented by:

$$N = p_1^{c1} \times p_2^{c2} \times p_3^{c3} \cdots \quad \text{Equation (2.31)}$$

where p_k is a prime number such as 2, 3, 5, and so forth. Thus, the FFT algorithm for a segment size of $81 = 3^4$ samples embodies the same computational advantages as for $64 = 2^6$ samples, and one should not feel tied to using only powers of 2 for the FFT size when using most signal-processing software packages, such as MATLAB.

Filters and Filter Banks

Frequency analysis is important in hearing aids because it forms the basis of algorithms such as multichannel compression. Frequency analysis can be provided by a Fourier transform or by a filter bank. The basic filter-bank structure is shown in Figure 2-3 for a group of filters in parallel. In a filter bank, the filters are chosen so that the band edges overlap, providing continuous coverage along the frequency axis. In an ideal filter bank, setting the gain in each filter to 0 dB will result in a ruler-flat magnitude frequency response for the summed output of the filter bank. An additional requirement is that an arbitrary selection of gains for the different filters will not cause any unexpected peaks or dips in the system frequency response. The behavior of a dynamic-range compression system can also be affected by the filter bank, and these effects are explored in Chapter 8. Thus, for every combination of filter band gains, the magnitude and phase responses of the filters must combine to give a smooth response.

FILTER DEFINITIONS

An idealized low-pass filter magnitude frequency response is sketched in Figure 2-6. The pass-band of the filter is the frequency region having gain close to 0 dB. For a low-pass filter, the pass band extends from 0 Hz to the band edge or filter cutoff frequency. The stop band is the region of signal attenuation, and the transition band links the pass band to the stop band. The transition band is characterized by its slope in dB/octave. In some filters, particularly those based on analog filter designs, there is no stop band; instead the transition band continues forever on its downward slope. The stop band in such a filter would be considered to be the frequency region having signal attenuation greater than some predefined value based on the problem being solved. The circuit elements used to design analog filters produce slopes that are integer multiples of 6 dB/oct.

For a high-pass filter the picture of Figure 2-6 would be flipped to produce its mirror image, with the pass band at high frequencies and the stop band at low frequencies. A band-pass filter passes a frequency region, defined by the lower and upper cutoff frequencies, with stop bands at frequencies below and above the pass band. The filters in a filter bank are often characterized by a set of crossover frequencies; for each pair of adjacent filters the crossover frequency is the upper cutoff frequency for the lower filter and also the lower cutoff frequency for the upper filter.

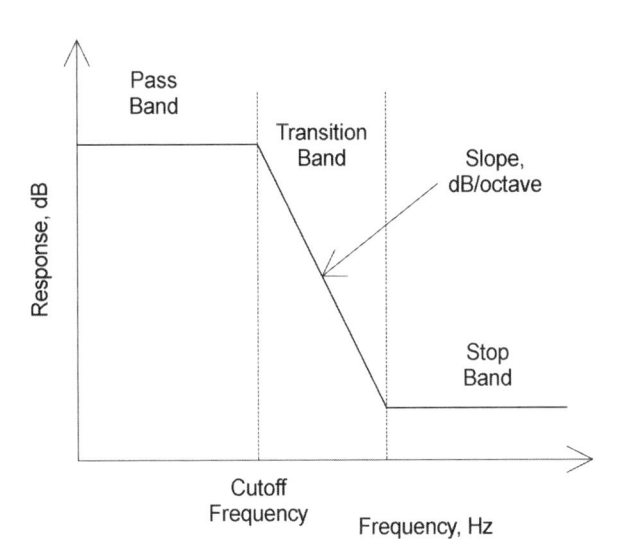

Figure 2-6. Idealized low-pass filter showing the pass band, transition band, and stop band.

RECURSIVE FILTERS

One way of designing the filters in the filter bank is to use digital signal processing to approximate the characteristics of analog filters. This approach produces a recursive or infinite-impulse response (IIR) filter. In an IIR filter, the current output sample depends on the current and past input samples and on the past output samples. Let $x(n)$ be the input sequence and $y(n)$ be the output sequence. The filter output is then given by:

$$y(n) = \sum_{k=0}^{K} b_k x(n-k) + \sum_{j=1}^{J} a_j y(n-j) \quad \text{Equation (2.32)}$$

This filter has K zeros (the terms where past input values are combined to form the current output) and J poles (the terms where the past output values are fed back to form the current output). The weights are chosen using a design rule to give the desired magnitude frequency response, and are often based on a digital transformation of an existing analog filter design such as a Butterworth or Chebychev filter.

As an example of an IIR filter bank, consider a combination of three filters. The system sampling rate is 16 kHz, so the highest frequency that can be represented is 8 kHz. The first filter is a three-pole Butterworth (maximally flat) low-pass filter that passes the frequencies up to 1000 Hz. The Butterworth low-pass filter design has no ripples, but instead proceeds monotonically from the gain of approximately 1 in the pass band to the continuous attenuation of the transition band. The second is a six-pole Butterworth band-pass filter that passes the frequencies from 1000 to 2500 Hz, and the third is a three-pole Butterworth high-pass filter that passes the frequencies above 2500 Hz. The filter magnitude frequency responses are plotted in Figure 2-7.

Because the digital filter design is based on an analog Butterworth filter, the response of each filter is down 3 dB at the frequencies that define its band edges. The filter outputs of a Butterworth low-pass/high-pass filter pair are 90 degrees out of phase at the crossover frequency, and for the same gain in both filters the outputs combine to give constant power and a flat magnitude frequency response. The low-pass and high-pass filters have identical phase responses, so their outputs can be summed for any combination of gains for the low-pass and high-pass filters and the system will always produce a smooth monotonic frequency response.

Signal Processing Basics 35

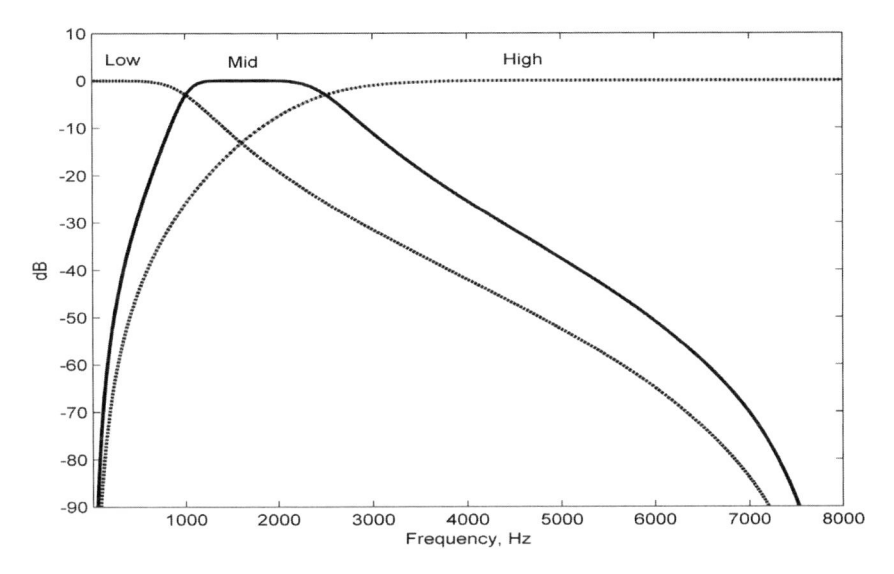

Figure 2-7. Individual frequency response curves for 3rd-order recursive (IIR) digital Butterworth filters having band edges at 1000 and 2500 Hz.

The filter interaction becomes much more complicated if more than two filters are combined to form the filter bank. The combined output of the three filters is plotted in Figure 2-8. The outputs of the three filters do not combine in the same way as for a simple pair of filters. The phase responses of the filters interact to produce peaks and valleys in the composite frequency response. The problem is that the three filters do not have identical phase (or group delay) responses. Changing the gain in each frequency band, as would occur in a compression system, will shift the locations of the peaks and valleys in frequency.

Another way to look at the system phase behavior is to compute the group delay. The group delay for the combination of three IIR filters is plotted in Figure 2-9. For most IIR filters, the group delay is proportional to the slope of the magnitude frequency response with frequency; the steeper the slope the greater the delay. The maximum delay occurs at the band edges. Filters at lower frequencies have steeper slopes and thus have greater group delay. Therefore, in Figure 2-9 there is a peak of about 1 msec in the delay at 1000 Hz and a second peak of about 0.5 msec at 2500 Hz. Reducing the order of the IIR filter will reduce the group delay, but at the expense of reducing the slope of the filter stop band.

36 Digital Hearing Aids

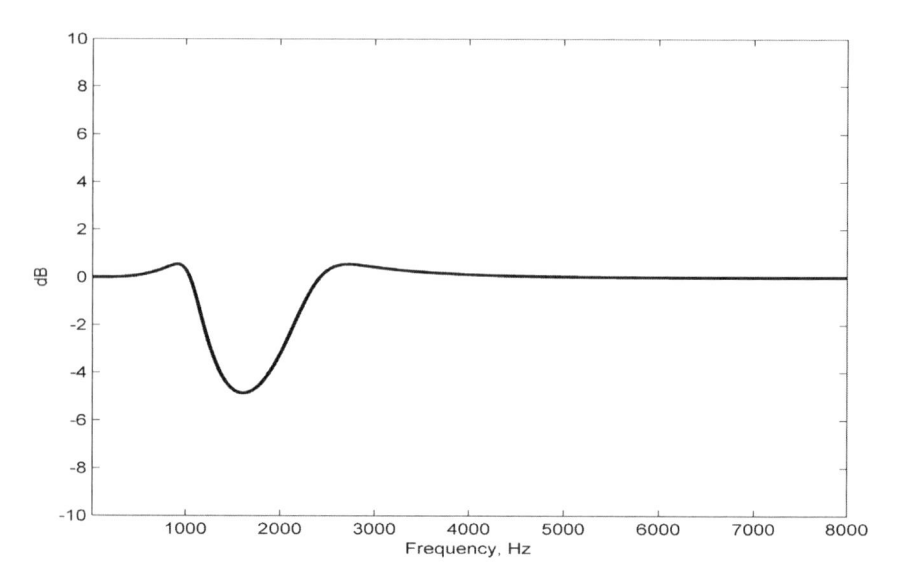

Figure 2-8. Composite frequency response for the combined output of the three filters presented in Figure 2-7. Each filter has a gain of 0 dB.

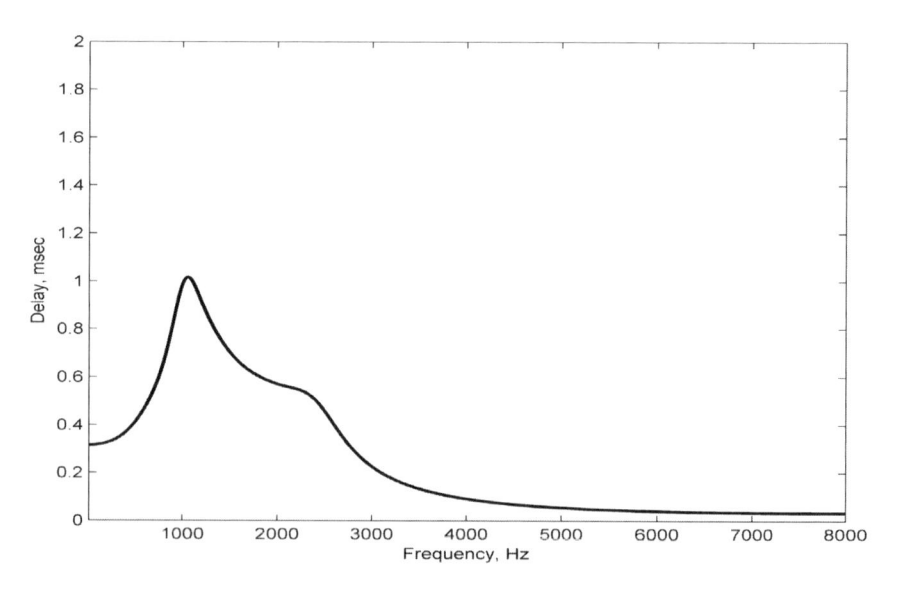

Figure 2-9. Group delay for the combined output of the three filters presented in Figure 2-7.

A naïve implementation of an IIR filter bank, as demonstrated in this section, results in unanticipated phase interactions that interfere with achieving the desired frequency response. These interactions shift depending on the filter gains, and could lead to audible processing artifacts in a system where the gain changes dynamically. We should point out, however, that there are analog design techniques that can lead to filter banks with a better match of the filter phase responses (Lerner, 1964) and which minimize the undesired filter interaction demonstrated here.

NONRECURSIVE FILTERS

In an ideal filter bank, every filter would have exactly the same phase response. If this were the case, the output of each filter would be in phase with the output of every other filter at every frequency. One could then compute the composite output by simply adding the magnitudes of the outputs of each filter without worrying about additional peaks or valleys introduced by phase interactions. This ideal can be realized in a digital filter bank by using linear-phase finite-impulse response (FIR) filters. A FIR filter is equivalent to a tapped delay line. In terms of Eq. (2.32), the output $y(n)$ depends only on weighted present and delayed samples of the input $x(n)$. There is no dependence on the past output samples $y(n)$ and the $\{a\}$ coefficients are all zero. The FIR filter is thus given by:

$$y(n) = \sum_{k=0}^{K} b_k x(n-k) \quad \text{Equation (2.33)}$$

A linear-phase FIR imposes the additional constraint that the set of coefficients $\{b\}$ has even symmetry, with $b_0 = b_K$, $b_1 = b_{K-1}$, and so on. The filter delay is then $K/2$ samples at all frequencies.

The output from a three-band linear-phase FIR filter bank is plotted in Figure 2-10. The filters have been designed to have band edges at 1000 and 2500 Hz, the same as for the IIR example discussed previously in this section, and each filter has a length of 129 samples. Although IIR filters are 3 dB down at the band edges, the FIR filters are 6 dB down. Each filter shown in Figure 2-10 has a nearly flat frequency response in its pass-band, stop-band attenuation of 60 dB or more, and narrow transition bands. The stop-band level means that the filter will have some response, albeit greatly reduced, to a signal that is at a frequency

38 Digital Hearing Aids

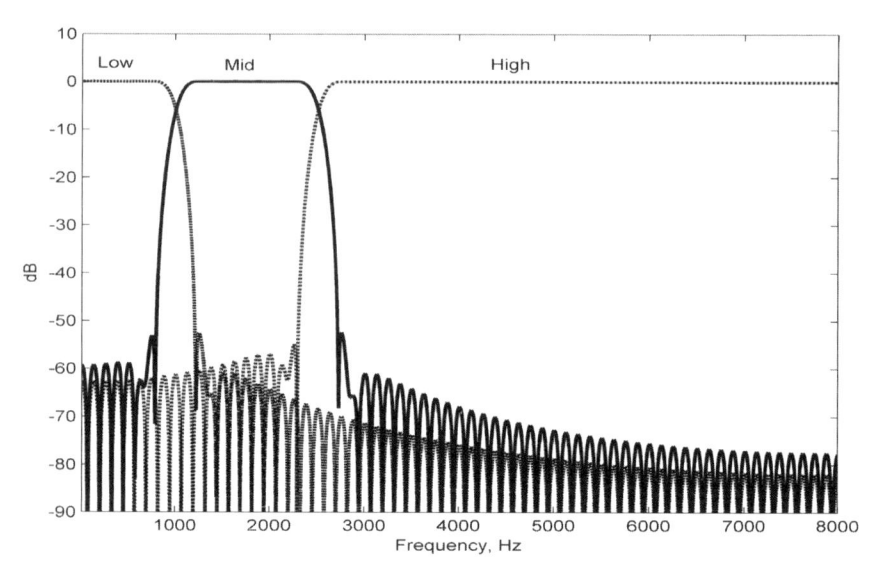

Figure 2-10. Individual frequency response curves for 127-point nonrecursive (FIR) filters having band edges at 1000 and 2500 Hz. The system sampling rate is 16 kHz.

out of its designated pass band. The FIR filters also have a large amount of ripple in the stop bands, the result of the finite filter length. Increased filter length can be used to reduce the ripple in the pass band, reduce the sidelobe levels, and/or reduce the width of the transition regions at the filter band edges.

The combined frequency response of the three FIR filters is plotted in Figure 2-11, and the group delay for the combined output is plotted in Figure 2-12. There is essentially no ripple in the magnitude frequency response, and the group delay is a constant 4 msec independent of frequency Thus, the linear-phase FIR filter satisfies the desire for a filter bank where the phase response of the filter can be ignored in summing the weighted outputs of the individual bands. However, the advantages of the FIR filter do not come without their cost. The group delay of the FIR filter, although independent of frequency, is substantially greater than the group delay plotted in Figure 2-9 for the IIR filter bank. Furthermore, the computational requirements for the linear-phase FIR filter are much greater than for the IIR filter; the 3rd-order low-pass IIR filter, for example, requires seven multiplications per output sample whereas the low-pass FIR filter requires 128 multiplications per output sample.

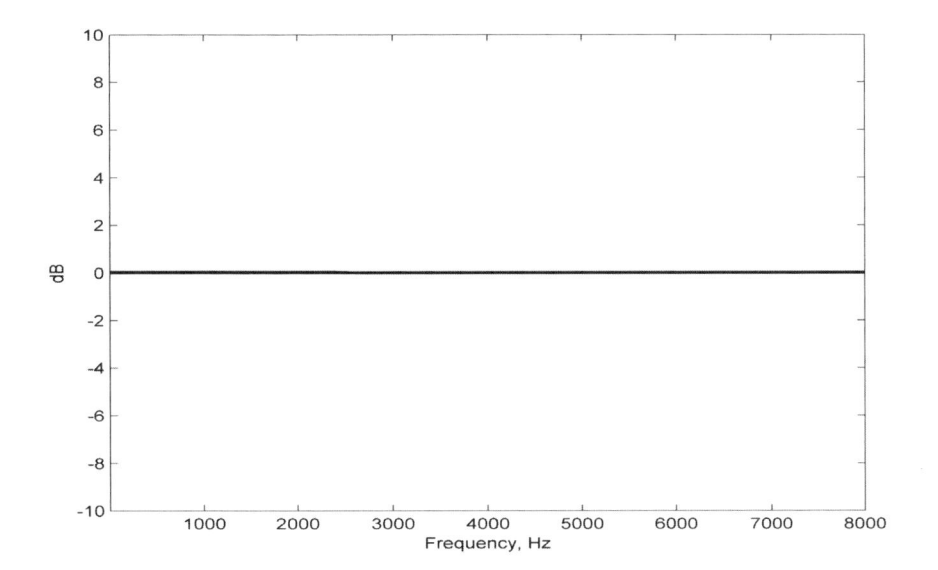

Figure 2-11. Composite frequency response for the combined output of the three filters presented in Figure 2-10.

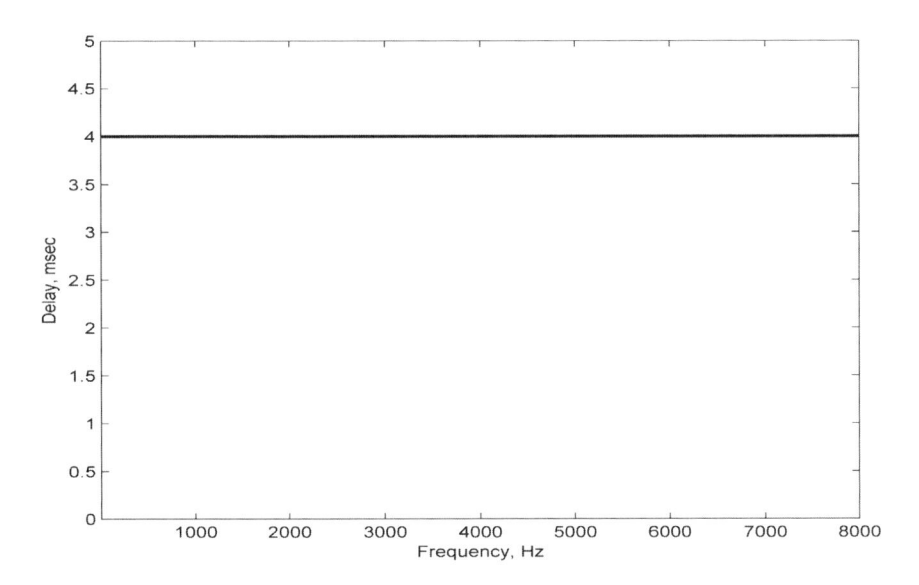

Figure 2-12. Group delay for the combined output of the three filters presented in Figure 2-10.

Thus, the design of a filter bank requires many tradeoffs between the allowable degree of filter interaction, the width of the filter transition bands, the filter side-lobe suppression, and the number of arithmetic operations per second permitted by the digital signal processor and battery in the hearing aid.

In the FIR filters used in the above example, the sampling rate in each frequency band is the same as for the original signal. But according to the Nyquist theorem, the sampling rate of the filter output can be reduced as the bandwidth is reduced. Not every output sample is needed at the original sampling rate; one only needs to sample at higher than twice the filter bandwidth. To reduce the number of operations per second needed to implement the frequency analysis, the signals in each frequency band can be processed at the reduced sampling rate within each frequency band (Vaidyanathan, 1993). The contents of the separate bands are then passed through a complementary filter bank and recombined at the original sampling rate. The ability to reduce the sampling rate in the separate frequency bands can thus be exploited to reduce the number of arithmetic operations per second needed in the digital hearing aid (Brennan & Schneider, 1998; Chau et al., 2004), but the basic behavior of the frequency analysis and group delay is the same as for the filter bank that maintains the original sampling rate in the separate frequency bands.

FREQUENCY RESOLUTION AND GROUP DELAY

In an FFT system, increasing the resolution of the analysis requires a larger FFT. In a filter-bank system, increasing the resolution of the analysis requires more filters, each having a narrower bandwidth. The narrower bandwidths require sharper transition bands at the edges of the filters, which in turn leads to an increase in the group delay. The FFT can only be computed after the complete data segment has been acquired, so a longer FFT in turn requires a longer delay while one waits for the data buffer to be filled. Thus, for both filter banks and FFTs, better frequency resolution results in longer delay.

Block Processing

Processing systems based on filtering can be implemented by operating on each data-sequence sample as it is acquired, or by accumulating a block of samples and then processing them all at once. An FFT system, on the other hand, requires that a complete block of data be acquired first, after which the FFT can be computed. One could, if desired, compute a new FFT every time a new data sample is acquired. However, the signal gain adjustments in a hearing aid do not generally need to updated for every sample, but rather can be updated at a slower rate, for example, once every millisecond. Thus, it is computationally more efficient to use a block implementation for both filters and FFT systems. A block of data is acquired (e.g., 1–2 msec), then the entire block is filtered or the frequency analysis performed on the entire block of data at once, after which the processing gains are computed for the entire block. The advantage of block processing is computational efficiency resulting from the reduced rate of updating the processing gains, but the price paid is additional time delay as the gains can not be computed until the data buffer has been filled.

The overlap-add technique is typically used for processing signal segments. The overlap-add procedure in the time domain using data windowing is illustrated in Figure 2-13. The input sequence is divided into segments each of length L samples. Each segment is multiplied by a smooth data window, such as a raised cosine function, also of length

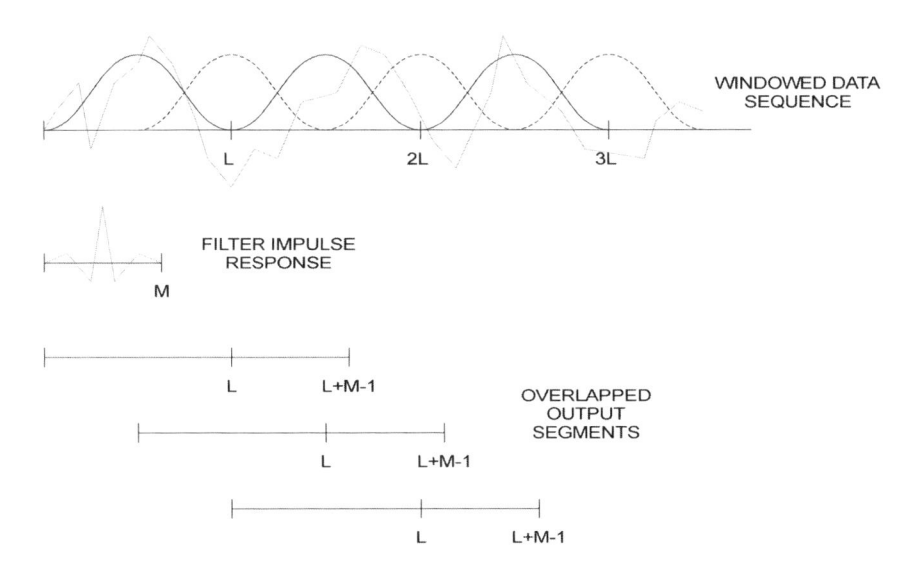

Figure 2-13. Overlap-add processing using windowed data segments.

L samples. The windowed segment is then convolved with the filter of length M samples. The output sequence from the convolution has a length of L+M-1 samples. A new windowed input segment is acquired every L/2 samples. The filtered output sequence is formed by summing all of the output segments that overlap for each L+M-1 sample interval.

For frequency-domain processing, the input sequence is again divided into windowed segments or blocks of length L samples. Each segment extended (padded) with zeros to give a total length of P > L+M-1 samples. The filter impulse response is M samples, and it is also padded with zeros to give a sequence of length P samples. The Fourier transform of the P-sample zero-padded input segment and the P-sample zero-padded filter segment are then computed. Most often the FFT algorithm is used for these computations. The two transforms are then multiplied together to effect the filtering in the frequency domain, and the resultant frequency response is inverse transformed to return to the time domain. The filtered time-domain sequences are then combined across processing segments using the overlap-add procedure as shown in Figure 2-13.

Digital System Concerns

The design of a digital hearing aid involves many tradeoffs in selecting and programming the signal processing that will be implemented. Because hearing aids are small, the signal processing is constrained by the space available in the device for the circuitry and by the power available from the small battery. Thus implementing an algorithm in a hearing aid can be much more difficult than programming the processing in the laboratory. Some of the practical concerns in designing processing for digital hearing aids are outlined in this section.

INTEGER ARITHMETIC

Most hearing aids use integer (fixed-point) arithmetic to reduce the size of the digital processor and its power consumption. Each signal sample is represented internally by a value having a limited number of allowed signal levels. The signal levels are quantized. For example, many hearing aids use 16-bit words to store each sample. The use of 16 bits gives 2^{16} possible integer values, ranging from −32767 to 32768. This is the same accuracy as used for audio compact disks, and the maximum dynamic range (peak level to root-mean-squared average quantization noise floor) of a 16-bit system is approximately 107 dB (Oppenheim et al., 1999). In a compact disk the 16-bit numbers are used purely for storing the digital signal. In a hearing aid, however, the 16-bit numbers are processed (multiplied and added) to produce the output, and the integer arithmetic introduces potential forms of distortion.

One problem is saturation. Assume that two positive numbers are being summed in a 16-bit system. If the two numbers are small, their sum will be less than 32768 and the addition will be correct. If the two numbers are large, however, then their sum could exceed 32768. Generally, the processor arithmetic saturates; if the true sum is greater than 32768, the result returned by the processor is set to 32768. Thus, the digital arithmetic provides internal peak clipping, and if the internal signal levels get to be too high, distortion will result. Bear in mind that a hearing aid may be programmed to provide up to 60 dB gain, which means multiplying the signal by a factor of 1000. If the largest output is 32768, then its internal representation must be less than or equal to 32 if saturation is to be avoided.

A second problem is numerical underflow. The system using 16-bit integer arithmetic has no intermediate values between 0 and 1. If the processing is programmed to attenuate a signal, then an value attenuated below 1 will be set to the next lower value, which is zero. If the signal is amplified at a later processing stage, the only signal value available will be zero, and it will be impossible to recover the original signal. It has been lost due to underflow. Thus, in implementing the signal processing in a hearing aid, one must pay close attention to the signal dynamics and scale the amplitude to minimize the chances of saturation and underflow.

QUANTIZATION NOISE

An additional processing concern is quantization noise. Quantization noise tends to be greater in recursive (IIR) than in nonrecursive (FIR) filters, and tends to be greater in fast Fourier transform (FFT) systems than in direct time-domain implementations. Often the amount of quantization noise depends on details of the signal-processing implementation that are beyond the scope of this book.

Quantization noise arises from using a limited number of bits to represent the numbers in the hearing aid. An analog 1-kHz sinusoid is plotted in Figure 2-14. A quantized version of the same signal is plotted in Figure 2-15. The signal in this example is quantized to 4 bits, which

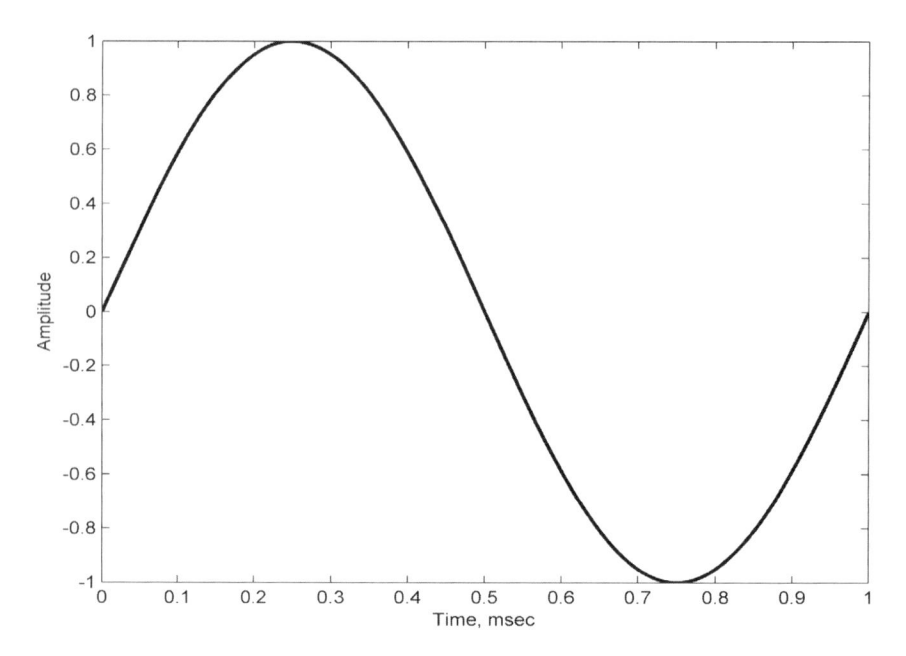

Figure 2-14. One period of a 1-kHz sinusoid.

gives $2^4 = 16$ levels that are used to represent the amplitude from -1 to 1. The quantized version of the signal can be represented as the analog amplitude plus an error term that gives the difference between the analog amplitude and its quantized representation. For example, consider two quantized numbers:

$$y_1 = x_1 + \varepsilon_1$$
$$y_2 = x_2 + \varepsilon_2$$

Equation (2.34)

The exact (analog) number is x_k. The approximation using the limited number of bits is y_k, and the error between the exact number and its digital representation is ε_k.

When the two digital numbers are added, the errors add as well, giving

$$y_1 + y_2 = (x_1 + x_2) + (\varepsilon_1 + \varepsilon_2) \quad \text{Equation (2.35)}$$

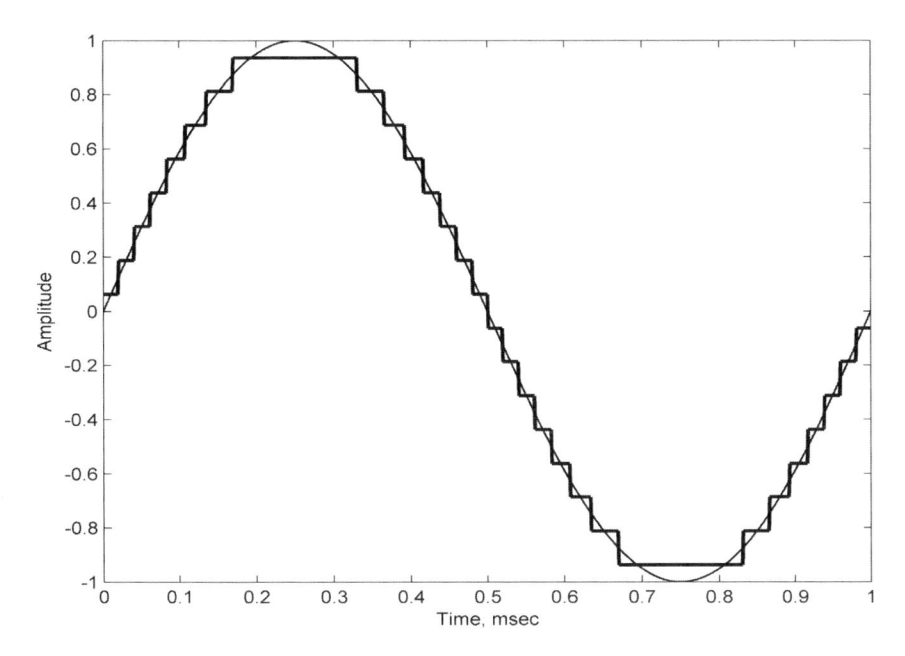

Figure 2-15. One period of a 1-kHz sinusoid (thin line) and the sinusoid quantized to 4 bits (thick line).

If two large numbers of equal amplitude but opposite sign are added, the correct values will cancel but the quantization error may still remain. Multiplication of the two numbers results in

$$y_1 y_2 = (x_1 x_2) + (x_1 \varepsilon_2) + (x_2 \varepsilon_1) + (\varepsilon_1 \varepsilon_2) \quad \text{Equation (2.36)}$$

If a large number is multiplied by a small number, the correct result may be small but the quantization error will be proportional to the larger number. Thus, as numbers are added or multiplied, the errors accumulate along with the correct answer. The greater the number of arithmetic operations the greater the total error, and audible noise can result. Controlling the amount of quantization noise in a hearing aid requires careful ordering and internal scaling of the arithmetic operations in the processing algorithms to keep the quantization noise at a minimum.

ALIASING DISTORTION

In any digital system, the highest frequency that can be represented is half the sampling rate, termed the Nyquist frequency. Thus, in a system using a 20-kHz sampling rate, the highest usable frequency is 10 kHz. Frequencies above 10 kHz are removed by a low-pass filter prior to the analog-to-digital (A/D) conversion. The anti-aliasing filter must meet two requirements: it must pass as much of the signal below the Nyquist frequency as possible, and attenuate as much as possible above the Nyquist frequency. No filter is perfect, and the anti-aliasing filter will occasionally permit signal components above the Nyquist frequency to leak into the hearing aid. Let the Nyquist frequency be represented by f_{max}. If the input is a tone at a higher frequency given by $f_{max} + \eta$ Hz, then the output from the A/D converter will be at $f_{max} - \eta$ Hz. For example, if the system has a 20-kHz sampling rate, an input at 12 kHz will be represented as a digital sinusoid at 8 kHz. The frequency of the digital representation is not harmonically related to the input frequency, and it can result in unpleasant distortion if the amplitude of the aliased frequency component is large enough.

Aliasing is illustrated in Figures 2-16 and 2-17. When the signal is sampled at a high rate, the sequence of samples gives a clear representation of the signal. For example, Figure 2-16 shows the 1-kHz sinusoid of Figure 2-14 after is has been sampled at a 20-kHz sampling rate. Reducing the sampling rate will still give an accurate representation of the signal as long as the Nyquist criterion is satisfied. If the 1-kHz sinusoid were sampled at 2 kHz, the resulting sequence of numbers would be {1, -1, 1, -1, . . .} from the positive and negative peaks of the waveform, which is sufficient to recreate the 1-kHz waveform at the output of the D/A converter. If the sampling rate drops below 2 kHz, however, the representation of the sinusoid becomes aliased. In Figure 2-17, the 1-kHz sinusoid is sampled at a 1.33-kHz rate as shown by the open circles. The recreated waveform linking these samples is shown by the dashed line, giving an aliased sine wave at 333 Hz.

TEMPORAL ALIASING

Another form of aliasing, distinct from the frequency aliasing described above, is temporal aliasing. In performing frequency-domain digital filtering, as described in a preceding section, it was assumed that the length of the data segment L and the length of the filter M were such that $L+M-1 \leq P$, where P is the size of the Fourier transform. If this con-

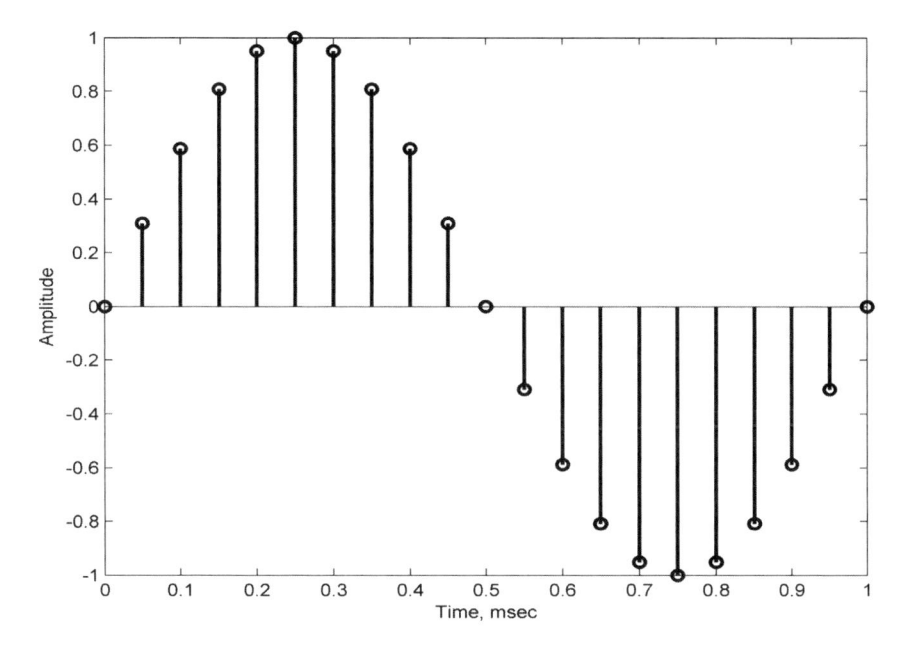

Figure 2-16. One period of a 1-kHz sinusoid sampled at 20 kHz.

dition is not met, that is either L or M is too long, then the total length of the equivalent convolution will exceed the transform size P. The result is that the convolution output that should lie beyond P samples is wrapped around to the beginning of the output sequence instead, producing temporal aliasing. Temporal aliasing is a pre-echo in which the end of a sound is heard before the beginning. If temporal aliasing occurs across a group of blocks, it can result in a buzzing distortion; the distortion components will be concentrated at the beginning of each block, producing a periodic pattern of distortion energy.

ALGORITHM COMPLEXITY

The size and power constraints imposed on the DSP in a hearing aid limit as well the algorithms that can be implemented. Signal processing developed in the laboratory is often developed without consideration of the number of arithmetic operations per second needed to process the signal, the amount of memory needed for the program and data, and the effects of digital word size. But all of these considerations are crucial in getting the algorithm to work effectively in a digital hearing aid. One

48 Digital Hearing Aids

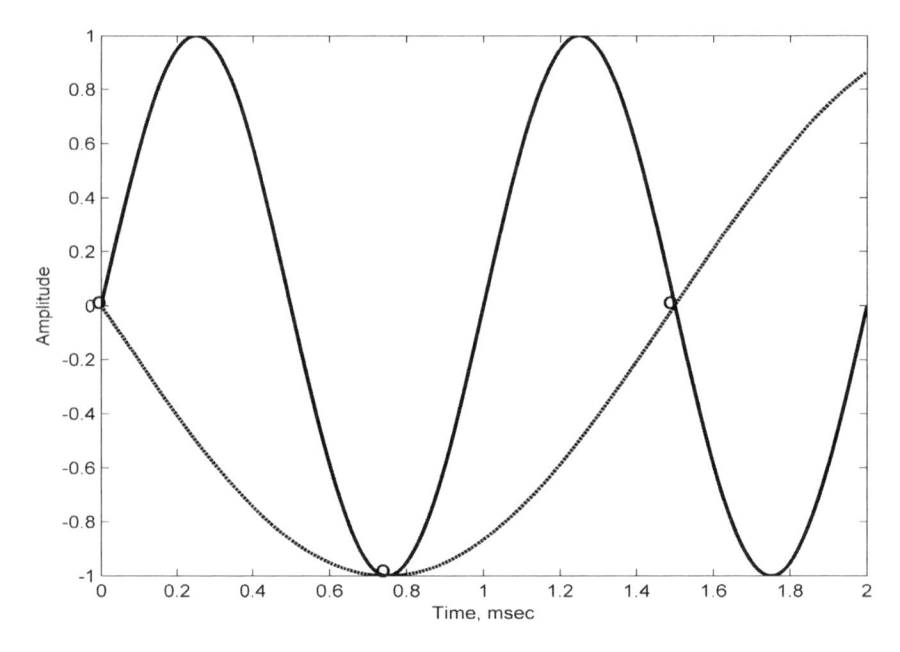

Figure 2-17. 1-kHz sinusoid (solid line) sampled at 1.33 kHz showing aliased component (dashed line) at 333 Hz.

might want a long filter to model the feedback path in a feedback-cancellation system, for example, but there may not be enough instructions per second available to implement the filter without stealing processing cycles from other essential operations, and there may not be enough data memory to store the filter coefficients.

Power and memory are at a premium in the hearing aid, and often compromises in the signal processing must be made to produce a practical implementation. The small word size can also introduce noise or distortion as it passes through the processing stages, and adjustments need to be made to the processing to remove them. An algorithm that works in the laboratory must therefore be converted into an algorithm that will work in a hearing aid. Simplicity can be more important in the final implementation than getting the last iota of optimal performance.

ALGORITHM INTERACTION

There are times when working with digital hearing aids that what one is hearing or measuring "Just doesn't make sense" in terms of the output expected from the processing algorithms. One culprit that should be kept in mind is algorithm interaction. A digital hearing aid normally has several algorithms running in parallel, for example dynamic-range compression, noise suppression, and spectral contrast enhancement. Each algorithm is trying to adjust the gain of the output signal, but the algorithms may not necessarily agree on what the gain should be at any given time. In addition, these algorithms are generally designed independently of each other. Putting them together into the hearing aid can, therefore, result in unanticipated interactions as each processing strategy tries to pull the gain in a different direction. The result of these interactions can be signal modulations that produce audible distortion or processing artifacts. One may protest that the manufacturer should test the devices for all potential interactions, but a modern digital hearing aid can have several hundred processing parameters; despite extensive evaluation protocols it may not be possible to test every possible combination.

Concluding Remarks

This chapter has presented a brief overview of important digital signal-processing concepts, and it is not intended as a substitute for a course in signal processing. The chapter presented basic ideas and operations, including linear systems, convolution, correlation, transfer functions, the discrete Fourier transform, and filters and filter banks. These operations form the signal-processing tools that will be applied in subsequent chapters as specific signal-processing algorithms are described.

References

Brennan, R., & Schneider, T. (1998). A flexible filterbank structure for extensive signal manipulations in digital hearing aids. *Proceedings of the 1998 IEEE International Symposium on Circuits and Systems*, pp. 569–572.

Chau, E., Sheikhzadeh, H., & Brennan, R. L. (2004). Complexity reduction and regularization of a fast affine projection algorithm for oversampled subband adaptive filters. *Proceedings of the 2004 International Conference on Acoustic Speech and Signal Processing*, Montreal, May 17 to 21.

Dillon, H. (2001). *Hearing aids*. New York: Thieme Medical Publishing.

Hartmann, W. M. (2004). *Signals, sound, and sensation (Modern acoustics and signal processing)*, Woodbury, NY: American Institute of Physics Press.

Lathi, B. P. (2004). *Linear systems*. New York: Oxford University Press.

Lerner, R. M. (1964). Band-pass filters with linear phase. *Proceedings of the IEEE International Symposium on Circuits Systems, 52,* 249–268.

Lyons, R. G. (1996). *Understanding digital signal processing*. Englewood Cliffs, NJ: Prentice-Hall.

McClellen, J., Schafer, R. W., & Yoder, M. (1997). *DSP first: A multimedia approach*. Upper Saddle River, NJ: Prentice-Hall.

Oppenheim, A. V., Schafer, R. W., & Buck, J. R. (1999), *Discrete-time signal processing* (2nd ed.). Englewood Cliffs, NJ: Prentice-Hall.

Peebles, P. Z. (1976). *Communication system principles*. Reading, MA: Addison-Wesley.

Rabiner, L. R., & Gold, B. (1975). *Theory and application of digital signal processing*. Englewood Cliffs, NJ: Prentice-Hall.

Vaidyanathan, P. P. (1993). *Multirate systems and filter banks*. Englewood Cliffs, NJ: Prentice-Hall.

3

The Electroacoustic System

THE SIGNAL PROCESSING built into a hearing aid is only part of the total electroacoustic system. It is very easy to consider the signal processing in isolation, ignoring the rest of the system, but the overall response depends not only on the signal processing but also on the transducers and acoustic factors that surround the signal processing. This chapter is a review of the important acoustic factors that affect hearing-aid performance in the ear. These acoustic factors include the head, ear, ear canal, the acoustic transducers, and the acoustic venting of the hearing aid. The sound pressure delivered to the tympanum is the product of all of the elements of the acoustic and electronic system.

This chapter begins with a presentation of the layers of signal processing that are present in a hearing aid inserted in the ear. The head, external ear, and ear canal all play important effects in modifying acoustic signals, and these effects are described next. The microphone used in the hearing aid affects the signal before the digital processing, and the receiver affects the signal after the processing, and these effects are discussed. The vent is an important factor in the acoustic response of the hearing aid, and the acoustics and effects of the vent and ear canal are described next. The chapter concludes with a discussion of the occlusion effect, in which the presence of the hearing aid in the ear modifies the user's perception of his or her own voice.

Hearing Aid System

A cross-section of an in-the-ear (ITE) hearing aid is presented in Figure 3-1. The circuit is what is normally considered to be the heart of the signal processing, as shown in Figure 3-2. However, the other items present also affect the signal. The microphone frequency response shapes the signal before it is processed by the circuit, and the receiver modifies the processed signal response after it leaves the circuit. These elements—the microphone, circuit, and receiver—are the electronic pieces of the hearing aid, and form the system shown in Figure 3-3. In addition, in a digital hearing aid the processing circuit includes the analog-to-digital converter (A/D) and the digital-to-analog converter (D/A), which can also modify the response going into and out of the digital processing.

Most hearing aids are vented for reasons of comfort; these reasons include the feeling of congestion in the ear, the buildup of moisture in the ear canal, and the occlusion effects discussed later in this chapter. The vent creates an additional acoustic filter that can have large effects on the low-frequency response of the hearing aid. Including the vent produces the system of Figure 3-4. The system now has a feedback loop

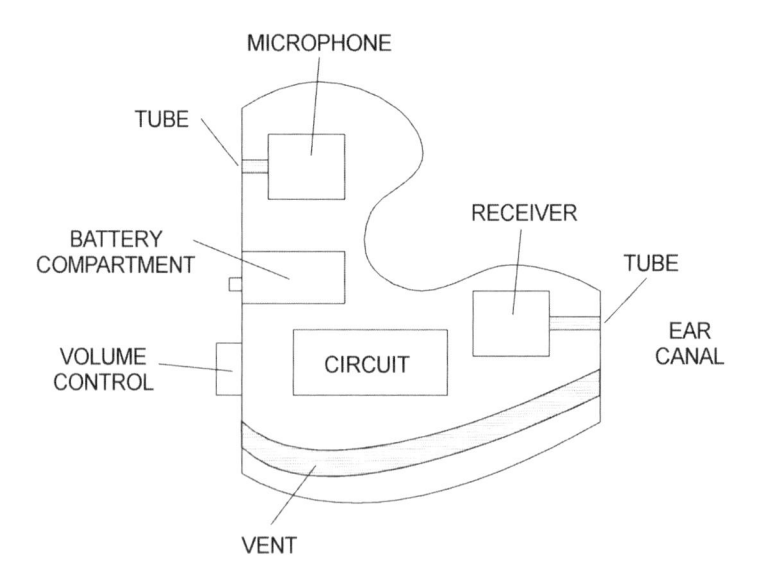

Figure 3-1. Cross-section of an in-the-ear (ITE) hearing aid showing the transducers and vent.

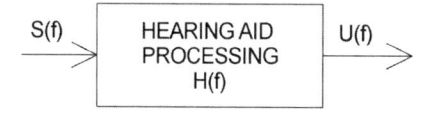

Figure 3-2. Block diagram showing the basic hearing-aid processing.

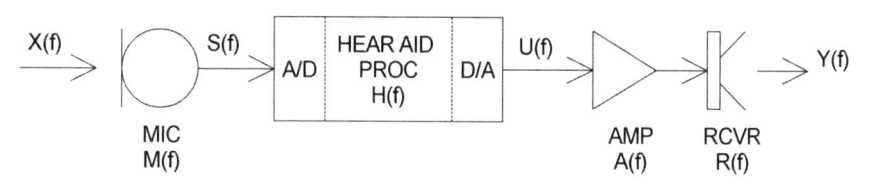

Figure 3-3. Block diagram showing the hearing-aid processing with the A/D and D/A converters added along with the microphone, amplifier, and receiver.

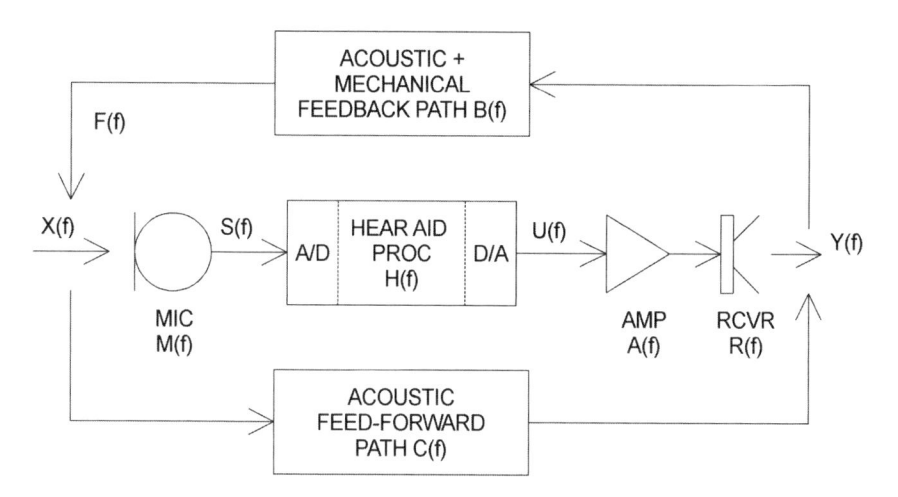

Figure 3-4. Block diagram showing the hearing aid with the vent acoustics.

going from the receiver through the vent to the microphone, plus a direct signal path going through the vent to the ear canal and which bypasses the hearing-aid processing entirely. The pressure in the ear canal is thus the combination of the desired signal processing plus the direct signal through the vent, and this whole system is modified by the potential presence of acoustic feedback.

There are still more acoustic factors that affect the hearing aid response. The receiver in an in-the-ear (ITE) hearing aid is connected to the outside world by a short length of tubing, and this tubing acts as an acoustic filter that further modifies the receiver output. In a behind-the-ear (BTE) hearing aid the hearing aid with the receiver sits behind the ear, and a long length of tubing is needed to connect the receiver to the ear. A long length of tubing acts as an acoustic resonator and can strongly affect the system frequency response. Some BTE hearing aids also have the electronics in the BTE case but place the receiver in the ear canal and connect to the receiver via wires; the acoustic behavior of the receiver in this system will be closer to that of an ITE device.

One more level of acoustic processing is the external ear and the head itself. If we consider a source of sound in front of the listener, for example, the head modifies the spectrum of the sound before it reaches the ear, and the outer ear and ear canal provide another level of acoustic modification before the sound reaches the eardrum. Put all of these effects together, and the simple ITE hearing aid of Figure 3-2 becomes the complicated system shown in Figure 3-5. The same degree of complexity also applies to a BTE. It is this system that describes the transformation of an external sound into the sound pressure at the eardrum. Even though the focus of this book is on digital signal processing, the effects of the transducers and acoustics cannot be ignored.

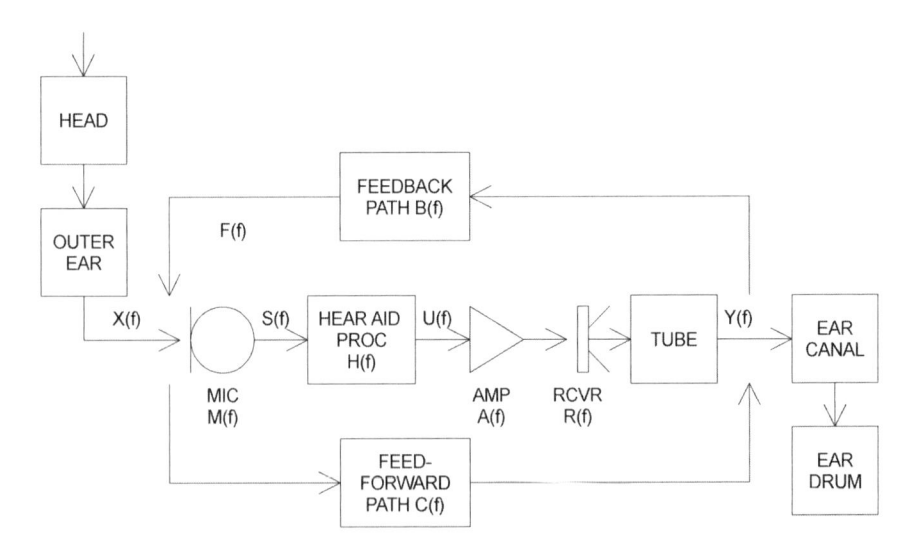

Figure 3-5. Block diagram showing the complete hearing aid in the ear.

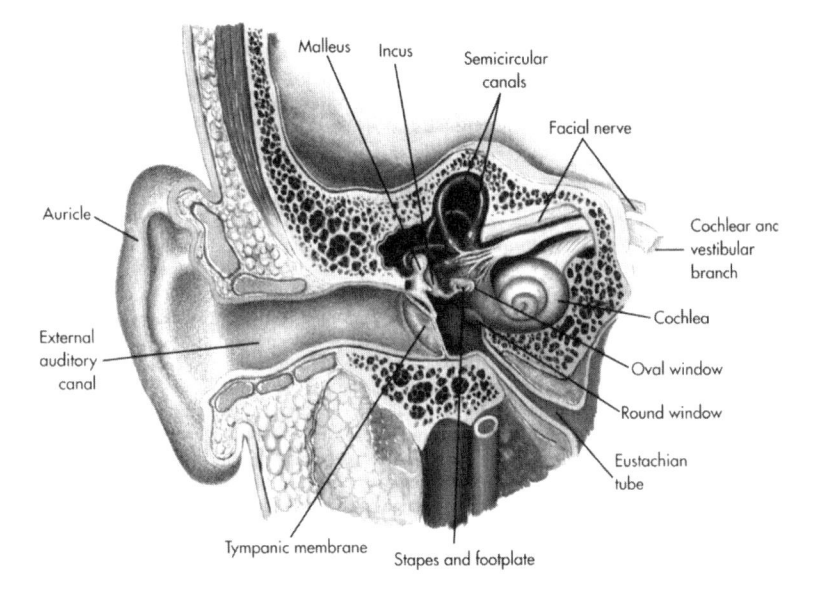

Figure 3-6. The external ear. Reprinted with permission from Acoustical Society of America.

Head and Ear

The anatomic structures of the head and ear provide complex analog signal processing, and the hearing aid can interfere with this anatomic system. A sketch of the external ear is provided in Figure 3-6. Both the auricle (or pinna) and the ear canal provide signal-processing functions. The simplest model of the ear canal, for example, is a pipe open at one end and closed at the other. The pipe will have a resonance when its length is equal to a quarter wavelength, three-quarters of a wavelength, and so on. The human ear canal is about 2.4 cm long, so the first resonance corresponds to a wavelength of 9.6 cm or a resonance frequency of 3600 Hz, which is in reasonable agreement with the 3.9-kHz value measured by Wiener and Ross (1946). Thus, the ear canal, considered in isolation, acts to amplify the high frequencies of speech. Blocking the ear canal with a hearing aid or earmold eliminates this amplification and reduces the high-frequency sensitivity of the ear.

The pinna, shown in Figure 3-7, is characterized by ridges inside and around its edge. The helix, the rim surrounding the concha, and the tragus are all reflecting surfaces for high-frequency sounds. When the

56 Digital Hearing Aids

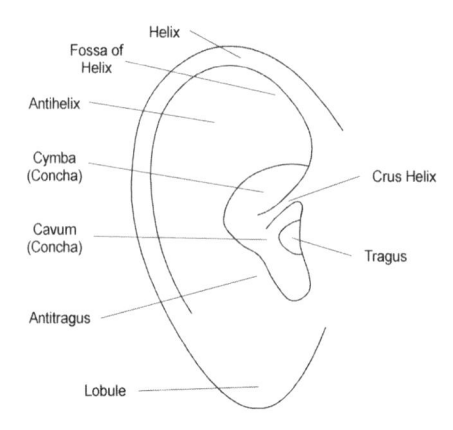

Figure 3-7. The pinna showing the components that are important for sound conduction.

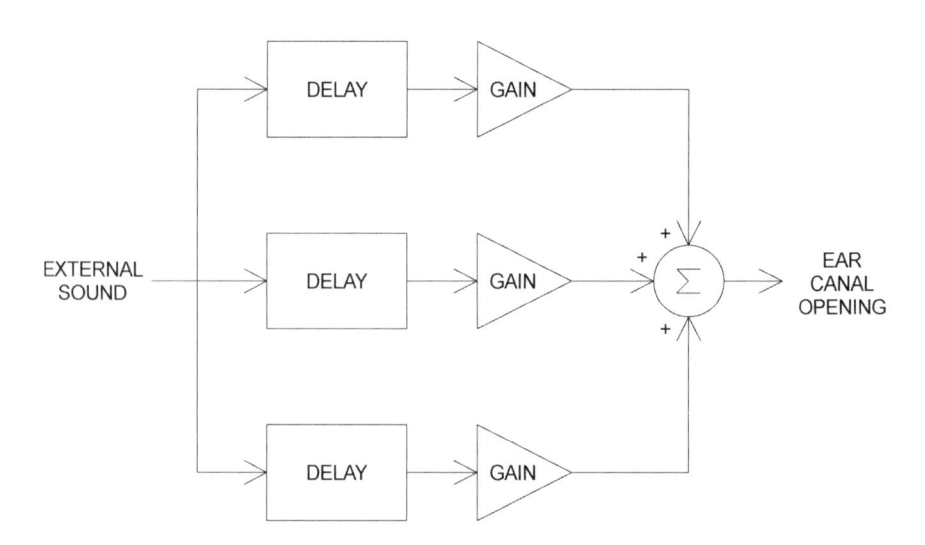

Figure 3-8. Pinna redrawn as an analog signal processing system.

sound originates from an external source, the reflection pattern changes with the location of the source relative to the head. A simple model of this reflection process (Batteau, 1967) is shown in Figure 3-8. Each ridge serves to reflect sound from the source into the opening of the ear canal,

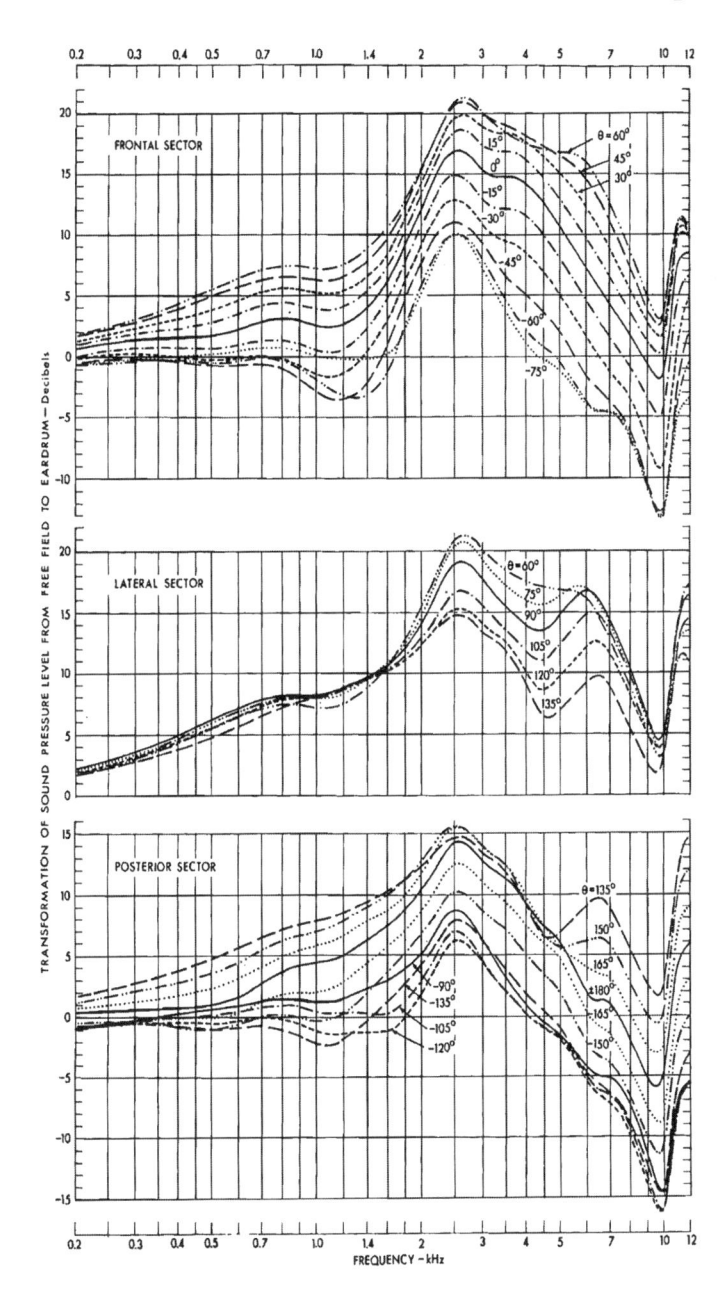

Figure 3-9. Transfer functions from free field to the eardrum as the azimuth of the sound source is moved around the head at an elevation of 0 degrees (from Shaw, 1974).

and this reflection is represented in the figure as a gain and time delay. The delayed and amplified versions of the signal combine to form an acoustic filter. One of the characteristics of this filter is a response notch that is positioned at approximately 6 kHz for a sound source directly in front of the listener and which increases in frequency to about 11 kHz as the sound source is elevated above the head (Langendijk & Bronkhorst, 2002; Rodgers, 1981; Wright et al., 1974). This notch serves as a vertical localization cue, but is lost if the pinna is filled with a hearing aid or the hearing aid is positioned behind the ear (of course, this pinna cue is also lost if it is rendered inaudible by the hearing impairment).

The transfer function from an external source to the ear canal includes the effects of the ear canal, pinna, and head. This head-related transfer function (HRTF) depends on the azimuth and elevation of the sound source. The dependence of the transfer function on azimuth for an elevation of 0 degrees is shown in Figure 3-9 (Shaw, 1974). The transfer function is close to 0 dB below about 1 kHz. The response for a source at 0 degrees (directly in front) shows little gain up to about 1.4 kHz, rises to a peak of about 17 dB at 2.6 kHz, and then drops to a deep notch at about 9.8 kHz. The magnitude of the peak response increases to over 20 dB as the source is moved around to the same side of the head as the test ear, reaching a maximum at 60 degrees, then drops by a small amount for the source at 90 degrees (perpendicular to the test ear), and continues to drop as the source moves behind the test ear.

Comparing the response for a source at 90 degrees (same side of the head as the test ear) to that for a source at −90 degrees (opposite the test ear) shows a difference of only about 2 dB at 1 kHz, increasing to about 10 dB at 2.6 kHz and 14 dB at 5 kHz. This difference between transfer functions from sources on opposite sides of the head is known as the head shadow. The head shadow is small at low frequencies because the head is small compared to the wavelength of sound; at 1 kHz, for example, the wavelength of sound is about 0.35 m (1 foot), so at frequencies below 1 kHz the sound will propagate around the head with little attenuation. At frequencies above 1 kHz the head becomes larger than a wavelength and casts an acoustic shadow. The head shadow can be important in speech perception because the high frequencies of the signal are much stronger at the ear on the same side of the head as the sound source than at the ear on the opposite side of the head.

A hearing aid changes the transfer function to the aided ear. Instead of going from the external sound source to the tympanum, the transfer

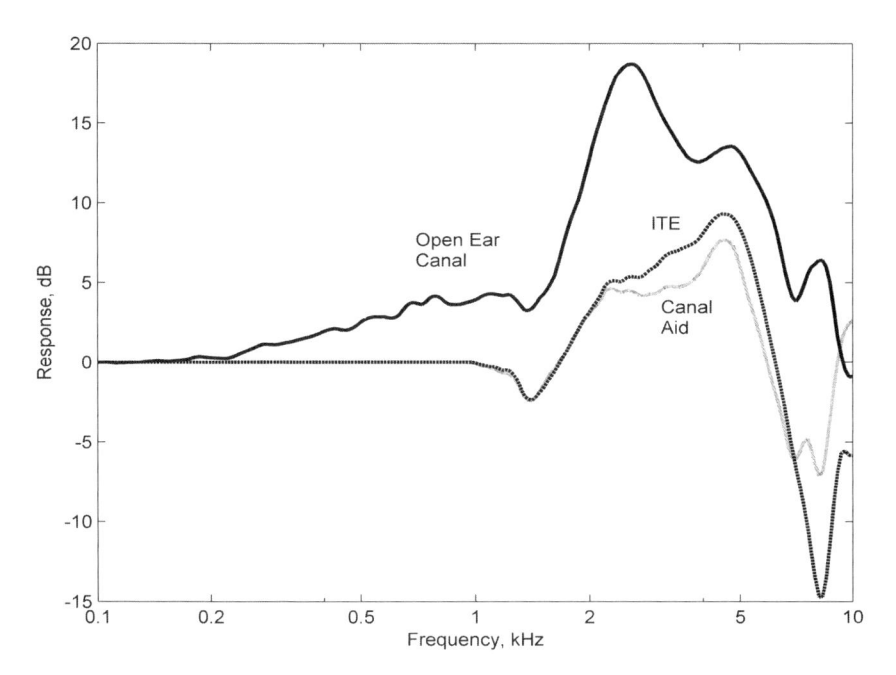

Figure 3-10. Free field to Zwislocki coupler transfer function for the open ear canal compared with the transfer function to the microphone in an in-the-ear (ITE) hearing aid and a canal aid. The source was at 0-deg azimuth.

function is now from the source to the hearing-aid microphone, which may be located within the pinna or placed behind the ear. These hearing-aid microphone positions preserve the gross effects of the shape of the head and head shadow, but the effects of the pinna are reduced or eliminated and the ear-canal resonance is also eliminated.

Figure 3-10 illustrates the difference in the HRTF that occurs when a hearing aid is placed in the ear. The solid line is the transfer function from a sound source directly in front of the KEMAR acoustic manikin to a microphone placed at the end of the ear canal. The dashed line is the transfer function from the same source to the microphone of an in-the-ear (ITE) hearing aid. The ITE blocks the ear canal opening and fills the bowl of the concha, but does not block the major ridges of the pinna. The dotted line is the transfer function to the microphone of a canal aid. The canal aid blocks the opening to the ear canal but leaves the pinna ridges and concha bowl unaffected. Both hearing aids eliminate the ear-canal resonance, and the signal at the hearing-aid microphones is about

15 dB lower than that for the open ear canal at the canal resonance frequency of about 2.5 kHz. Both hearing aids have a response peak at about 4.5 kHz, and a similar peak appears in the open canal response. One would assume that this 4.5-kHz peak is due to reflections within the pinna that are unaffected by the presence of the hearing aids. At low frequencies the open ear canal has a small amount of gain, rising to about 4 dB at 1 kHz, and this gain is also absent from the hearing-aid responses. A hearing aid thus substantially changes the HRFT, and part of the gain needed in a hearing aid is compensation for the loss of amplification that had been provided by the anatomic structure of the external ear.

There are also situations where we choose to modify the acoustic environment surrounding the head and ear. A telephone handset, for example, presents a reflecting surface that changes position as the handset is brought up to the ear. Putting on a hat or scarf can also place reflecting surfaces close to the hearing-aid microphone. These surfaces

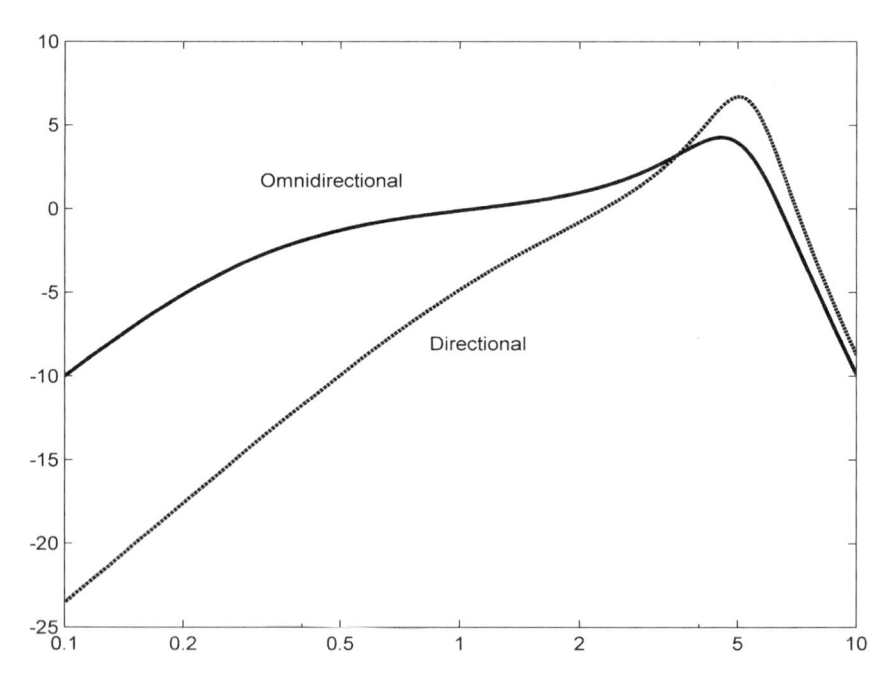

Figure 3-11. Frequency response for a Knowles Electronics EA1842 omnidirectional microphone and a Knowles Electronics EA1868 directional microphone.

modify the sound field at the microphone in complicated ways, and can affect the frequency response at the microphone input and can alter the behavior of signal processing algorithms such as the feedback cancellation discussed in Chapter 7.

Microphone and Receiver

The microphone in a hearing aid can be omnidirectional or it can be designed to have a directional spatial response pattern that favors sounds coming from the front and attenuates sounds coming from the rear. The properties of directional microphones are explored in more detail in Chapter 4. The frequency response of a Knowles Electronics EA1842 omnidirectional hearing-aid microphone is plotted in Figure 3-11 along with the frequency response of a similar directional microphone for a sound source in front of the hearing aid. The omnidirectional micro-

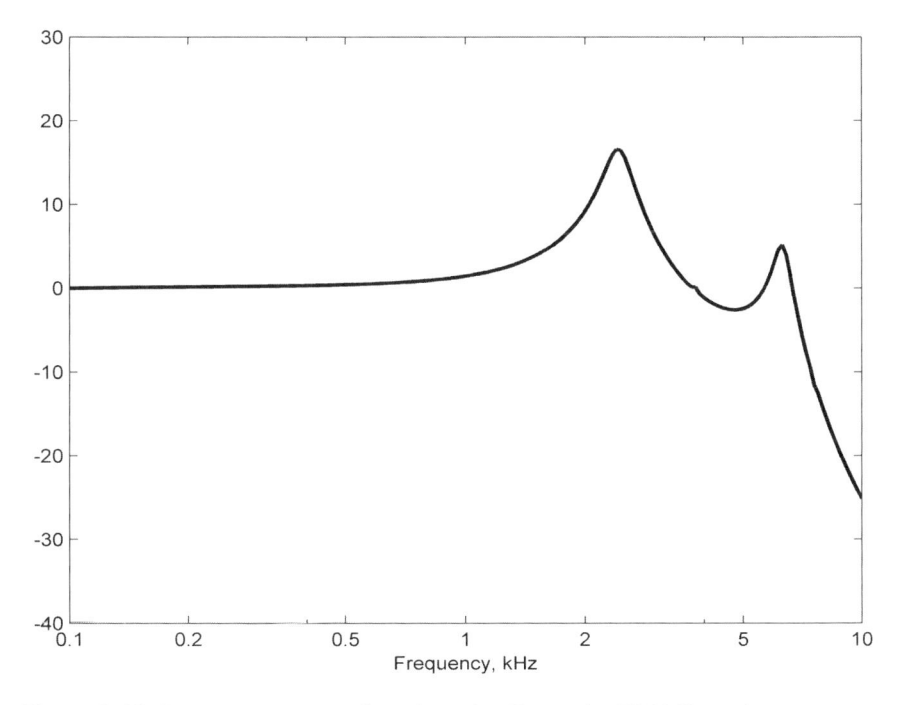

Figure 3-12. Frequency response for a Knowles Electronics ED1913 receiver.

phone response has a gradual low-frequency roll-off below about 300 Hz, a small response peak at about 5 kHz, and has a high-frequency roll-off above 5 kHz. The directional microphone has a slight increase in output near the 5-kHz resonance peak, but at low frequencies it has a frequency response that rises with increasing frequency at a rate of 6 dB/octave. Thus, the spatial noise rejection of a directional microphone comes at the expense of reduced low-frequency response.

The magnitude frequency response of a hearing-aid receiver is plotted in Figure 3-12. The receiver has a flat frequency response at low frequencies, and then rises to a resonance peak at about 2.4 kHz. The receiver has been designed to provide a mechanical resonance to replace the ear-canal resonance that is lost when the hearing aid is placed in the ear. A second resonance peak occurs at about 6.3 kHz, and the receiver response falls rapidly at frequencies above the second resonance. Adding a damping screen at the output port of the receiver will reduce the quality factor (Q) of the resonances and give a smoother response, but the peak output level will not be as high. The Q of an acoustic system is discussed in more detail later in this chapter.

Vent Acoustics

The hearing-aid signal processing is part of a larger electroacoustic system, and one of the most important aspects of this larger system is the vent. The vent contributes to acoustic feedback, as discussed in Chapter 7, and the feedback and the techniques used for feedback prevention can have a strong effect on the high-frequency response of the hearing aid. In this section we consider the effects of the vent on the low-frequency response of the hearing aid.

The vent interacts with the residual volume of the ear canal to form a resonant system, much like a mass-spring resonator. The behavior of this system can be described using acoustic circuit elements to give the equivalent mass of the air in the vent and the spring constant of the air in the ear canal. The resulting acoustic behavior acts to provide an acoustic short circuit that reduces the gain of the hearing aid at frequencies below the vent resonance frequency. No matter what type of signal processing is designed into the hearing aid or the amount of low-frequency amplification provided for the hearing loss, the processing effects are greatly reduced at low frequencies in a vented fitting.

ACOUSTIC ELEMENTS

The behavior of the vent-ear canal system can be described using acoustic circuit elements to give the equivalent acoustic mass and compliance (Beranek, 1954; Kinsler & Frye, 1962). The acoustic compliance is the inverse of the spring constant. The acoustic mass of the air in the vent is given by:

$$M_{vent} = \frac{\rho_0 L}{\pi a^2} \; kg/m^4 \quad \text{Equation (3.1)}$$

where ρ_0 is the density of air (1.18 kg/m³), a is the radius of the vent, and L is its length. Note that the acoustic mass increases with the length of the vent but, perhaps counterintuitively, increases as the radius is decreased—the smaller the vent radius the greater the acoustic mass.

The compliance is related to the volume of the residual air in the ear canal:

$$C_{canal} = \frac{V}{\rho_0 c^2} \; m^4/kg \quad \text{Equation (3.2)}$$

where V is the volume of air in m³ and c is the speed of sound (345 m/sec). The compliance is proportional to the enclosed volume of air. The compliance of the air in the ear canal is only part of the story, however, as there is also the compliance of the tympanic membrane. These compliances sum, giving the total compliance of the ear canal as:

$$C_{total} = C_{canal} + C_{tymp} \quad \text{Equation (3.3)}$$

The average compliance of the tympanum in a normal adult corresponds to an acoustic volume of about 0.8 mL (ASLHA, 1990).

The resonance frequency of the acoustic mass-spring system is given by:

$$\omega_0^2 = \frac{1}{M_{vent}[C_{canal} + C_{tymp}]} \quad \text{Equation (3.4)}$$

Converting from radians to Hz results gives the resonance frequency:

$$f_0 = \frac{1}{2\pi}\frac{1}{\sqrt{M_{vent}[C_{canal}+C_{tymp}]}} \quad \text{Equation (3.5)}$$

Thus increasing the mass or increasing the compliance reduces the resonance frequency of the vent-ear canal system.

An additional consideration is the Q of the resonance, which is the ratio of the resonance frequency to the bandwidth of the resonance peak. A high Q corresponds to a response having a sharp narrow peak. The Q depends on the acoustic resistance as well as the mass and compliance. Acoustic resistance can be provided by a damping element such as a piece of cotton or a sintered metal disk inserted into a tube, or by the local turbulence of the airflow along the walls of the tube. For an acoustic resistance R_{vent}, the quality factor is given by:

$$Q = \frac{1}{R_{vent}}\sqrt{\frac{M_{vent}}{C_{canal}+C_{tymp}}} \quad \text{Equation (3.6)}$$

Increasing the damping reduces the system Q. The Q also increases with increasing acoustic mass (smaller vent radius) but decreases with increasing acoustic compliance (larger residual ear canal volume).

Consider an example of a vented ITE hearing aid. The vent is assumed to be 22 mm in length with a radius of 1.2 mm. The hearing aid blocks much of the ear canal, but leaves a residual segment between the receiver and the tympanum having a length of 12 mm and a radius of 3.75 mm, which is the radius of the ear canal in the KEMAR acoustic manikin (Burkhard & Sachs, 1975). The mass of the air in the vent is given by Eq. (3.1):

$$M_{vent} = \frac{\rho_0 L}{\pi a^2} \, kg/m^4 = \frac{(1.18)(0.022)}{\pi(.0012)^2} = 5740 \quad \text{Equation (3.7)}$$

The compliance of the residual air volume in the ear canal is given by *Eq. (3.2)*:

$$C_{canal} = \frac{V}{\rho_0 c^2} m^4/kg = \frac{\pi(.012)(.00375)^2}{(1.18)(345)^2} = 3.77 \times 10^{-12}$$

Equation (3.8)

while the compliance of the tympanum is also given by *Eq. (3.2)* for the equivalent volume:

$$C_{tymp} = \frac{V}{\rho_0 c^2} m^4/kg = \frac{0.8 \times 10^{-6}}{(1.18)(345)^2} = 5.70 \times 10^{-12}$$

Equation (3.9)

The resonance frequency is then given by *Eq. (3.5)*:

$$f_0 = \frac{1}{2\pi} \frac{1}{\sqrt{M_{vent}[C_{canal}+C_{tymp}]}} = \frac{1}{2\pi} \frac{1}{\sqrt{(5740)[3.77 \times 10^{-12} + 5.70 \times 10^{-12}]}} = 683\ Hz$$

Equation (3.10)

VENT SIZE

The vent has a strong effect on the low-frequency response of the hearing aid in the ear. Figure 3-13 shows the transfer function from free field to ear canal for a simulated ITE hearing aid (Kates, 1988a, 1988b) mounted on the KEMAR manikin (Burkhard & Sachs, 1975). The simulation uses tubes of varying lengths and radii to model the vent and ear canal (Egolf, 1977), and the acoustic impedance of the tympanum is represented by a Zwislocki coupler (Zwislocki, 1970). The simulated transducers are a Knowles EA1842 microphone and a Knowles ED1913 receiver. The simulation was adjusted to allow sound to enter the ear canal through the vent and to give the interaction between the vent and ear canal. However, perfect feedback cancellation was assumed to eliminate the acoustic feedback effects at high frequencies caused by the vent. The hearing aid was set to have a gain of 30 dB at 1 kHz.

The effects of varying the vent radius are plotted in Figure 3-13. The curves range from no vent ($a = 0$) to a large vent ($a = 1.2$ mm). Increas-

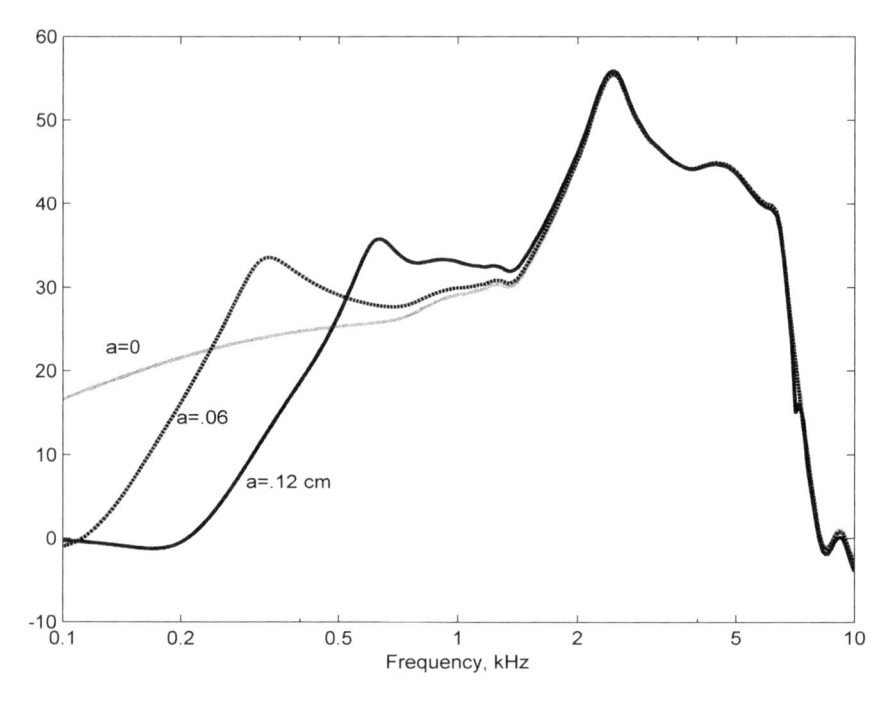

Figure 3-13. Frequency response for a simulated ITE hearing aid in the ear as the vent radius *a* is varied.

ing the vent radius reduces the acoustic mass of the vent, as given by Eq. (3.1). The reduced acoustic mass increases the vent-ear canal resonance frequency given by Eq. (3.5) and also reduces the Q of the vent-ear canal resonance given by Eq. (3.6). The vent interacts with the residual volume of air in the ear canal to produce a high-pass acoustic filter. As the vent radius is increased the cutoff frequency of this filter also increases as it is controlled by the resonance frequency given by Eq. (3.5). The resonance frequency for a vent radius of 1.2 mm is about 630 Hz, which is in reasonable agreement with the value calculated previously for the same vent and ear canal parameters, but with the tympanum represented by a simple compliance instead of the Zwislocki coupler. Compared to the hearing aid without a vent, the vented ITE loses essentially all of the amplification below the vent-ear canal resonance frequency, but gains amplification at and above the resonance frequency due to the Q of the acoustic filter.

The vent provides an acoustic modification of the hearing-aid fre-

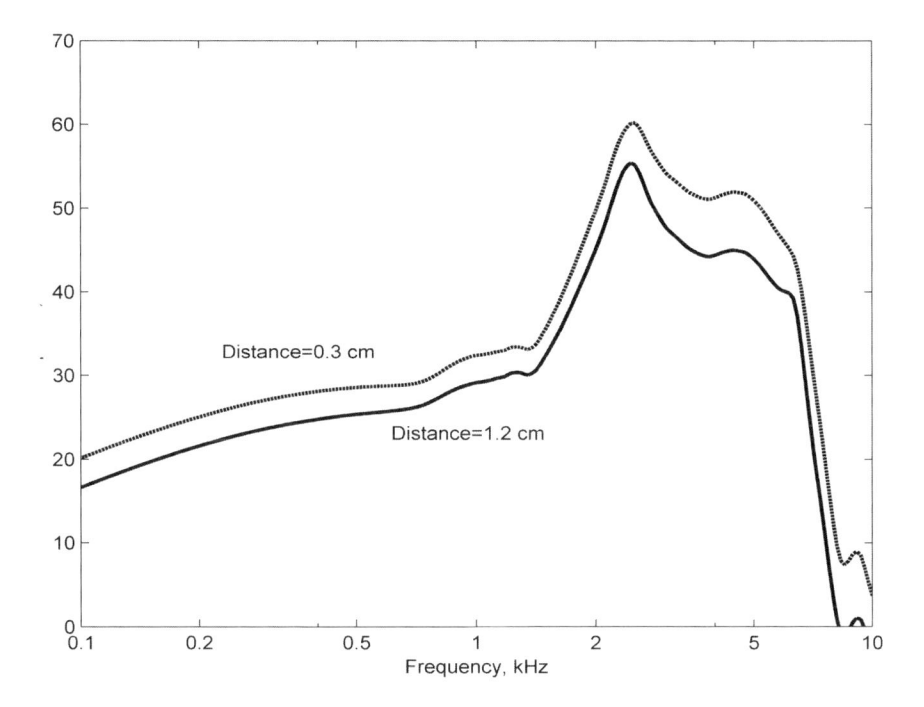

Figure 3-14. Frequency response for a simulated ITE hearing aid in the ear as the distance from the hearing-aid receiver to the ear drum is varied.

quency response. No matter what signal processing is provided at low frequencies, the vent will remove signal power for all frequencies below the vent-ear canal resonance frequency and will provide additional amplification for about an octave above the vent-ear canal resonance frequency. Because of the vent effects, the amplification achieved in the ear may differ significantly from that shown on the computer screen for the fitting software unless the vent is explicitly incorporated into the calculations.

RESIDUAL EAR-CANAL VOLUME

The pressure developed in the ear canal when a hearing aid is used depends on the acoustic compliance of the residual volume of air, the compliance of the ear-canal walls, and the acoustic impedance of the tympanum. One factor in a hearing-aid fitting is the depth to which the hearing aid or earmold is placed within the ear canal. A deeper fitting reduces the residual volume of air and will increase the sound pressure generated in the ear canal (Egolf et al., 1986; Kates, 1988a). This effect is illustrated in Figure 3-14 for the same simulated hearing aid as used in Figure 3-13. The vent has been removed. The indicated distance is the distance from the end of the KEMAR ear canal to the end of the hearing aid or earmold. Reducing this distance by filling more of the ear canal with the hearing aid reduces the residual volume and increases the pressure in the ear canal for the same receiver and gain setting. Note that the simulation assumes that the ear canal is a perfectly rigid tube and ignores the compliance of the walls of the ear canal.

The above example shows that inserting the hearing aid deeper into the same ear increases the sound pressure level. A related question is whether the sound pressure level at the tympanum can be predicted by measuring the residual ear-canal volume. The example worked previ-

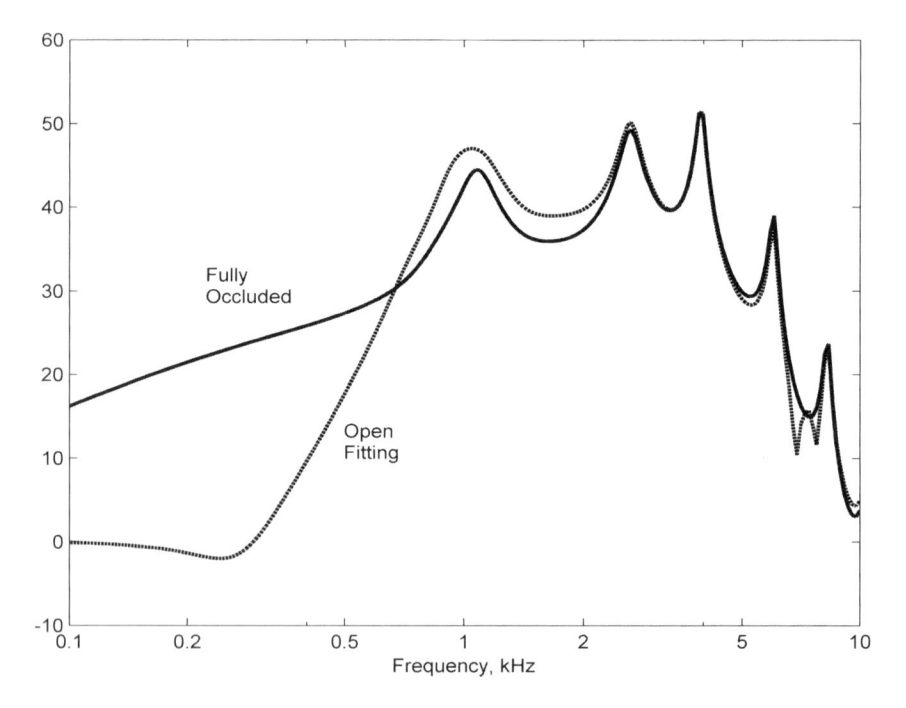

Figure 3-15. Frequency response for a simulated BTE hearing aid in the ear for an earmold that completely blocks the ear canal opening and for an earmold that leaves the ear canal completely open.

ously indicates that the average compliance of the tympanum (Eq. 3.9) is about 50% greater than that of the air in the ear canal (Eq. 3.8) for a nominal fitting depth. Reducing the residual volume of air in the ear canal to zero will still leave the compliance of the tympanum. The change in the total compliance is only about 40% as the residual volume of air is reduced to zero.

Individual variation in the compliance of the tympanum, and in the walls of the ear canal, is thus an important factor in attempting to predict the hearing aid sound pressure at the tympanum. The variation in the compliance of the tympanum will tend to dominate the variation in the total compliance of the combined ear canal plus tympanum, and this variation is apparent in measurements of in situ hearing-aid sound pressure levels. A small but statistically significant correlation has been observed between the residual ear-canal volume and the sound pressure at the tympanum measured using a probe-tube microphone (Cooper et al., 1988), and a somewhat larger correlation obtained when the residual ear-canal volume is combined with the compliance of the tympanum (Bergman & Bentler, 1990).

OPEN BTE FITTING

An open fitting refers to a behind-the-ear (BTE) hearing aid in which the sound is conducted into the ear canal through a tube without an earmold, or where the earmold is just a skeleton that holds the tube in place. A BTE hearing aid was simulated by increasing the length of the tube that connects the receiver to the ear canal. The tube was made 60 mm long and had a diameter of 0.6 mm. In Figure 3-15, the response of a BTE with an unvented earmold that completely blocks the ear canal is compared to an open fitting in which the ear canal is completely unoccluded. The ear canal functions as the vent in a completely open fitting. The hearing aid gain was set to 30 dB at 1 kHz.

At low frequencies, the effect of the vent on the BTE frequency response is very similar to its effect on the ITE response illustrated in Figure 3-13. The open fitting reduces the system response beyond the vent-ear canal resonance frequency. Because the radius of the vent in the open fitting is that of the ear canal, the open fitting represents the highest possible vent-ear canal resonance frequency and thus the greatest amount of low-frequency signal attenuation. The hearing aid is effective only above 700 Hz in this simulation, so an open fitting only provides amplification at high frequencies.

The receiver tube is itself a resonator, and it introduces multiple peaks and valleys into the system frequency response at high frequencies. Adding acoustic damping to the receiver tube can reduce the magnitude of the peaks and valleys. With modern digital hearing aids one tends to adjust the system frequency response by adjusting the gain-versus-frequency characteristic of a multichannel digital amplifier. But in the days of one-channel analog hearing aids, acoustic modification of the receiver tubing was one of the few techniques available for modifying the system frequency response (Killion, 1981; Libby, 1982) and tubing modifications can still be appropriate for digital instruments. The reader is referred to Dillon (2001) for a more complete treatment of earmold designs and the effects of tubing.

Occlusion Effect

The hearing aid or earmold blocks the ear canal. The occlusion effect refers to the increase in low-frequency sound pressure within the blocked ear canal when the hearing-aid user is talking. The user's own voice is the source of sound, and it enters the ear canal via bone conduction and the flexing of the cartilaginous walls of the ear canal (Killion et al., 1988). The occlusion effect is not caused by the hearing-aid amplification, but rather by the acoustic effects of blocking the ear canal. To demonstrate the occlusion effect, vocalize a continuous vowel, such as "eeee," and place your fingers in your ears while vocalizing. The high frequencies in the sound will be attenuated, but the low frequencies will appear to be amplified in comparison with the open ear canals.

The intensity and spectrum of the bone-conducted excitation was measured by Won and Berger (2005) for one female subject. They compared the sound pressure measured on the skull using a piezo-electric transducer to the signal at a microphone in front of the person singing various notes and glides. The transfer function relating the signal at the piezo-electric transducer to that at the microphone shows approximately 12 dB gain at very low frequencies, dropping to a valley of 0 or negative dB at around 500 Hz, and then rising to a resonance peak of between 5 and 15 dB at around 2 kHz. The high-frequency resonance peak may be due to the vocal training of the subject, as Western classical voice training encourages singers to recognize and exploit the acoustic resonances of the head and skull. However, the bone-conducted sound also has a substantial low-frequency component, and this component would be expected to be present in the speaking voices of both genders and would form the dominant component of the ear-canal excitation.

Blocking the ear-canal opening increases the sound pressure level from the talker's own voice within the ear canal. In comparison with an open ear canal, the sound pressure level in a completely occluded ear canal can be up to 25 dB greater (Kuk et al., 2005), and most of the additional sound intensity occurs below 500 Hz (Killion et al., 1988). The data of Killion et al. (1988) also suggest that the occlusion effect may be greater in males than in females, possibly due to the lower fundamental frequency of the male voice. The perceived intensity of the occlusion effect will also depend on the vowel being used to demonstrate it as the first formant of the vowel defines the frequency region having the greatest sound power.

There are two ways to reduce the occlusion effect in a hearing aid. One is to insert the hearing aid deeply into the ear canal (Killion et al., 1988). The deep insertion goes past the cartilaginous wall of the ear canal and seats the hearing aid tip in the bony portion. The bony portion of the ear canal doesn't flex as much as the cartilaginous portion during vocalization and thus produces less sound pressure in the ear canal and results in a reduced occlusion effect.

The second way to reduce the occlusion effect is to vent the hearing aid shell or earmold. Increasing the vent diameter leads to a reduction in the measured occlusion effect and a corresponding reduction in its perceived intensity (Kiesling et al., 2005; Kuk et al., 2005). Kiesling et al. (2005) found a very high correlation between the acoustic mass of the vent and the subjects' perception of occlusion. Remember from *Eq. (3.1)* that the acoustic mass is inversely proportional to the cross-sectional area of the vent, so an increased acoustic mass corresponds to a reduced diameter. The greatest acoustic mass occurs as the vent diameter shrinks to zero giving an unvented earmold, whereas the smallest acoustic mass occurs in an open fitting. An open fitting causes essentially no occlusion effect. But an open fitting also provides little low-frequency amplification, as shown in Figure 3-15. So here is yet another tradeoff in hearing-aid design—the annoyance of the occlusion effect versus the amount of low-frequency gain.

Concluding Remarks

A hearing-aid is a complex electroacoustic system. The acoustics of the head, ear, transducers, and vent all affect the sound pressure at the tympanum. The design of the hearing-aid signal processing is generally taken to mean the circuit (analog or digital) situated within the hearing aid, but the acoustics can strongly affect the processing performance. A directional microphone, for example, imposes a very different frequency response at the input to the hearing aid than an omnidirectional microphone. The receiver has a response peak that partially replaces the ear canal resonance lost when the hearing aid or earmold is placed in the ear, but the detailed structure of the HRTF is not duplicated when a hearing aid is used and much of the head and ear transfer function is lost. The vent can greatly reduce the low-frequency gain of the hearing aid, and the sound pressure obtained in the ear may differ from that predicted by the hearing-aid fitting software if the vent is not taken into account. The occlusion effect is caused by a bone-conduction path within the head that exists in addition to the external acoustic path, and fitting a hearing aid may well require a compromise between the desired low-frequency gain and a vent large enough to ameliorate the occlusion effect.

References

American Speech-Language-Hearing Association. (1990). Guidelines for screening for hearing impairments and middle ear disorders. *Asha, 32* (Suppl. 2), 17–24.

Batteau, D. W. (1967). The role of the pinna in human localization. *Proceedings of the Royal Society of London, 168* (Series B), 158-180.

Beranek, L. L. (1954). *Acoustics*. New York: McGraw-Hill.

Bergman, B. M., & Bentler, R. A. (1990). *Relating hearing aid output to measurements of volume and immitance*. Paper presented at the American Speech-Language-Hearing Association meeting, Seattle, November 18, 1990.

Burkhard, M. D., & Sachs, R. M. (1975). Anthropometric manikin for acoustic research. *Journal of the Acoustical Society of America, 58*, 214–222.

Cooper, W. A., Larson, V. D., Balfour, P. B., Copps, T. E., & Brooks, B. A. (1988). *Ear canal SPL as a function of residual volume*. Paper presented at the American Speech-Language-Hearing Association meeting, Boston, November 18–21, 1988.

Dillon, H. (2001), Hearing aid earmolds, earshells, and coupling. In *Hearing aids*, (pp. 117–158). New York: Thieme.

Egolf, D. P. (1977). Mathematical model of a probe-tube microphone. *Journal of the Acoustical Society of America, 61,* 200–205.

Egolf, D. P., Haley, B. T., & Larson, V. D. (1986). The constant-volume-velocity nature of hearing aids: Conclusions based on computer simulations. *Journal of the Acoustical Society of America, 79,* 1592–1602.

Kates, J. M. (1988a). A computer simulation of hearing aid response and the effects of ear canal size. *Journal of the Acoustical Society of America, 83,* 1952–1963.

Kates, J. M. (1988b). Acoustic effects in in-the-ear hearing aid response: Results from a computer simulation. *Ear and Hearing, 9,* 119–132.

Kiesling, J., Brenner, B., Jespersen, C. T., Groth, J., & Dyrlund Jensen, O. (2005), Occlusion effect of earmolds with different venting systems. *Journal of the American Academy of Audiology, 16,* 237–249.

Killion, M. C. (1981). Earmold options for wideband hearing aids. *Journal of Speech and Hearing Disorders, 46,* 10–20.

Killion, M. C., Wilbur, L. A., Gudmundsen, G. I. (1988). Zwislocki was right...*Hearing Instruments, 39*(1), 14–18.

Kinsler, L. E., & Frye, A. R. (1962). *Fundamentals of acoustics* (2nd ed.). New York: Wiley.

Kuk, F., Keenan, D., & Lau, C. -C. (2005). Vent configurations on subjective and objective occlusion effect. *Journal of the American Academy of Audiology, 16,* 747–762.

Langendijk, E. H. A., & Bronkhorst, A. W. (2002). Contribution of spectral cues to human sound localization. *Journal of the Acoustical Society of America, 112,* 1583–1596.

Libby, E. R. (1982). In search of transparent insertion gain hearing aid responses. In G. A. Studebaker & F. H. Bess, Eds., *The Vanderbilt Hearing-Aid Report.* Upper Darby, PA: Monographs in Contemporary Audiology.

Rodgers, C. A. P. (1981). Pinna transformations and sound reproduction. *Journal of the Audio Engineering Society, 29,* 226–233.

Shaw, E. A. G. (1974). Transformation of sound pressure level from the free field to the eardrum in the horizontal plane. *Journal of the Acoustical Society of America, 56,* 1848–1861.

Wiener, F. M., & Ross, D. A. (1946). The pressure distribution in the auditory canal in a progressive sound field. *Journal of the Acoustical Society of America, 18,* 401–408.

Won, S. Y., & Berger, J. (2005). Estimating transfer function from air to bone conduction using singing voice, Paper 1259. *Proceedings of the International Computer Music Conference*, Barcelona, Sept. 5–9, 2005.

Wright, D., Hebrank, J. H., & Wilson, B. (1974). Pinna reflections as cues for sound localization. *Journal of the Acoustical Society of America, 56*, 957–962.

Zwislocki, J. J. (1970). *An acoustic coupler for earphone calibration.* Syracuse University, New York: Report LSC-S-7.

4
Directional Microphones

DIRECTIONAL MICROPHONES are implemented in many digital hearing aids. A common listening situation has the listener looking at the talker, and noise or speech coming from other directions interferes with the conversation. The objective of using a directional microphone is to preserve the desired signal coming from in front of the listener while attenuating noise and interference coming from beside or behind the listener. A directional microphone provides spatial processing in which the physical separation between the desired signal source and the sources of interference is exploited to improve the signal-to-noise ratio (SNR).

This chapter introduces directional microphones and explains their basic behavior. The simplest directional microphone is equivalent to two omnidirectional microphones whose outputs are combined in a fixed proportion, and the properties of this simple system are explored in this chapter. More complicated systems can be built by combining the outputs of more than two microphones, or by combining the outputs in ways that change over time to produce an adaptive system. These complex microphone systems are discussed in the next chapter.

Hearing-Aid Microphones

MICROPHONE CONSTRUCTION

An omnidirectional microphone responds to the fluctuations in acoustic pressure at one point in space, and it is equally sensitive to sounds coming from all directions. There are many ways to design such a microphone, and the design involves tradeoffs between the microphone sensitivity, size, and internal noise level. The basic microphone, illustrated in Figure 4-1, is a membrane that moves in response to pressure fluctuations (Beranek, 1954). Attached to the membrane is a coil of wire that moves in a magnetic field. The motion of the coil induces a current that flows in proportion to the movement of the membrane. The larger the membrane, the greater the force that will be generated for equal motions of the air and the more sensitive the microphone will be to small changes in pressure. Brownian motion of the air molecules will cause

MICROPHONES

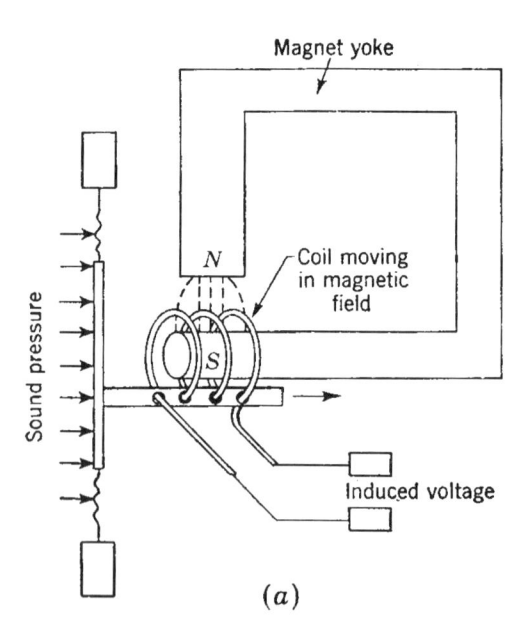

FIGURE 4-1. General design of an omnidirectional pressure microphone (Reprinted with permission from Beranek, L. L. (1954). *Acoustics*, New York: McGraw-Hill. Copyright 1954, Acoustical Society of America.).

random fluctuations of the membrane even in the absence of a pressure signal, and this random motion establishes a background noise level. A large membrane can average the random pressure over a greater surface area than a small membrane, and will thus have a lower noise level. These factors, taken together, mean that a larger microphone will produce a larger output for a given sound pressure level and will have a lower internal noise level than a smaller microphone using the same design technology. In designing a microphone for a hearing aid, the goal is to achieve the smallest microphone that has the necessary sensitivity and internal noise level for monitoring speech and environmental sounds.

An omnidirectional microphone designed for hearing aids is illustrated in Figure 4-2. The coil and magnetic structure are not shown; the structure in a hearing-aid microphone differs mechanically from that shown in Figure 4-1 so that the microphone can be made as small as possible while preserving an adequate membrane surface area. Sound pressure enters through the port and displaces the membrane. The volume of air behind the membrane acts as a spring that resists the membrane motion, and the motion induces current in a coil that is sensed and amplified by a transistor pre-amplifier to give the microphone output signal.

A directional microphone designed for hearing aids is shown in Figure 4-3. The directional microphone has two ports, one connected to the top of the membrane, as in the omnidirectional microphone shown

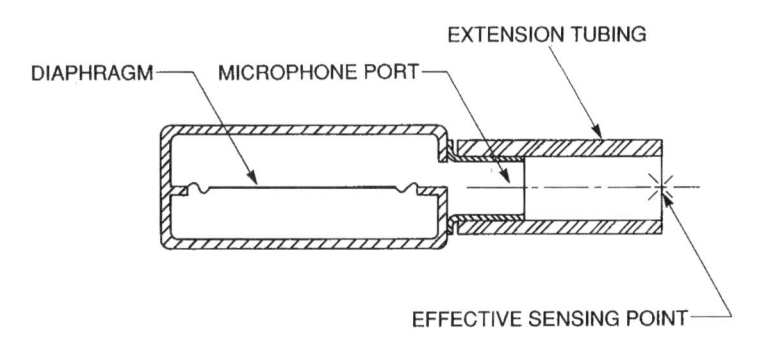

FIGURE 4-2. Cross-section drawing of an omnidirectional hearing-aid microphone (from Knowles Electronics Technical Bulletin TB21, 1980).

78 Digital Hearing Aids

in Figure 4-2, and the other connected to the underside of the membrane through an acoustic time-delay network. The membrane moves in response to the difference between the pressure at the upper surface and the pressure at the lower surface. If the pressure is the same at the two surfaces of the membrane, for example in a uniform static pressure, then the microphone output is zero. If a pressure wave is propagating across the microphone it will arrive at the two ports at different times, and the output signal will depend on the direction of arrival of the pressure wave, its frequency, and the built-in time delay.

DIRECTIONAL MICROPHONES AND SPATIAL SIGNAL PROCESSING

To understand the spatial behavior of the directional microphone, it helps to redraw the two-port system of Figure 4-3 as an equivalent system using a pair of omnidirectional microphones. This equivalent system is shown in Figure 4-4. The front microphone in Figure 4-4 represents the front microphone port that generates the pressure at the upper surface of the membrane in Figure 4-3. The rear microphone in Figure 4-4 represents the rear microphone port that generates the pressure at the underside of the membrane. The acoustic time delay net-

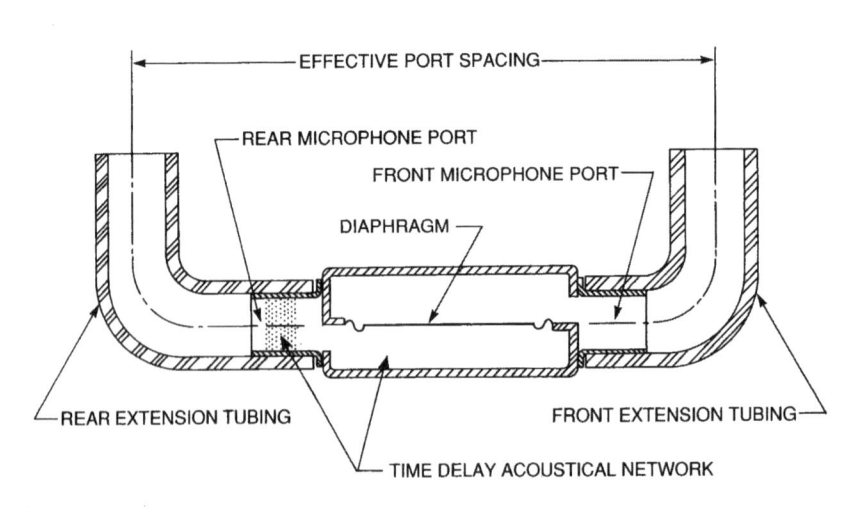

Figure 4-3. Cross-section drawing of a directional hearing-aid microphone (from Knowles Electronics Technical Bulletin TB21, 1980).

work in Figure 4-3 is replaced by a time-delay block having a delay of τ sec in Figure 4-4. The pressure difference in Figure 4-3 is given in Figure 4-4 by subtracting the delayed rear microphone output from the front microphone signal. The pair of omnidirectional microphones are separated by distance d, and it is assumed that there is a plane wave propagating over the pair of microphones from an azimuth given by the angle θ.

The output of the directional microphone can be expressed in terms of the microphone separation d, the angle of arrival θ, and the rear microphone time delay τ and gain b. The time it takes for the plane wave to propagate from the front microphone to the rear microphone is given by:

$$\delta(\theta) = \frac{d}{c}\cos\theta \qquad \text{Equation (4.1)}$$

where c is the speed of sound (approximately 345 m/sec). If the angle of arrival θ is less than ±90 degrees, $\cos(\theta) > 0$ and the signal wavefront will arrive at the front microphone before it reaches the rear microphone.

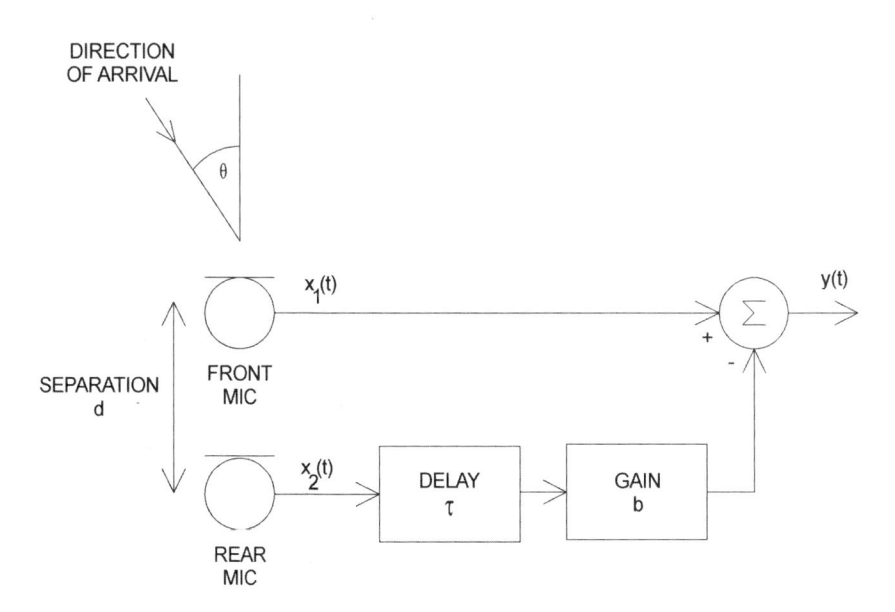

Figure 4-4. Directional microphone as a spatial signal-processing system.

80 Digital Hearing Aids

For θ = ±90 degrees, $\cos(\theta) = 0$ and the signal will arrive at the two microphones at the same time. And when 270 < θ < 90 degrees, $\cos(\theta) < 0$ and the signal will arrive at the rear microphone before it reaches the front microphone.

Let the external signal be denoted by $s(t)$, the output from the front microphone in response to this signal by $x_1(t)$, and the output from the rear microphone by $x_2(t)$. Taking the propagation delay into account, the outputs from the two microphone are:

$$x_1(t) = s(t)$$
$$x_2(t) = s\left(t - \frac{d}{c}\cos\theta\right) \quad \text{Equation (4.2)}$$

The two microphone outputs are then combined to form the directional microphone output $y(t)$:

$$y(t) = x_1(t) - bx_2(t - \tau) \quad \text{Equation (4.3)}$$

A directional microphone normally has $b = 1$, and an omnidirectional microphone can be represented using Eq. (4.3) by setting $b = 0$ to eliminate the rear microphone signal. Substitute Eq. (4.2) into Eq. (4.3) to get

$$y(t) = s(t) - bs\left(t - \frac{d}{c}\cos\theta - \tau\right) \quad \text{Equation (4.4)}$$

Note that the rear microphone signal now has two time delays: the delay caused by the sound wave propagating across the pair of microphones, followed by the delay τ inserted by the directional microphone processing.

The signal $s(t)$ can be any waveform, such as speech or music. However, a particularly useful signal for our analysis is a sinusoid at frequency ω having unit power, giving $s(t) = \sqrt{2}\cos(\omega t)$. For this choice of signal, the microphone output $y(t)$ can be expanded using the trigonometric identity $\cos(\xi - \phi) = \cos(\xi)\cos(\phi) + \sin(\xi)\sin(\phi)$:

Directional Microphones

$$y(t) = \sqrt{2}\cos(\omega t) - b\sqrt{2}\cos(\omega t)\cos\left[\omega\left(\frac{d}{c}\cos\theta + \tau\right)\right] - b\sqrt{2}\sin(\omega t)\sin\left[\omega\left(\frac{d}{c}\cos\theta + \tau\right)\right]$$

Equation (4.5)

The terms in Eq. (4.5) can be rearranged to give a cosine frequency-dependent term and a sine frequency-dependent term:

$$y(t) = \sqrt{2}\left\{1 - b\cos\left[\omega\left(\frac{d}{c}\cos\theta + \tau\right)\right]\right\}\cos(\omega t) - \sqrt{2}\left\{b\sin\left[\omega\left(\frac{d}{c}\cos\theta + \tau\right)\right]\right\}\sin(\omega t)$$

Equation (4.6)

The magnitude of the directional microphone output power, averaged over time, is then:

$$|Y(\omega,\theta)|^2 = \left\{1 - b\cos\left[\omega\left(\frac{d}{c}\cos\theta + \tau\right)\right]\right\}^2 + \left\{b\sin\left[\omega\left(\frac{d}{c}\cos\theta + \tau\right)\right]\right\}^2$$

Equation (4.7)

Expanding the squared quantity in the first bracket, and using the identity $\cos^2\varphi + \sin^2\varphi = 1$, leads to:

$$|Y(\omega,\theta)|^2 = (1 + b^2) - 2b\cos\left[\omega\left(\frac{d}{c}\cos\theta + \tau\right)\right] \quad \text{Equation (4.8)}$$

For most hearing-aid applications, the spacing between the microphones is small compared to the wavelength of sound. Under these conditions, the argument of the cosine function in Eq. (4.8) will be close to zero and we can use the first two terms of the Taylor series expansion to approximate $\cos\varphi \approx 1 - \varphi^2/2$. Making this substitution in Eq. (4.8) leads to:

$$|Y(\omega,\theta)|^2 \approx \left(1+b^2\right) - 2b\left[1 - \frac{\omega^2}{2}\left(\frac{d}{c}\cos\theta + \tau\right)^2\right] \quad \text{Equation (4.9)}$$

Separating the terms that do not involve the frequency ω from those that have a frequency dependence then gives:

$$|Y(\omega,\theta)|^2 \approx (1-b)^2 + b\left[\omega^2\left(\frac{d}{c}\cos\theta + \tau\right)^2\right] \quad \text{Equation (4.10)}$$

For the expected situation of b = 1, the first term becomes zero, giving the approximation:

$$|Y(\omega,\theta)| \approx \omega\left(\frac{d}{c}\cos\theta + \tau\right) \quad \text{Equation (4.11)}$$

Eq. (4.11) describes the low-frequency magnitude response of a directional microphone. The response can be separated into a frequency term times a directional term. The frequency term is simply ω. The directional term is the sum of the propagation delay from the front to the rear microphone plus the rear microphone delay, and these time delays do not depend on frequency. The microphone directional response pattern therefore depends solely on the microphone spacing d and the rear microphone delay τ. The microphone response patterns that result from varying these two parameters are described in the next section, and the microphone frequency response behavior is discussed in the subsequent section.

Directional Response Patterns

MICROPHONE SPACING AND TIME DELAY

The directional microphone response given by *Eq. (4.11)* is a function of the microphone spacing d and the rear microphone delay τ. The influence of these two factors can be combined by setting $\tau = \beta(d/c)$, that is, expressing the rear microphone delay in terms of the microphone spacing. The directional microphone response given by *Eq. (4.11)* then becomes:

$$|Y(\omega,\theta)| \approx \omega \frac{d}{c}(\cos\theta + \beta) \quad \text{Equation (4.12)}$$

The frequency dependence is given by ω, the term d/c is a constant that scales the magnitude of the response, and changing the rear microphone time delay by adjusting β changes the microphone directional pattern.

Consider the directional pattern for $\beta = 0$. The directional pattern for this situation is proportional to $cos(\theta)$. For a wave arriving from the front, $\theta = 0$, giving $cos\,\theta = 1$, and the response has a maximum. A wave arriving from 90 degrees has $cos\,\theta = 0$, and the response has a null. A wave arriving from 180 degrees has $cos\,\theta = -1$, and the response has another maximum in its magnitude response, but the phase of the response has been inverted.

Consider now a directional microphone with $\beta = 1$, so that the rear microphone delay is equal to the time it takes for a wave to propagate from rear microphone to the front microphone. For a signal arriving from 180 degrees, $cos\,\theta = -1$ while $\beta = 1$. These two values cancel, resulting in a null facing the rear. This behavior can also be understood in terms of Figure 4-3. A signal from 180 degrees reaches the rear microphone d/c sec before it reaches the front microphone. The rear microphone signal is then delayed d/c sec before it reaches the underside of the diaphragm, which is exactly the same amount of time that it takes the signal to propagate forward to reach the top of the diaphragm. The pressure waveforms at the top and underside of the diaphragm are therefore identical, so the net diaphragm motion is zero and there is no microphone output.

Often, in describing microphone directional patterns, the response is normalized to give a gain of 1 in the forward direction corresponding to $\theta = 0$. The normalization is equivalent to removing the frequency dependence in *Eq. (4.12)*, giving:

$$\frac{|Y(\omega,\theta)|}{|Y(\omega,0)|} \approx \alpha + (1-\alpha)\cos\theta \quad \text{Equation (4.13)}$$

where $0 \leq \alpha \leq 1$. The directional pattern given by *Eq. (4.13)* can be interpreted as the sum of an omnidirectional pattern and a cosine (also called a "figure-eight" or dipole) directional pattern. The first term in *Eq. (4.13)* is just α, and this can be interpreted as the relative weight given to the omnidirectional portion of the total response, and the second term is the cosine portion of the response with a weight of $(1-\alpha)$. Comparing *Eq. (4.13)* to *Eq. (4.12)* shows that the same directional response can be described either in terms of the rear microphone time delay or as a weighted sum of an omnidirectional plus a cosine response.

Several common response patterns are summarized in Table 4-1 and are illustrated in Figure 4-5. The response patterns shown are (A) cosine, (B) hypercardioid, (C) supercardioid, and (D) cardioid response. Cardioid, by the way, refers to the pattern being heart-shaped (think of the heart on a Valentine's Day card). In progressing from the cosine pattern to the cardioid pattern, the rear microphone time delay in *Eq. (4.12)* is increased from 0 to d/c, and the relative weight a for the omnidirectional part of the response in *Eq. (4.13)* is increased from 0 to 0.5. Going from cosine to cardioid, one can see that the size of the rear lobe of the response pattern shrinks and the width of the front lobe increases, whereas the null in the response pattern shifts from ±90 degrees for the cosine pattern to 180 deg for the cardioid pattern.

Table 4-1. Summary of Some Directional Responses That Can Be Achieved with Two Microphones.

Pattern	Rear Mic Delay	a	DI, dB
Omnidirectional	–	1	0
Cosine	0	0	4.8
Hypercardioid	d/3c	0.25	6.0
Supercardioid	2d/3c	0.4	5.7
Cardioid	d/c	0.5	4.8

The rear microphone delay corresponds to τ in Figure 4-3. The directional response is given by $R(\theta) = \alpha + (1-\alpha)\cos(\theta)$. DI is the directivity index.

MICROPHONE MISMATCH

The ideal directional patterns shown in Figure 4-5 all assume that the rear microphone gain $b = 1$ and that the front and rear microphones have identical magnitude and phase responses. What happens if the front and rear microphones don't exactly match? The changes to a cardioid directional response are plotted in Figure 4-6 as the rear microphone gain is decreased from 1 to 0.9. The microphone output is given by Eq. (4.8), normalized so that the microphone gain for a signal arriving from 0 degrees is 0 dB. The expected cardioid response is obtained for $b = 1$. Setting $b = 0.98$, a reduction of just 0.18 dB, begins to fill in the rear null in the response and the null depth goes from perfect cancellation to a level of about -18 dB re: 1. A further reduction in b to 0.95, a reduction of 0.45 dB, fills in the rear null to the point where it is about -12 dB re: 1. Setting $b = 0.9$, which gives a reduction of 0.92 dB in the rear microphone output level, almost completely removes the rear null. Increasing the value of b to be greater than 1, rather than the decrease illustrated here, causes similar changes in the directional response of the microphone system.

The cardioid microphone response pattern requires perfect cancellation of the front and rear microphone signals to achieve the response null at 180 degrees. A mismatch between the two microphones fills in the null with the difference in output between the rear and front microphones. Microphones are usually selected from the same manufacturing batch when building the hearing aid to give the best match between the mechanical components. However, even a small mismatch can interfere with achieving the desired directional response, and the mismatch can increase over time as the microphones age.

Frequency Response

MAGNITUDE FREQUENCY RESPONSE

The magnitude frequency response for a directional microphone for a sound source located directly in front of the microphone is given by Eq. (4.8) with $\theta = 0$. An omnidirectional microphone has $b = 0$, resulting in a frequency response that is flat across frequency. An ideal directional microphone has $b = 1$, and can be approximated at low frequencies using Eq. (4.12). The magnitude of the response of a directional microphone at low frequencies is proportional to d/c. The output of the directional

86 Digital Hearing Aids

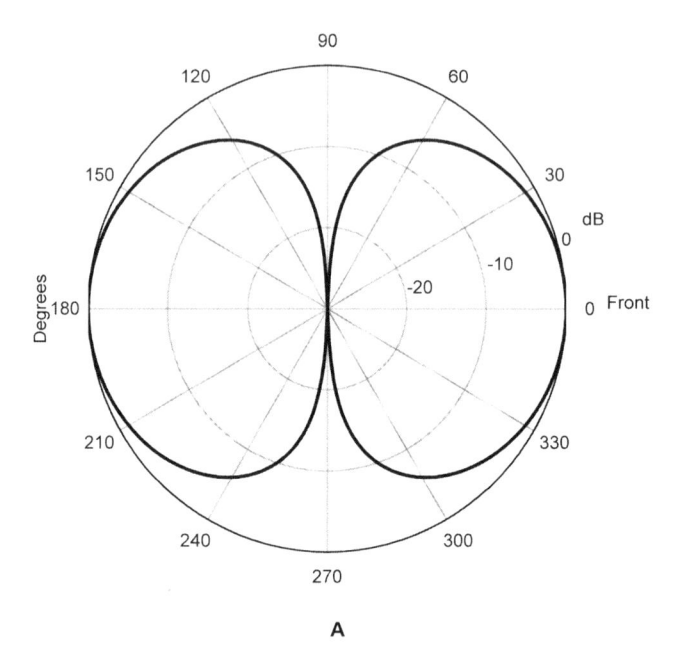

Figure 4-5. Microphone directional patterns as the rear microphone time delay is varied: **A.** dipole ($\tau = 0$), **B.** hypercardioid ($\tau = d/3c$), **C.** supercardioid ($\tau = 2d/3c$), and **D.** cardioid ($\tau = d/c$). The spacing between the microphones is 1 cm, and the input is a sinusoid at 500 Hz.

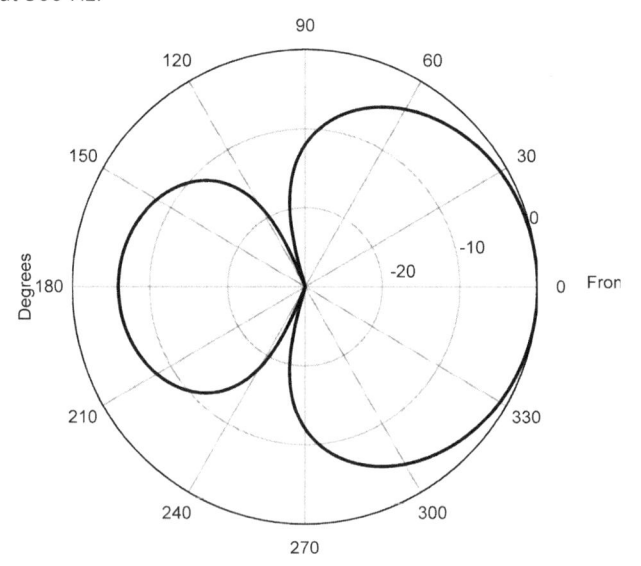

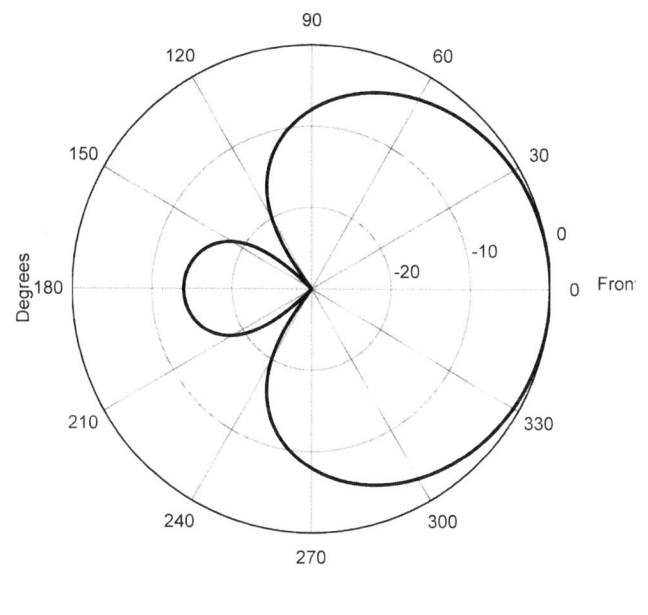

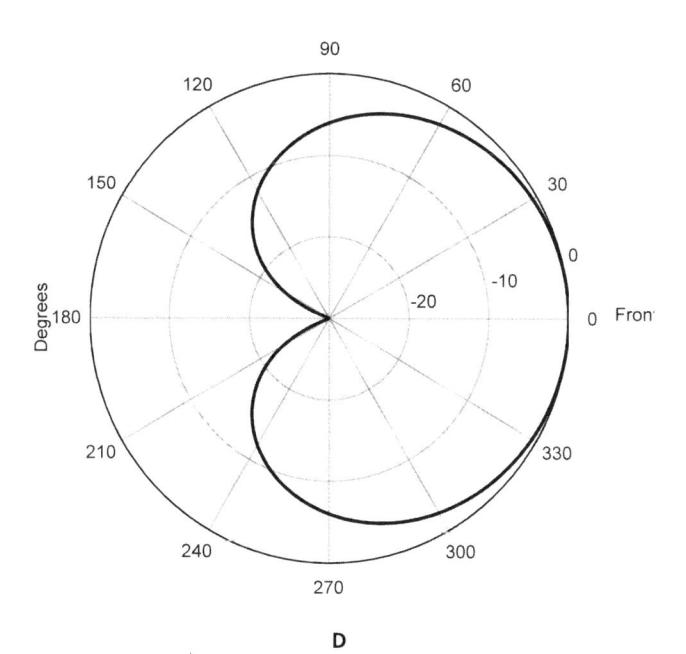

Directional Microphones 87

C

D

88 Digital Hearing Aids

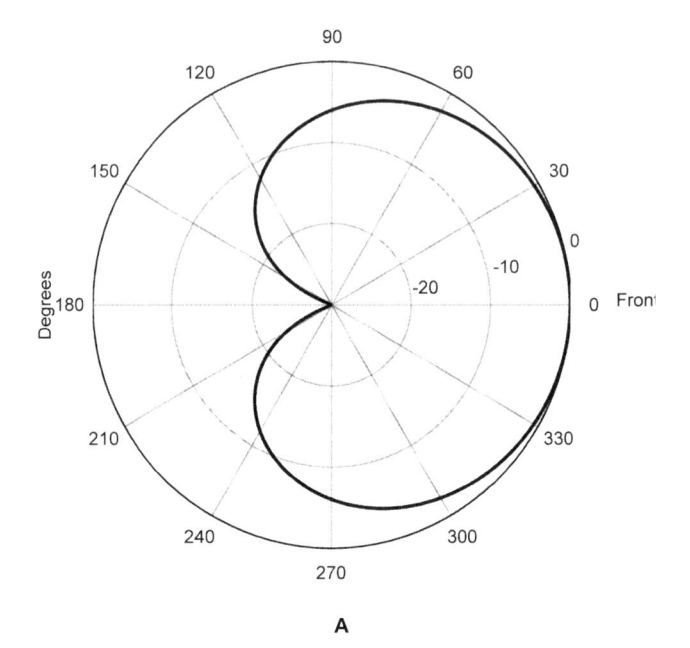

Figure 4-6. Cardioid microphone directional patterns as the rear microphone gain b is varied: **A.** b = 1.00, **B.** b = 0.98, **C.** b = 0.95, and **D.** b = 0.90. The spacing between the microphones is 1 cm, and the input is a sinusoid at 500 Hz.

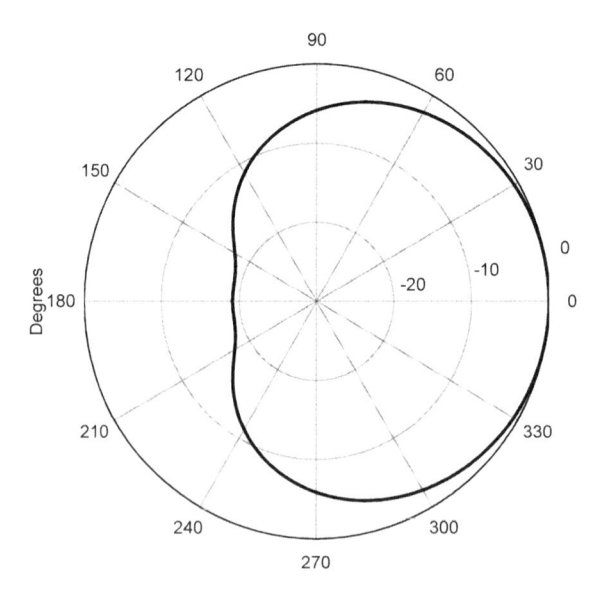

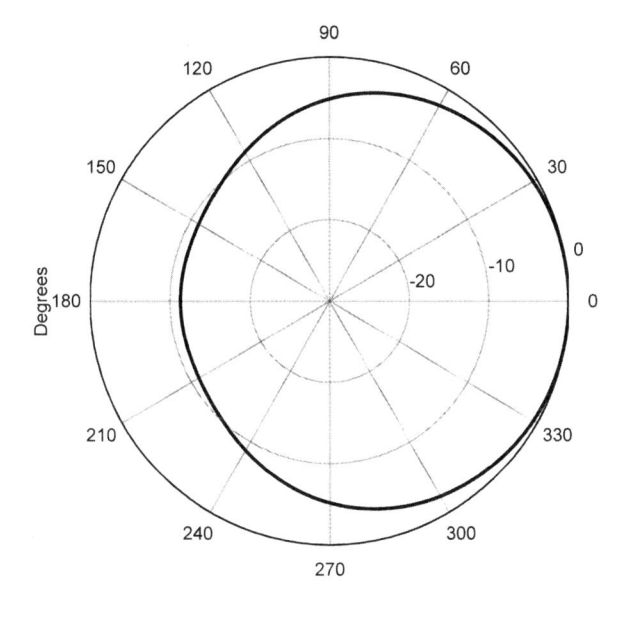

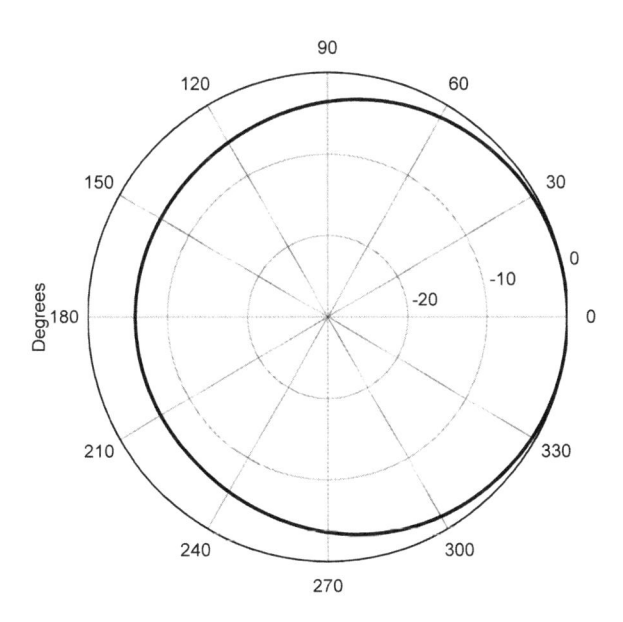

Directional Microphones **89**

C

D

microphone is proportional to ω, which means that the magnitude frequency response has a rising slope of 6 dB/octave. Furthermore, the output is proportional to the microphone spacing d, which means that reducing the separation between the directional microphones will reduce the output level. At high frequencies the microphone separation starts to approach the wavelength of sound, so the low-frequency approximation of Eq. (4.12) is no longer valid and the exact solution of Eq. (4.8) must be used.

Changing the value of β in Eq. (4.12) can change the directional response along a continuum ranging from dipole to cardioid. However, the magnitude of the response is still proportional to $\omega d/c$ no matter what value of β is chosen. Thus, any directional microphone, no matter which directional response pattern is chosen, will have the same frequency response slope of 6 dB/octave at low frequencies.

The magnitude frequency response of an ideal omnidirectional microphone is compared to the output of a cardioid microphone in Figure 4-7. The cardioid microphone response is shown for two different microphone spacings. The separation of 1 cm is typical of a BTE hearing aid, whereas the reduced separation of 0.5 cm might be found in some ITE or miniature BTE devices. The cardioid responses show the 6-dB/octave slope, with the output from the 0.5-cm spacing 6 dB below that for the 1-cm spacing. Reducing the microphone separation extends the directional response behavior out to higher frequencies, but the reduced output means that additional microphone amplification will be required to achieve the same output level and microphone noise will be more of a problem. At high frequencies, the directional microphone response is approximately the same as for the omnidirectional microphone, after which the output from the directional microphone starts to decrease.

MICROPHONE MISMATCH

The low-frequency directional microphone response changes if there is microphone mismatch. To understand this effect, refer back to Eq. (4.10). Perfectly matched microphones correspond to $b = 1$, and the first term in Eq. (4.10) becomes zero. The magnitude frequency response is then given by the second term in the equation, which is proportional to ω and which results in a 6-dB/octave slope. But if $b \neq 1$, the first term does not become zero. At very low frequencies, the second term in the equation approaches zero but the first term remains greater than zero. Thus, at a low enough frequency, the magnitude frequency response

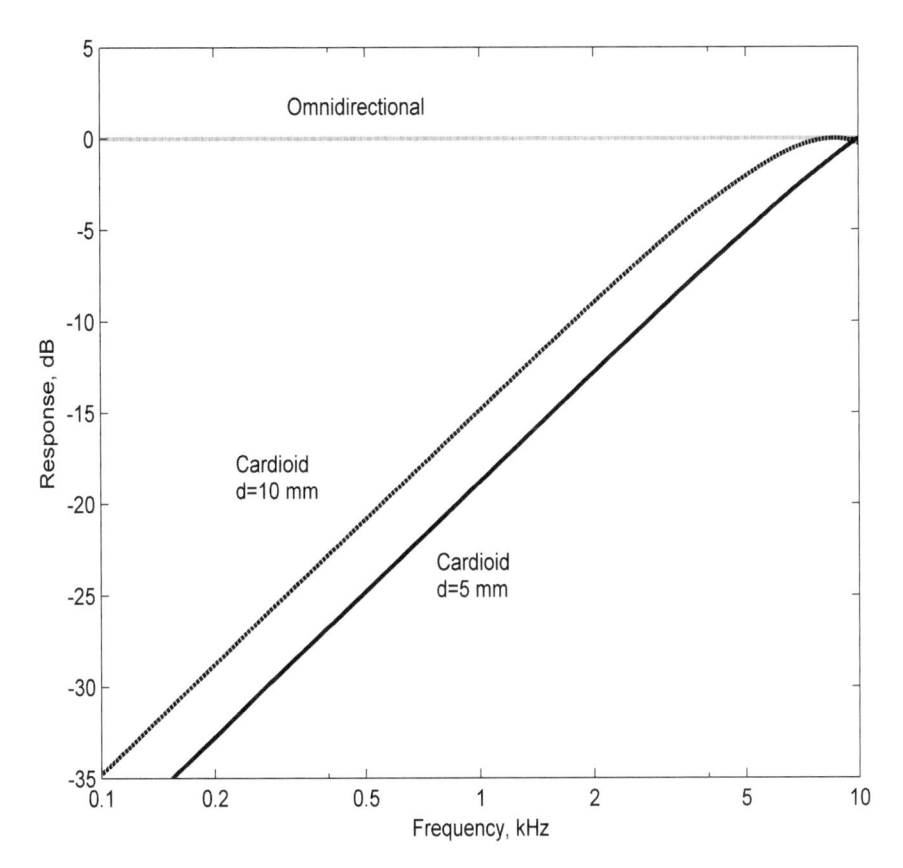

Figure 4-7. On-axis frequency response for an ideal omnidirectional microphone and for a cardioid directional microphone as the separation between the two microphones is changed.

flattens out. This effect is illustrated in Figure 4-8 for a cardioid microphone having perfect matching of the front and rear ($b = 1$) and having mismatch giving a reduced rear-microphone output ($b = 0.9$). The mismatch causes the frequency response below about 400 Hz to approach an asymptote of about −25 dB re: 1, thus providing some residual low-frequency output from the directional microphone.

INTERACTION WITH VENTS

In a vented hearing aid, the sound pressure at the ear drum is the sum of the signal produced in the ear canal by the hearing-aid receiver and

92 Digital Hearing Aids

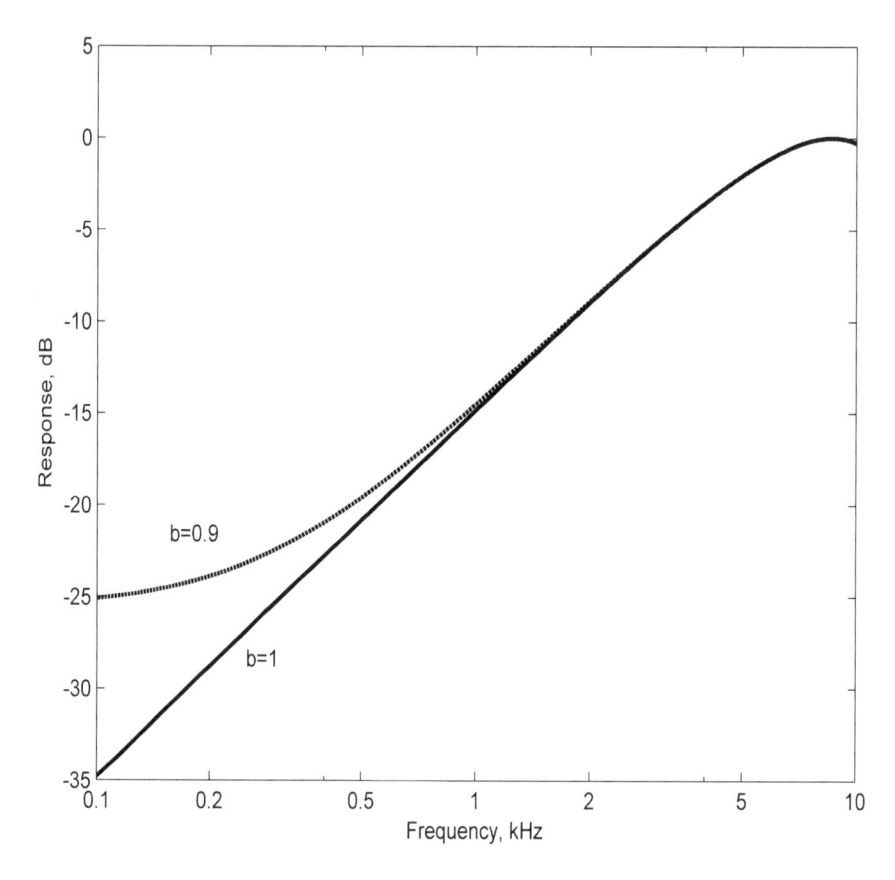

Figure 4-8. On-axis frequency response for a cardioid directional microphone having perfect microphone matching ($b = 1$) and microphone mismatch with the rear microphone output reduced ($b = 0.9$).

the unamplified signal that enters the ear canal through the vent. The unamplified signal has an omnidirectional response pattern as the head shadow is not a factor at low frequencies. Furthermore, as shown in Chapter 3, the presence of the vent greatly attenuates the amplified signal level at frequencies below 200 Hz for a small vent diameter, ranging up to 500 Hz for a large vent diameter. Thus, at low frequencies there is a substantial omnidirectional signal component that is entering the ear canal via the vent even if a directional microphone is being used in the hearing aid. As a result, the benefit of using a directional microphone to suppress the response to external noise sources will disappear in a vented fitting at sufficiently low frequencies.

MICROPHONE NOISE

An additional concern is the internal noise of the microphone. Every microphone produces a small amount of noise caused by the random motion of the air molecules hitting the diaphragm and random currents within the transduction circuitry. The design of most high-quality omnidirectional hearing-aid microphones results in an equivalent background noise level of about 25 dB SPL (Knowles, 2005), which is close to that experienced by the unaided human ear (Killion, 1976). Thus, the noise produced by an omnidirectional hearing-aid microphone is nearly inaudible.

Now consider the on-axis frequency response of the directional microphones shown in Figure 4-7. In many hearing-aid applications, the flat frequency response of the omnidirectional microphone is wanted, not the sloping response of the directional microphone. An example would be a hearing aid where the user can switch between omnidirectional and directional modes. It is desirable in such a hearing aid that the amplified frequency response remain constant independent of which mode is selected. Thus, when the directional mode is selected, additional low-frequency amplification is needed to compensate for the reduction in low-frequency output from the directional microphone.

At 500 Hz, for example, the cardioid microphone with 1-cm spacing will need a boost of about 23 dB to match the output from the omnidirectional microphone. This equalization amplification will increase the low-frequency signal level from the desired sound source in front of the listener, but it will also amplify the random microphone noise by the same amount. Thus, a directional microphone rejects environmental noise that is external to the microphone, but equalizing the frequency response to match that of an omnidirectional microphone can greatly increase the effective internal noise level. An equalized directional microphone will therefore improve the net SNR only if the intensity of the internal noise, after equalization, is less than the intensity of the external noise.

Microphones on the Head

The directional patterns derived above assumed that the microphones were situated far from any surfaces that could affect sound propagation from the source to the microphone. The directional patterns are based on the assumption that the time delay from the front microphone to the rear microphone is the propagation delay that occurs in free space, and that the amplitude of the pressure wave at the rear microphone is the same as at the front microphone. Mounting the microphone on the head violates these assumptions and changes the directional response. Two problems that can occur are diffraction and local reflections. In diffraction, the sound propagates around a surface, so the path taken by the acoustic wave is no longer the direct path from the source to the microphone. Local reflections can scatter the wave propagating from a distant source so that several apparent sources appear close to the microphone. The microphone may have a null in its response pattern in the direction of the distant source, but can not cancel all of the local scatterers.

When a microphone is placed in or over an ear, both diffraction and local scatterers affect the microphone response. Diffraction occurs as the sound propagates around the head (Wiener, 1947). For example, if the sound source is on the opposite side of the head from the microphone, the sound will propagate from the source to the head, and will then proceed to propagate around the circumference of the head until it reaches the microphone. At higher frequencies, as discussed in Chapter 3, the edges of the pinna and the ridges within the concha reflect sound and can change the amplitude and phase of the pressure at a microphone positioned within the concha, ear canal, or behind the ear.

The transfer functions from a sound source in front of the KEMAR manikin to microphone locations along side the head were measured by Kuhn and Burnett (1977). These transfer functions show the effects of both diffraction and local scatterers. Several different contours were used, as shown in Figure 4-9. Contours 1, 2, and 3 are particularly relevant for BTE hearing aids as different positions along each contour roughly correspond to the microphone port locations in a directional microphone. The origin of the coordinate system used for the measurements is the center of the ear canal opening. The positions along the contours that are most relevant for BTE hearing aids are thus from 0 to 2 cm along these three contours. Contours 1, 2, and 3 are spaced 5 mm apart in the vertical direction, and are displaced from the side of the head, with contour 1 a distance of 2 mm from the side of the head, contour 2 a distance of 4 mm, and contour 3 a distance of 7 mm.

The reference measurement was made at the location along contour 2 directly above the ear canal opening, but with the manikin removed to give the free-field pressure. The measured sound pressure levels along

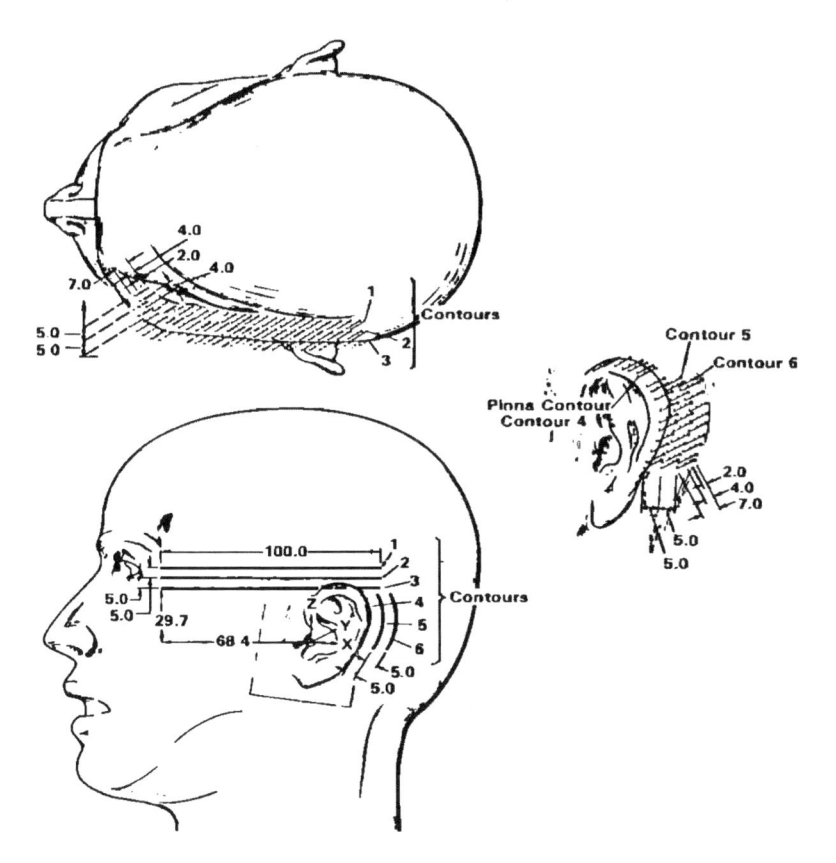

Figure 4-9. Contours along the side of the KEMAR manikin used to measure the transfer function from a source in front of the manikin to a microphone location (from Kuhn & Burnett, 1977).

contours 1, 2, and 3 are plotted in Figure 4-10. A value of 0 dB means that the sound pressure level measured on the side of the head was the same as that measured at a point given by a distance of 0 on contour 2, but with the dummy head removed. The plots of Figure 4-10 indicate that as the microphone position is moved from 0 to 3 cm (toward the rear of the head starting from just above the ear canal opening) the sound pressure level decreases, and the magnitude of the change increases with increasing frequency. Consider the pressures measured distances of 0 and 1 cm along the contours, which correspond to the front and rear port openings (or separate microphone locations) in a typi-

96 Digital Hearing Aids

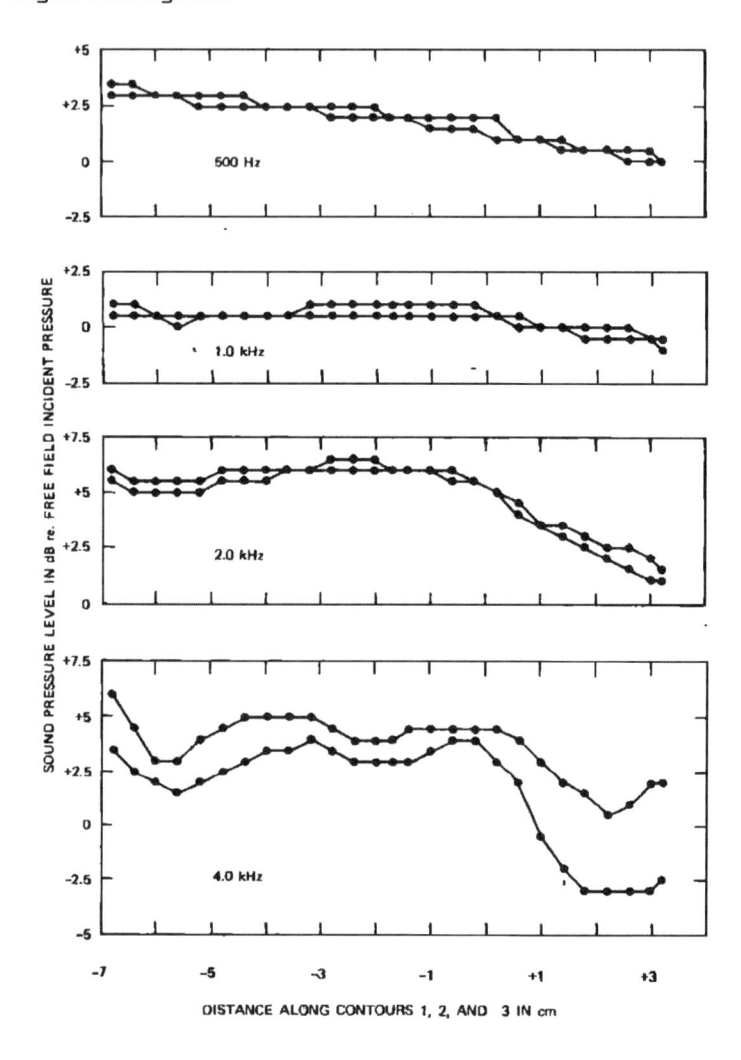

Figure 4-10. Pressure measures along side the head of the KEMAR manikin for contours 1, 2, and 3 (from Kuhn & Burnett, 1977).

cal BTE hearing aid using a directional microphone. The differences in pressure between distances of 0 and 1 cm are less than 0.5 dB at 500 Hz, but increase to over 5 dB at 4 kHz. If the directional microphone pattern was designed with the hearing aid mounted on a stand, then putting the hearing aid on the head amounts to an instant mismatch between the front and rear microphones and will change the directional pattern.

Directional Microphones 97

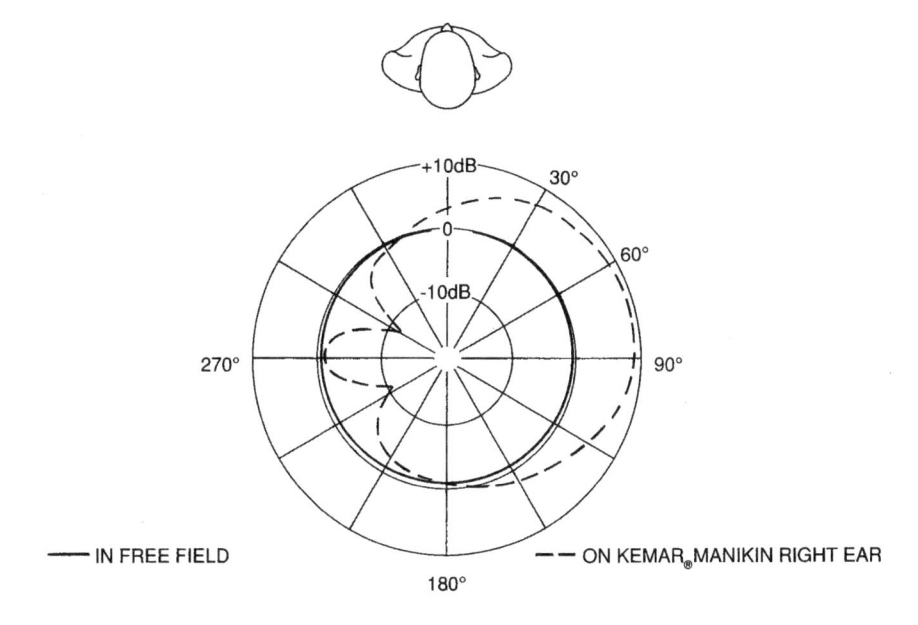

Figure 4-11. Directional responses at 2 kHz measured in free field and on KEMAR for an omnidirectional hearing-aid microphone (from Knowles Electronics Technical Bulletin TB-21, 1980).

The changes in the microphone directional patterns that occur when the microphone is mounted on the head are illustrated in Figures 4-11 and 4-12 (Knowles, 1980). Figure 4-11 is for an omnidirectional microphone, and it shows that the head affects the directional response even for a single microphone. The microphone in free space has uniform sensitivity with azimuth, but the same microphone mounted on the right ear has a peak in sensitivity at about 75 degrees. Sound coming from the opposite side of the head is attenuated, and there are two nulls in the directional pattern caused by the presence of the head. The same basic behavior is observed for the directional microphone in Figure 4-12. The directional microphone response in free space has a peak at 0 degrees and a null at 180 degrees, producing the designed cardioid pattern. On the head, the response peak shifts to about 50 degrees, the single rear null is replaced by a pair of nulls at about 180 and 230 degrees, and the response to sound from the opposite side of the head is attenuated. Most directional microphones used in hearing aids are designed assuming free space conditions as this greatly simplifies the design procedure, but the responses found when the microphone is

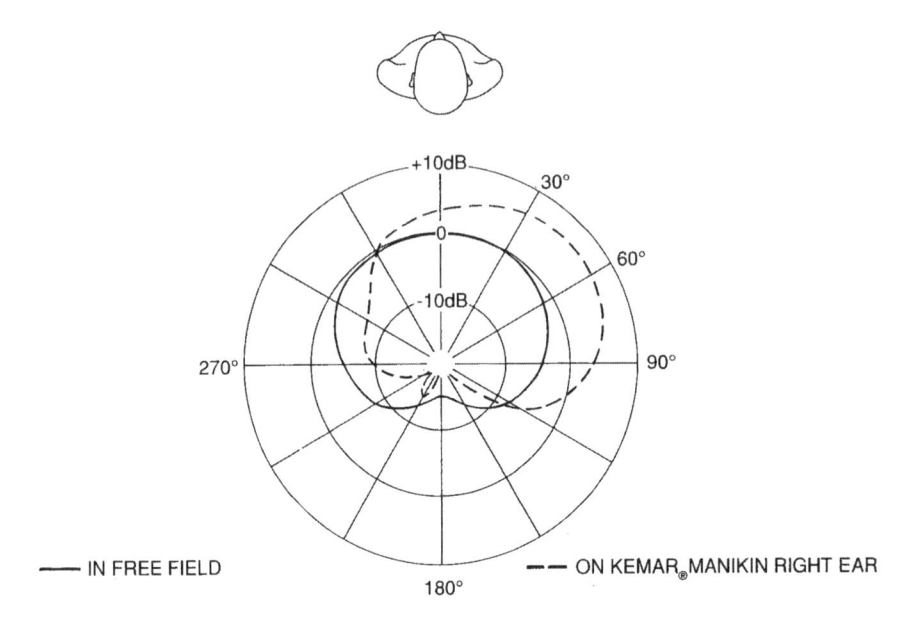

Figure 4-12. Directional responses at 2 kHz measured in free field and on KEMAR for an cardioid hearing-aid microphone (from Knowles Electronics Technical Bulletin TB-21, 1980).

mounted on the head indicate that the diffraction around the head should be considered in order to get the desired directional patterns in real life.

Microphone Performance Indexes

Many different microphone directional patterns can be realized using the same basic system. The directional patterns range from dipole through hypercardioid and supercardioid to cardioid. Which directional pattern is "best," and how can they be compared? The preference for one directional pattern over the others depends on the assumptions made about the desired sound source and the characteristics of the interference. A performance index is a single number that summarizes the microphone performance for a specific set of assumed signal and noise conditions.

FRONT-TO-BACK RATIO

One set of assumptions is that the desired source of sound is in front of the microphone and the interference comes from a single source behind the microphone. The improvement in SNR when the directional microphone is used will then be the ratio of the sound pressure level resulting from the front source at 0 degrees to the pressure resulting from the rear interference at 180 degrees. This improvement in SNR is termed the front-to-back ratio (FBR).

The FBR is really a measure of the depth of the rear null in the microphone response pattern. A cardioid pattern, with a null at exactly 180 degrees, will have an infinite FBR as there is no output for a sound source at 180 degrees. The limitation of the FBR is that it indicates nothing about the microphone response for sources at azimuths other than 0 and 180 degrees. It measures the directional behavior at just these two angles, and ignores everything else. If we know that a microphone is designed to have a cardioid pattern, then FBR can give an indication of how well the design was realized and how closely the front and rear microphones have been matched. But the FBR provides very little information about an arbitrary directional pattern and how well it will suppress interference.

DIRECTIVITY INDEX

A more realistic set of assumptions is that the desired source of sound is in front of the microphone and the interference is coming uniformly from all directions. These assumptions more accurately describe the problem of listening in a reverberant room or in a noisy situation like a restaurant where there are interfering talkers arrayed all around the listener.

Assume that the microphone response has been normalized so that the sound from a source directly in from of the microphone is passed with a gain of 0 dB. This normalization is provided by *Eq. (4.13)*, where the directional response has been divided by the output for a signal arriving from 0 degrees. The directivity index (DI) is then the ratio in dB of the microphone power due to the front source to the output power caused by noise coming uniformly from all directions in azimuth and elevation (Beranek, 1954). The uniform noise is termed an isotropic noise field.

For a microphone used in free space (not on the head), the DI can be computed by first measuring the output power from an omnidirectional microphone in an isotropic noise field. The noise field can be produced, for example, by placing several loudspeakers in a reverberation chamber. The omnidirectional microphone is then replaced by a directional microphone and the output power measured again. The DI is the ratio of the output from the omnidirectional microphone to the output from the directional microphone, expressed in dB. The DI indicates how much better the directional microphone is at reducing the noise level than an omnidirectional microphone. For a microphone used on the head, one can measure the microphone output power for a source at 0 degrees in an anechoic chamber, and then compare this output to the output power measured for the same microphone/head combination in the isotropic noise field of the reverberation chamber.

The directivity indexes for several different directional patterns are presented in Table 4-1. These DI values indicate that under ideal conditions a directional microphone can reduce the background noise level by up to 6 dB. The hypercardioid response does the best job, closely followed by the supercardioid response pattern. The cardioid and cosine patterns offer identical performance of 4.8 dB. The cardioid pattern, which might intuitively appear to be the best given its deep null at 180 degrees, is not as effective as the hypercardioid response. The reason is that whereas the cardioid pattern has a deep rear null, its main lobe is wider than that of the hypercardioid pattern and thus passes more noise power coming from the sides. The hypercardioid pattern offers the optimum tradeoff between front lobe beamwidth and rear lobe suppression.

The DI values for hearing aids mounted on the head, plotted in Figure 4-13, differ from the ideal values given in Table 4-1. The diffraction around the head, as shown in Figures 4-11 and 4-12, changes the shape of the directional pattern and shifts the angle giving the maximum of the directional response. BTE devices with omnidirectional microphones actually have a negative DI because of this shift in the angle of the response maximum. The response to azimuths in the right hemisphere are all above 0 dB in Figure 4-11, so the microphone output for the isotropic noise field is greater than the output for the on-axis sound source at 0 degrees. ITE devices with omnidirectional microphones offer some directional benefit above 1 kHz; the similarity between the omnidirectional ITE and the KEMAR open ear response suggests that this benefit is due to the directional nature of the local reflections from the pinna at high frequencies. The directional microphones give the highest DI values. A directional microphone in an ITE shell is more effective than a directional microphone in a BTE case, although at low frequencies the directional BTE is substantially better than the unaided KEMAR ear.

Directional Microphones **101**

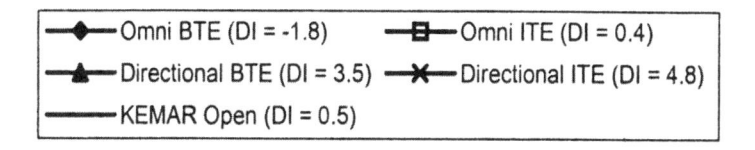

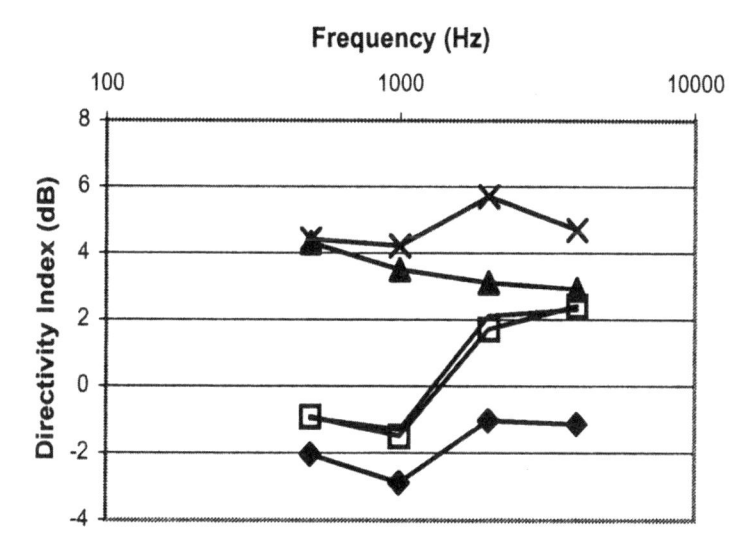

── Omni BTE (DI = -1.8)   ── Omni ITE (DI = 0.4)
── Directional BTE (DI = 3.5)   ── Directional ITE (DI = 4.8)
── KEMAR Open (DI = 0.5)

Figure 4-13. Directional Index (DI) as a function of frequency for five different conditions. The DI measurements are based on horizontal polar patterns measured on the KEMAR manikin. All hearing-aid conditions reflect an average across 8 to 12 hearing aids from different manufacturers (from Ricketts & Mueller, 1999).

UNIDIRECTIONAL INDEX

The unidirectional index (UI) is the ratio of the microphone response to signals coming uniformly from the front hemisphere to signals coming uniformly from the rear hemisphere. This metric is based on the assumptions that the desired signal is coming from in front of the listener and that the interference is coming from behind the listener. The UI is therefore intermediate between the FBR and the DI. The UI responds to noise coming from the rear of the listener while avoiding the sensitivity of the FBR to the depth of the null at 180 degrees, and it allows for a desired sound source to be at an azimuth other than 0 degrees. However, the UI assumes that the noise is only coming from the rear, which is a less realistic assumption for many listening situations than the isotropic noise field assumed in the DI. Although the hypercardioid response pattern has the highest DI, the supercardioid response gives the highest UI (Borwick, 1990).

THE AI-DI

As shown in Figure 4-13, the DI for hearing aids varies with frequency. For a source in front of the microphone and a isotropic noise field, the DI gives the improvement in SNR due to the directional microphone. Changes in SNR can be linked to changes in speech intelligibility through the speech intelligibility index (SII) (ANSI S3.5, 1997), formerly called the articulation index (AI). In the SII, the SNR is computed in separate frequency bands, and a weighted sum across frequency of the SNR values in dB is used to predict speech intelligibility. The weights give the importance of each frequency band for speech intelligibility.

Greenberg et al. (1993) proposed using the same procedure to compute an AI-weighted DI. Compute the DI in each frequency band, and then sum the DI values in dB across frequency using the AI (or now the SII) weights. Ricketts et al. (2005) investigated several different sets of weights used to combine the DI values across frequency for omnidirectional and directional microphones in hearing aids. They found that the weights chosen did not have a significant effect on the predicted benefit of the directional microphone. Their result may be due in part to the narrow range of DI values that were found for the directional microphones; in the limit, if all of the DI values are the same independent of frequency, then all of the weighting schemes considered yield the same answer. However, the AI-DI may still be relevant for the microphone arrays considered in the next chapter which can have much larger DI values and greater variation of DI with frequency.

Rooms and Reverberation

The directivity index implicitly assumes that all sound coming from in front of the listener is beneficial and all sound coming from other directions is deleterious. However, the situation in rooms is more complicated. Even if the desired source of sound is directly in front of the listener, the sound is reflected by the floor, walls, and ceiling of the room. The sound arrives at the ear or microphone from multiple directions and with different delays. Although later reflections are deleterious, reflections that arrive within a short delay relative to the direct sound are actually beneficial and can improve speech intelligibility.

CRITICAL DISTANCE

The sound field caused by someone talking in a room consists of the direct sound from the talker plus the reverberation. The intensity of the sound from the talker falls off with increasing distance, but the reverberant field is assumed to be uniform in intensity everywhere within the room. If the talker is close to the listener, the direct sound will be more intense than the reverberation. As the talker moves away from the listener, the intensity of the direct sound will decrease, but the intensity of the reverberation remains constant.

The critical distance is defined as the distance between talker and listener at which the direct sound and reverberation are equal in intensity. The greater the amount of reverberation in a room, that is, the longer the reverberation time, the smaller the critical distance. The critical distance is thus a useful way of summarizing the relationship between the source intensity and the reverberation at the listener's location. If the source is within the critical distance the source intensity is greater than the reverberation, and if the source is beyond the critical distance the reverberation dominates.

EARLY REFLECTIONS

The amount of reverberation in a room does not completely describe the effects of the reverberation on speech intelligibility. In particular, the integration of a short echo with the direct sound can improve speech perception. Haas (1949) found that an echo occurring within 1 to 30 msec of the direct sound improved speech intelligibility consistent with combining the powers of the direct sound and the reflection. Furthermore, Haas found that the echo occurring within 1 to 30 msec must be at least 10 dB more intense than the direct sound in order to be perceived as a separate event. Lochner and Berger (1964) found that the auditory integration time was also about 30 msec for an echo having an intensity equal to that of the direct sound. An echo 5 dB less intense than the direct sound resulted in an integration time of about 40 msec, whereas an echo 5 dB more intense than the direct sound resulted in a greatly reduced amount of auditory integration. In simulating a room environment, Lochner and Berger (1964) found that echoes occurring within 30 msec of the direct sound contributed to speech intelligibility in a manner consistent with combining the signal powers. Longer delays reduced the benefit in intelligibility. Significantly longer reflection delays, in excess of 350 msec, reduce speech intelligibility much in the manner of additive noise (Bolt & MacDonald, 1949).

Nábělek and Robinette (1978) conducted an experiment similar to that of Lochner and Berger (1964), but used hearing-impaired as well as normal-hearing subjects. The Nábělek and Robinette results show that the power summation of the direct and delayed signals applies to speech intelligibility for hearing-impaired as well as for normal-hearing listeners. Improvements in intelligibility based on increased total signal power were found for delays shorter than 20 msec, and the benefit of the delayed sound gradually decreased with increasing delay; essentially no benefit was observed for a 160-msec delay, the longest used in the study. They concluded that the effect of a single reflection is similar for hearing-impaired and normal-hearing subjects for both monaural and binaural sound presentation.

COMBINING NOISE AND REVERBERATION

An accurate prediction of speech intelligibility in a room needs to take into account the power in the direct sound from the source and the beneficial early reflections, as well as the power in the background noise and the deleterious late reflections (Bistafa & Bradley, 2000). Work in architectural acoustics has led to several metrics that combine noise and reflections in predicting speech intelligibility in rooms, and one of the most useful is U_{50} (Bradley et al., 1999):

$$U_{50} = 10 \log_{10} \left[\frac{Direct + Early}{Noise + Late} \right] \quad \text{Equation (4.14)}$$

where each term gives the power in the corresponding portion of the sound field in the room. The early reflections are defined as those occurring within 50 msec of the arrival of the direct sound from the source, and the late reflections are those that arrive after 50 msec.

A directional microphone will have different effects on U_{50} depending on the listening environment. Consider two situations, one outdoors and the other in a lecture hall where the talker is far from the listener. We assume that outdoors there are no reflections, that the noise comes uniformly from all directions, and that the desired source of sound is in front of the microphone. Given these assumptions, the *Early* and *Late* reflection terms in *Eq. (4.14)* are both zero and U_{50} reduces to:

$$U_{50} \approx 10\ log_{10}\left[\frac{Direct}{Noise}\right] \quad \text{Equation (4.15)}$$

The directional microphone will pass the direct sound without any attenuation. However, the noise will be attenuated by an amount given by the DI. The result is an improvement in U_{50} that is identical to that given by the DI of the microphone.

In the lecture hall, we assume that the talker is far enough from the listener that the early reflections contain much more speech power than the direct sound. That is, the talker is substantially beyond the critical distance for the room. For this situation, U_{50} is approximated by:

$$U_{50} \approx 10\ log_{10}\left[\frac{Early}{Noise + Late}\right] \quad \text{Equation (4.16)}$$

We further assume that the early reflections, late reflections, and noise all arrive uniformly from all directions. Given these assumptions, the directional microphone will reduce the power of the early reflections, late reflections, and noise all by the amount given by the DI. The DI thus scales the numerator and denominator of *Eq. (4.16)* by exactly the same amount, and there is no change in U_{50}. Thus outdoors the directional microphone benefits are those predicted by the DI, but in a reverberant environment with the talker far from the listener, the directional microphone will have essentially no benefit at all (Kates, 1997).

Benefit in the Real World

A directional microphone can improve the signal-to-noise ratio (SNR) when the source of the noise is spatially separated from the source of the speech. A directional microphone in a hearing aid is assumed to improve speech intelligibility under nearly all listening conditions. Laboratory experiments, conducted in a sound booth and using a limited number of interfering sources, generally show a significant improvement in speech recognition in comparison with omnidirectional microphones (Hawkins & Yacullo, 1984; Ricketts & Dahr, 1999; Valente et al., 1995). However, the benefit of directional microphones under real-world conditions is often much less than that observed under laboratory conditions. These results run counter to the expectation that directional microphones should be helpful in all listening situations.

Ricketts et al. (2003) used the Profile of Hearing Aid Benefit (PHAB) as a self-assessment measure to determine the benefit of directional microphones in a hearing aid. The PHAB (Cox et al., 1991) is a 66-item inventory questionnaire that assesses hearing aid benefit in a variety of everyday listening conditions. Rickets et al. (2003) developed 24 additional questions in the style of the PHAB to address spatial hearing concerns. The hearing aids used in the Rickets et al. (2003) study were Siemens "Music" behind-the-ear (BTE) devices, which have a user switch to change between omnidirectional and directional microphone modes. Fifteen adults with a range of hearing losses were first fitted with the BTE with the switch locked in either the omnidirectional (O) or directional (D) mode, and they completed the questionnaires after two weeks of daily use. The switches were then moved to the opposite microphone mode, and the questionnaires again completed after two weeks of daily hearing-aid use. For the final 2-week period, the subjects were allowed to choose the microphone mode and instructed to switch between modes (OD) in order to determine which one was "best" under a variety of listening conditions.

Rickets et al. (2003) found that under laboratory conditions, the D and OD microphone modes yielded statistically significant improvements in speech intelligibility compared to the O mode, with no significant difference between the D and OD modes. The real-world evaluations using the PHAB showed that the OD mode was significantly better than the O mode, with no significant difference between the D and OD modes. However, the OD mode was rated higher than the D mode for the background noise (BN) subscale of the PHAB. The new questions on spatial performance, with subscales for sound front and sound behind/localization, showed a statistically significant benefit for the D and OD modes when compared to the O mode. Performance for the OD mode was better than for the D mode on both spatial subscales. The OD mode was significantly better than the D mode for the sound behind/localization subscale, and the D mode was worse than the O mode for this subscale.

These results indicate that the users felt that they performed better when they were allowed to adjust the microphone mode. Furthermore, the directional microphone did not always give better perceived performance than the omnidirectional microphone. Thus, the choice of an omnidirectional or directional microphone should be based on the specific listening situation.

   The specific conditions under which a directional microphone is preferable to an omnidirectional microphone have also been investigated by Walden and colleagues (Cord et al., 2002; Cord et al., 2004; Surr et al., 2002; Walden et al., 2004). In the Surr et al. (2002) paper, 11 experienced hearing-aid users were fitted with GN ReSound Canta 7 BTE hearing aids, which have an omnidirectional and an adaptive directional microphone mode. For 6 weeks the subjects were required to keep a journal in which they described at least one situation each day for which one microphone mode worked better than the other. For most listening situations, there was no clear preference of one microphone mode over the other. Although the directional mode was preferred in about two-thirds of the conditions, the preference was generally small.

   Walden et al. (2004) performed a similar experiment using 17 hearing-impaired listeners fitted with GN ReSound Canta 750D in-the-ear (ITE) instruments. The listening conditions were analyzed using a binary tree structure based on the absence or presence of background noise, the signal location, the signal distance, reverberation, and the noise location. They found that, for the average adult with impaired hearing, the majority of active listening time in daily living is in the presence of background noise. The vast majority of this listening time is typically with the source in front of the listener and the noise spatially separated from the signal source. The directional mode was generally preferred when background noise was present to the sides or rear, the signal near to the listener, and the reverberation low. The omnidirectional mode was generally preferred when the signal was far from the listener or when reverberation was high.

   The results of these studies are summarized in Walden et al. (2003):

1. Directional microphones work better in the test booth than they do in everyday listening situations.
2. Environmental acoustics often limit the effectiveness of directional microphones in everyday listening.

3. Directional microphones work effectively only when a specific set of environmental conditions exist. Generally, everyday benefit should be expected only when the signal source is located in front of and relatively near to the listener and the noise sources are spatially separated from the signal source.
4. The omnidirectional mode is the appropriate default setting for most hearing-impaired patients.

The effectiveness of directional microphones for indoor listening situations appears to depend strongly on the amount of reverberation (Ricketts & Mueller, 1999). Reduced benefit for directional microphones is found for increasing levels of reverberation (Hawkins & Yacullo, 1984; Ricketts & Dahr, 1999), and reduced benefit in reverberation is also found as the distance between the sound source and the listener is increased (Ricketts & Hornsby, 2003). These results are fully consistent will the U_{50} analysis provided above.

Concluding Remarks

Directional microphones provide an effective yet simple form of spatial signal processing. Signals originating in front of the listener are passed with maximum intensity, whereas signals originating from other directions are attenuated. The directional microphone is formed by subtracting the sound pressure at the rear microphone or port, with an appropriate delay, from the sound pressure at the front. The time delay can be realized using an acoustic time-delay circuit or electronically; the resulting microphone behavior is identical for either approach. Adjusting the time delay from 0 to d/c yields free-field directional patterns along a continuum from cosine to cardioid.

Directional microphones, although beneficial in many situations, are not a perfect solution. A directional microphone, no matter which directional pattern is implemented, has an on-axis frequency response with a rising slope of 6 dB/octave at low frequencies. Achieving a flat frequency response in a directional microphone requires low-frequency amplification to compensate for this inherent slope. The low-frequency boost amplifies the internal noise of the microphone, so there is a tradeoff between the attenuation of noise from external sources versus the increase in level of the internal microphone noise. Most directional microphones are designed to optimize the free-field response pattern, but the microphones are used on the head, and the acoustic effects of the head shift the locations of the response peak and nulls. A further consideration is the listening environment. In a reverberant environment, with a talker far from the listener, most of the useful signal power is in the early reflections and not in the direct sound. The directional microphone attenuates both the early reflections and the noise and late reflections, and can result in no net improvement in intelligibility for this common listening situation.

References

ANSI S3.5. (1997). *American National Standard: Methods for the calculation of the speech intelligibility index.* New York: American National Standards Institute.

Beranek, L. L. (1954). *Acoustics.* New York: McGraw-Hill.

Bistafa, S. R., & Bradley, J. S. (2000). Reverberation time and maximum background-noise level for classrooms from a comparative study of speech intelligibility metrics. *Journal of the Acoustical Society of America, 107,* 861–875.

Bolt, R. H., & MacDonald, A. D. (1949). Theory of speech masking by reverberation. *Journal of the Acoustical Society of America, 21,* 577–580.

Borwick, J. (1990). *Microphones: Technology and technique.* Boston: Focal Press.

Bradley, J. S., Reich, R. D., & Norcross, S. G. (1999). On the combined effects of signal-to-noise ratio and room acoustics on speech intelligibility. *Journal of the Acoustical Society of America, 106,* 1820–1828.

Cord, M. T., Surr, R. K., Walden, B. E., & Dyrlund, O. (2004). Relationship between laboratory measures of directional advantage and everyday success with directional microphone hearing aids. *Journal of the American Academy of Audiology, 15,* 353–364.

Cord, M. T., Surr, R. K., Walden, B. E., & Olson, L. (2002). Performance of directional microphone hearing aids in everyday life. *Journal of the American Academy of Audiology, 13,* 295–307.

Cox, R. M., Alexander, G. C., & Gilmore, C. (1991). Objective and self-report measures of hearing aid benefit. In G. A. Studebaker, F. H. Bess, & L. B. Beck (Eds), *The Vanderbilt Hearing-Aid Report II* (pp. 201–214). Parkton: MD: York Press.

Greenberg, J. E., Peterson, P. M., & Zurek, P. M. (1993). Intelligibility-weighted measures of speech-to-interference ratio and speech system performance. *Journal of the Acoustical Society of America, 94,* 3009–3010.

Haas, H. (1949). Über den Einfluss eines Einfachechos auf die Hörsamkelt von Sprache available in translation as Haas, H. (1972). The influence of a single echo on the audibility of speech. *Journal of the Audio Engineering Society, 20,* 146–159.

Hawkins, D. B., & Yacullo, W. S. (1984). Signal-to-noise ratio advantage of binaural hearing aids and directional microphones under different levels of reverberation. *Journal of Speech and Hearing Disorders, 49,* 278–286.

Kates, J. M. (1997). Relating change in signal-to-noise ratio to array gain for microphone arrays used in rooms. *Journal of the Acoustical Society of America, 101,* 2388–2390.

Killion, M. (1976). Noise of ears and microphones. *Journal of the Acoustical Society of America, 59,* 424–433.

Knowles. (1980). *EB directional hearing aid microphone application notes,* Technical Bulletin TB-21. Itasca, IL: Knowles Electronics, Inc.

Knowles. (2005). *EM series microphone data sheet,* Issue 05-0801. Itasca, IL: Knowles Electronics, Inc.

Kuhn, G. F., & Burnett, E. D. (1977). Acoustic pressure field alongside a manikin's head with a view towards in situ hearing-aid tests. *Journal of the Acoustical Society of America, 62,* 416–423.

Lochner, J. P. A., & Berger, J. F. (1964). The influence of reflections on auditorium acoustics. *Journal of Sound Vibrations, 1,* 426–454.

Nábělěk, A. K., & Robinette, L. (1978). Influence of the precedence effect on word identification by normally hearing and hearing-impaired subjects. *Journal of the Acoustical Society of America, 63,* 187–194.

Ricketts, T., & Dahr, S. (1999). Aided benefit across directional and omni-directional hearing aid microphones for behind-the-ear hearing aids. *Journal of the American Academy of Audiology, 10,* 180–189.

Ricketts, T., Henry, P., & Gnewikow, D. (2003). Full time directional versus user selectable microphone modes in hearing aids. *Ear and Hearing, 24,* 424–439.

Ricketts, T., Henry, P., & Hornsby, B. W. Y. (2005). Application of frequency importance functions to directivity for prediction of benefit in uniform fields. *Ear and Hearing, 26,* 473–486.

Ricketts, T. A., & Hornsby, B. W. Y. (2003). Distance and reverberation effects on directional benefit. *Ear and Hearing, 24,* 472–484.

Ricketts, T., & Meuller, H.G. (1999). Making sense of directional microphone hearing aids. *American Journal of Audiology, 8,* 1059–1069.

Surr, R. K., Walden, B. E., Cord, M. T., and Olson, L. (2002). The influence of environmental factors on hearing aid microphone preference. *Journal of the American Academy of Audiology, 13,* 308–322.

Valente, M., Fabry, D. A., & Potts, L. G. (1995). Recognition of speech in noise with hearing aids using dual microphones. *Journal of the American Academy of Audiology, 6,* 440–449.

Walden, B. E., Surr, R. K., & Cord, M. T. (2003). Real-world performance of directional microphone hearing aids. *Hearing Journal, 56,* 40–46.

Walden, B. E., Surr, R. K., Cord, M. T., & Dyrlund, O. (2004). Predicting hearing aid microphone preference in everyday listening. *Journal of the American Academy of Audiology, 15,* 365–394.

Wiener, F. M. (1947). Sound diffraction by rigid spheres and circular cylinders. *Journal of the Acoustical Society of America, 19,* 444–451.

5

Adaptive and Multimicrophone Arrays

A MICROPHONE ARRAY is a system of two or more microphones whose outputs are filtered and combined to give the array output signal. The array behavior is determined by the number of microphones, the physical extent of the array, and the type of filters used. The directional microphone discussed in Chapter 4 can be considered to be a two-microphone array in which no filter is applied to the front microphone output and the filter applied to the rear microphone output is a fixed time delay. The directional microphone was treated separately as it can be realized with purely acoustic means, and can thus be considered to be a simple building block when assembling a hearing aid. The arrays treated in this chapter rely on electronic signal-processing means to achieve their performance, however, and thus combine the microphone acoustics with digital signal processing. In this chapter the treatment of microphones is extended to include adaptive two-microphone arrays, multimicrophone arrays, and adaptive multimicrophone arrays.

In an adaptive array, the filters attached to each microphone change over time in response to changes in the spatial characteristics of the interference. An adaptive array can be built using just two microphones, and this approach is typically taken in hearing aids due to considerations of cost, size, and power consumption. The array performance can often be improved by increasing the size of the array or the number of microphones, and several approaches to the design of multimicrophone arrays are discussed as well. These larger arrays may not be practical in many hearing-aid applications, but this situation may change as microphone size and digital power consumption are reduced in the future.

Two-Microphone Adaptive Array

The simplest array consists of just two microphones. In this section we consider a two-microphone array built into a single hearing-aid case. As with the directional microphone considered in Chapter 4, the two microphones are close together relative to the wavelength of sound at the highest frequencies of interest. An alternative is to place the two microphones on opposite sides of the head, and this configuration is treated later in this chapter.

ADAPTIVE DELAY

A diagram of the two microphone array, copied from the previous chapter, is presented in Figure 5-1. The front and rear microphones are assumed to have omnidirectional patterns, and the directional response is created by subtracting a delayed version of the rear microphone signal from the front microphone signal. The result is a directional pattern with a single null. The azimuth of the null can move from 90 degrees to 180 degrees as the delay in increased from 0 to d/c sec, where d is the separation between the microphones and c is the speed of sound. The rear microphone gain $b = 1$. The directional pattern is symmetric along the axis of the array, so a null at θ degrees will have a matching null at $360-\theta$ degrees. The symmetry includes rotation around the axis of the array, so a null at 90 degrees in an array pointing forward means that there is also a null pointing down at the floor and up to the ceiling.

An adaptive two-microphone system is shown in Figure 5-2. This system uses a variable time delay to steer the direction of the null. Adjusting the delay from 0 to d/c sec moves the response null from 90 to 180 degrees. If there is a single interfering source of sound, then steering the null to the azimuth of the interference will maximally attenuate it and give the highest possible SNR.

The delay in this example is controlled by the output of the micro-

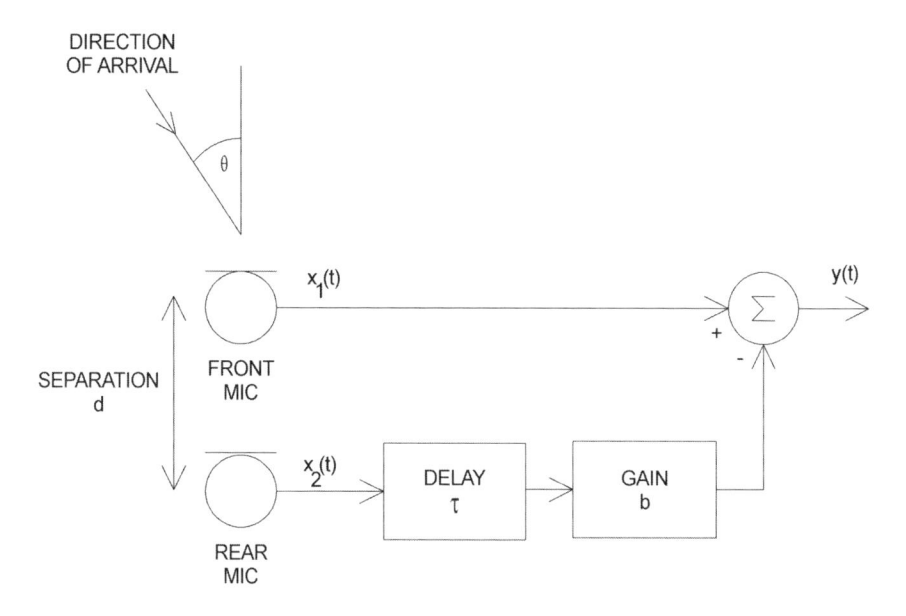

Figure 5-1. Directional microphone as a spatial signal-processing system.

phone array. The objective is to maximize the SNR. However, the array does not know what portion of the output is the desired signal and what portion is interference. So, an assumption is embedded into the array processing, which is that the desired signal is coming from directly in front of the array (0 deg). The signal processing is then designed to minimize the output power from the array, with the constraint that a signal coming from directly in front is passed without any attenuation (Monzigo & Miller, 1980).

An adaptive delay is conceptually simple, but there is a serious problem with building a digital implementation of this system. In a digital system the signal is sampled at discrete intervals. The allowable time delays are quantized in units of the sampling period. The exact delay needed to steer the null in the direction of the interference may not be available among the set of allowable delays. A second problem is that the equations used to adapt the system require smoothly varying outputs and are incompatible with quantized delay values. A different approach is needed to build a system that is compatible with the digital processing constraints.

116 Digital Hearing Aids

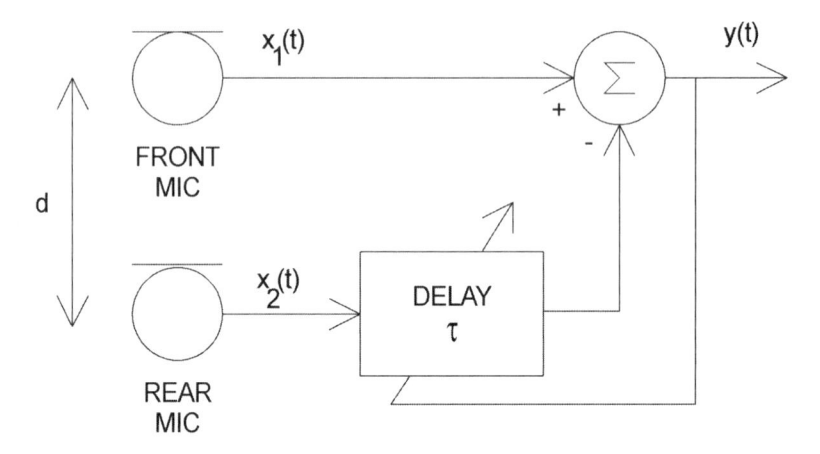

Figure 5-2. Directional microphone with an adaptive time delay.

ADAPTIVE GAIN

The adaptive delay can be replaced with an adaptive gain by reconfiguring the microphone connections using the system shown in Figure 5-3. The system starts with a pair of omnidirectional microphones. However, the microphone outputs $x_1(n)$ and $x_2(n)$ are combined with delays to give a pair of cardioid response patterns (Elko, 2000; Luo et al., 2002). One cardioid pattern faces forward, and is thus most sensitive to sounds originating in front of the array. The second cardioid pattern faces the rear; the null in the cardioid response thus faces forward and this microphone output is least sensitive to sounds originating in front of the array. One can consider the output $c_1(n)$ to be predominantly the desired signal and output $c_2(n)$ to be predominantly interference, given the assumption that the desired source of sound is in front of the array. The interference output $c_2(n)$ is then weighted and subtracted from the desired signal output $c_1(n)$ to remove as much of the interference as possible from the array output.

The directional pattern of this adaptive array is controlled by adjusting the rear cardioid gain b. The array output is given by:

$$y(n) = c_1(n) - bc_2(n) \quad \text{Equation (5.1)}$$

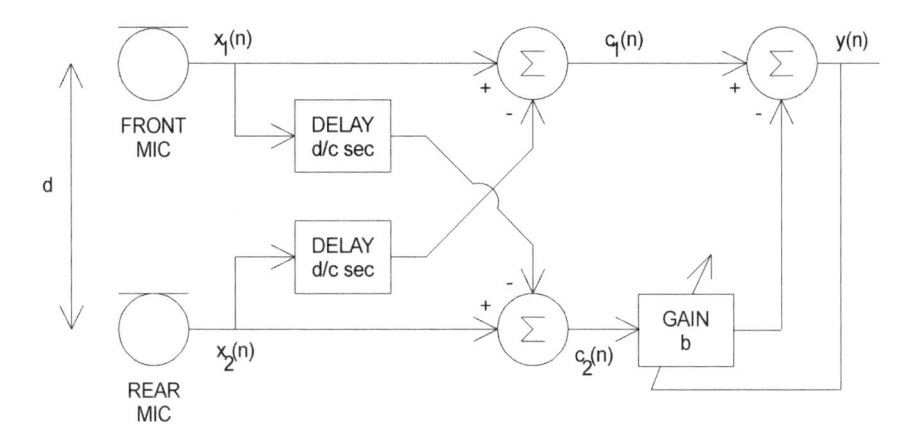

Figure 5-3. Adaptive directional microphone using front-facing and rear-facing cardioid response patterns. The overall directional pattern is controlled by the adaptive gain b.

Consider, for example, $b = 0$. In this case the output $y(n) = c_1(n)$, which is just the response of the front-facing cardioid pattern. Thus setting $b = 0$ gives a null at 180 degrees. Now consider the output for $b = 1$, which gives $y(n) = c_1(n) - c_2(n)$. A signal coming from an azimuth of 90 degrees will be halfway around the response pattern for the front-facing cardioid, and also halfway around the response pattern for the rear-facing cardioid. The amplitudes and phases of the signals $c_1(n)$ and $c_2(n)$ output by the two cardioid patterns will be identical, and these two outputs will cancel when combined to form $y(n)$. Thus, setting $b = 1$ gives a null at 90 degrees.

Generalizing from these two examples, adjusting the gain b to lie between $0 \leq b \leq 1$ steers the null in the response pattern to lie between 180 and 90 degrees. Increasing b to be greater than 1 will move the null around into the front hemisphere of the response pattern where it could possibly cancel the desired signal, so the maximum value of b is limited to 1. Making b negative will cause the rear null in the cardioid response to be filled in, reducing the depth of the null. In the limit of $b = -1$, the response is reduced to that of an omnidirectional microphone. So to preserve the directional null in the response pattern, the minimum value of b is limited to 0.

The adaptive system adjusts the gain b to minimize the power in the array output $y(n)$. The gain update uses least-mean-squared (LMS) adaptation (Haykin, 1996). The adaptive gain update equation is given by (Luo et al., 2002):

$$b(n+1) = b(n) + \frac{\mu}{\sigma_y^2} c_2(n) y(n) \quad \text{Equation (5.2)}$$

where μ controls the rate at which the gain is updated and σ_y^2 is the average power in the array output $y(n)$. The gain update is based on the cross-correlation between the array output $y(n)$ and the rear-facing cardioid output $c_2(n)$. If the signal $c_2(n)$ is similar to $y(n)$, the output $y(n)$ is assumed to contain interference from the side and the gain b is increased toward 1 to try to cancel the interference. If the source of interference is behind the array, then the interference will be present in signal $c_2(n)$ and present with a minus sign in signal $y(n)$. The cross-correlation of $c_2(n)$ with $y(n)$ will then be negative, which will drive the gain $b(n)$ toward zero until the interference is canceled by the rear-facing null in the output directional pattern. The update is normalized by the output signal power σ_y^2 so that the azimuth of the null will change at the same rate independent of the intensity of the desired signal.

ADAPTIVE FILTER

The adaptive gain steers a single null in the array directional response pattern. The direction of the null is the same at all frequencies, which is consistent with the assumption that there is a single source of interference. In the real world there may be many sources of interference, for example, conversations from surrounding tables in a restaurant. With two microphones the array can provide only a single response null, but the array benefit may be improved if the azimuth of the null is allowed to vary with frequency.

One approach is to divide the cardioid output signals $c_1(n)$ and $c_2(n)$ into separate frequency bands using a filter bank (McKinney & DeBrunner, 1996) or an FFT (Kates & Weiss, 1996; Larson et al., 2004; Lockwood et al., 2004). A system using a filter bank is shown in Figure 5-4. The gain b is adapted independently in each frequency band, so the response null can be steered in one direction at low frequencies and in a different direction at high frequencies, depending on the location of the dominant interference source at each frequency.

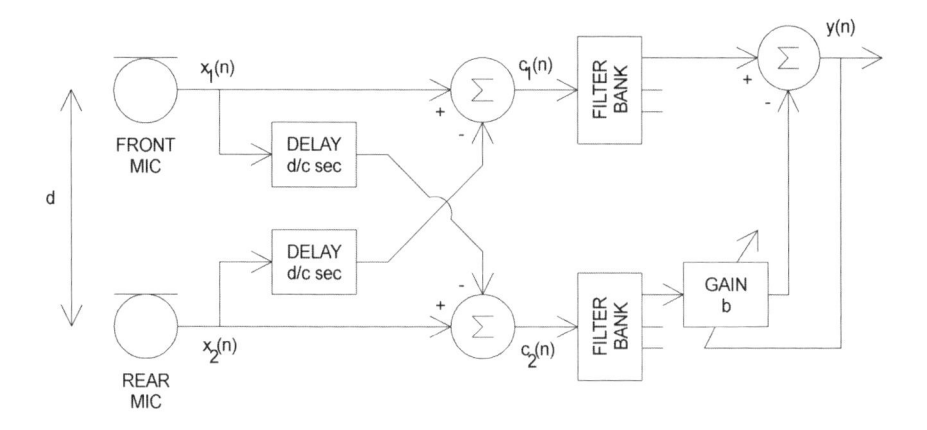

[Figure: Block diagram showing FRONT MIC producing $x_1(n)$ and REAR MIC producing $x_2(n)$, separated by distance d. Each signal passes through a DELAY d/c sec, cross-combined with summers to produce $c_1(n)$ and $c_2(n)$, each passed through a FILTER BANK. The $c_2(n)$ path goes through GAIN b, and is subtracted from the upper branch summer to yield $y(n)$.]

Figure 5-4. Adaptive directional microphone using front-facing and rear-facing cardioid response patterns. The overall directional pattern is controlled by the adaptive gain *b* in each frequency band.

An equivalent system is shown in Figure 5-5, in which the adaptive gain *b* is replaced by an adaptive filter. The adaptive finite-impulse response (FIR) filter has many filter coefficients, and the magnitude transfer function (gain versus frequency) of the filter can provide the equivalent of different gains *b* as a function of frequency. Every filter has a corresponding time delay, and the delay in the upper branch of the block diagram aligns signal $c_1(n)$ with the delayed output of the adaptive filter in the lower branch. The longer the adaptive filter, the finer the frequency resolution but the greater the processing delay.

Desloge et al. (2004) evaluated the two-microphone array shown in Figure 5-5 as a function of the number of the amount of reverberation, the number of interfering sources, and the adaptive filter length. They found that the adaptive processing was most effective outdoors and least effective in a household environment, and that the processing effectiveness decreased as the distance from the desired source of sound to the array was increased. For a single interfering source in an indoor reverberant environment, the average benefit of the adaptive array is about 0.5 to 2 dB in comparison with a cardioid microphone. A similar benefit was found for multiple interfering sources. Increasing the length of the adaptive filter from 32 to 2048 taps at the 22.05-kHz sampling rate improved the adaptive array performance for the single-interferer

120 Digital Hearing Aids

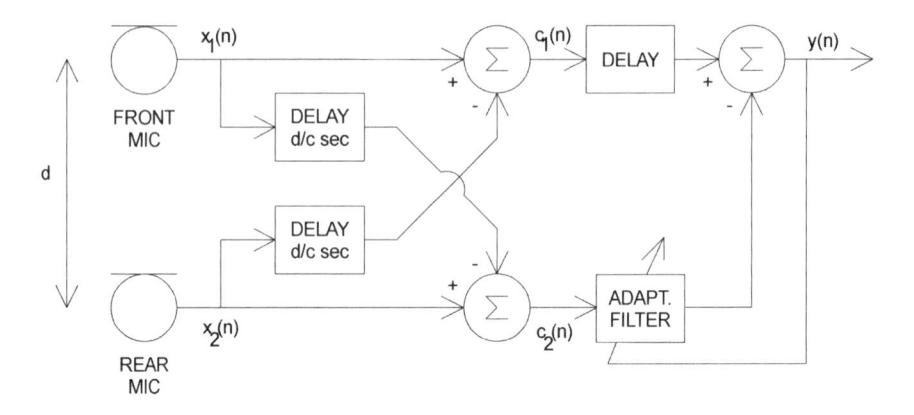

Figure 5-5. Adaptive two-microphone array using front-facing and rear-facing cardioid response patterns. The overall directional pattern is controlled by the adaptive filter.

case by 2 to 4 dB, but provided only a 0.5-dB improvement for the multiple-interferer situation. The array performance for multiple sources of interference is similar to the performance for a single source of interference in a reverberant room; both of these situations involve interference arriving at the array from multiple directions (sources or reflections), and point out the limitations of using an array consisting of just two microphones and which can provide only a single steerable null in the directional response pattern.

The two-microphone arrays that have been investigated so far combine the omnidirectional microphone outputs to produce forward- and rear-facing cardioid response patterns. The microphone outputs can also be combined in other ways. One approach, shown in Figure 5-6, uses a front cardioid microphone combined with a rear omnidirectional microphone (Maj et al., 2004). A fixed filter is applied to the output of the rear omnidirectional microphone. This filter is designed in an anechoic chamber using speech-shaped noise produced by a loudspeaker 1 m in front of the array. The fixed filter matches the front and rear microphone outputs and ensures that there is no signal present in the noise reference path for a desired source of sound directly in front of the array (Vanden Berghe & Wouters, 1998). The resultant noise reference has a directional response pattern very similar to that of a rear-facing cardioid microphone. The adaptive filter is allowed to

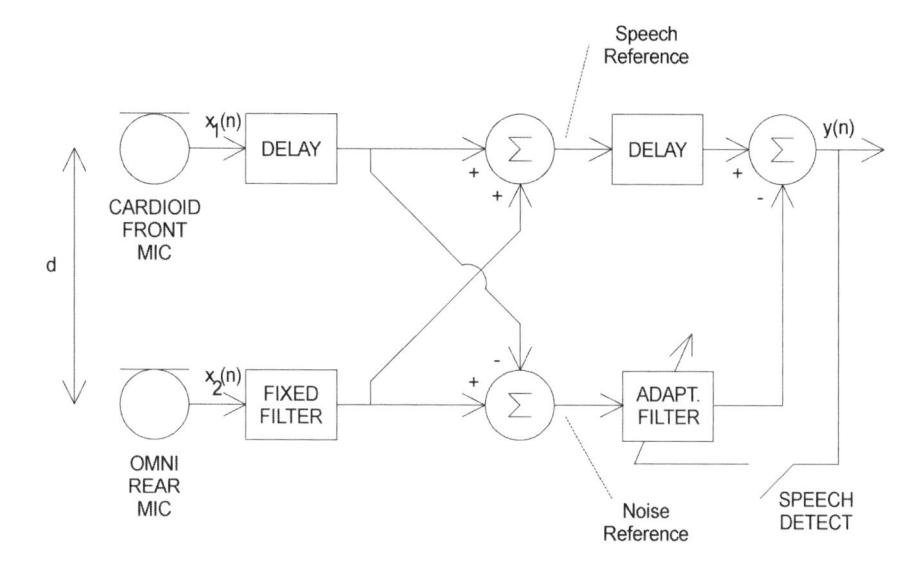

Figure 5-6. Adaptive two-microphone array a combination of directional and omnidirectional microphones and an adaptive filter to control the directional pattern (after Maj et al., 2004).

adapt when speech is absent and held constant when speech is present. When speech is absent the array output $y(n)$ is predominantly noise, and the LMS adaptation adjusts the adaptive filter to minimize the array output power.

The array performance under ideal conditions is shown in Figure 5-7. The omnidirectional microphone has a uniform response, whereas the hardware cardioid microphone shows a reduction in its rear sensitivity of about 13 dB. The adaptive system shows a much greater reduction in sensitivity to sounds coming from the sides and rear than does the cardioid microphone. The directivity index (DI) is about −0.5 dB for the omnidirectional microphone, 4 dB for the cardioid microphone, and 11 dB for the adaptive system. However, testing a microphone with just a single source of interference in an anechoic environment is a highly artificial situation; the real world generally consists of multiple sources of interference and often includes reverberation.

The array performance mounted on a dummy head under reverberant conditions is shown in Figure 5-8. The null in the cardioid response pattern has been filled in by the reverberation, and the adaptive system has a much broader response than was found in the anechoic chamber.

122 Digital Hearing Aids

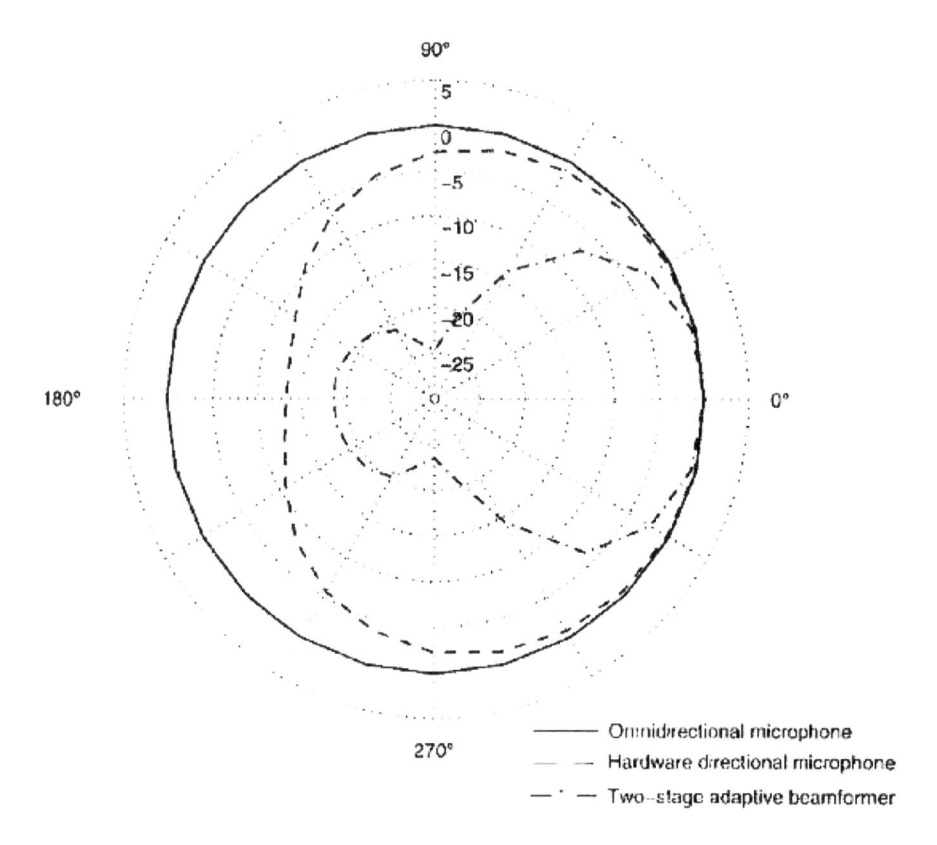

Figure 5-7. AI-weighted directional patterns produced by the two-microphone array of Figure 5-6. The response was measured with the microphone array in free field in an anechoic chamber for a speech source in front of the array (from Maj et al., 2004). The hardware directional microphone had a cardioid polar pattern.

The DIs for the reverberant test condition are substantially lower than for the anechoic measurements as they include both the effects of the dummy head and the reverberation. The adaptive array, when compared to an omnidirectional microphone, improved the SNR by about 11 dB for a single source of interference at 90 degrees, but the benefit was greatly reduced in diffuse noise.

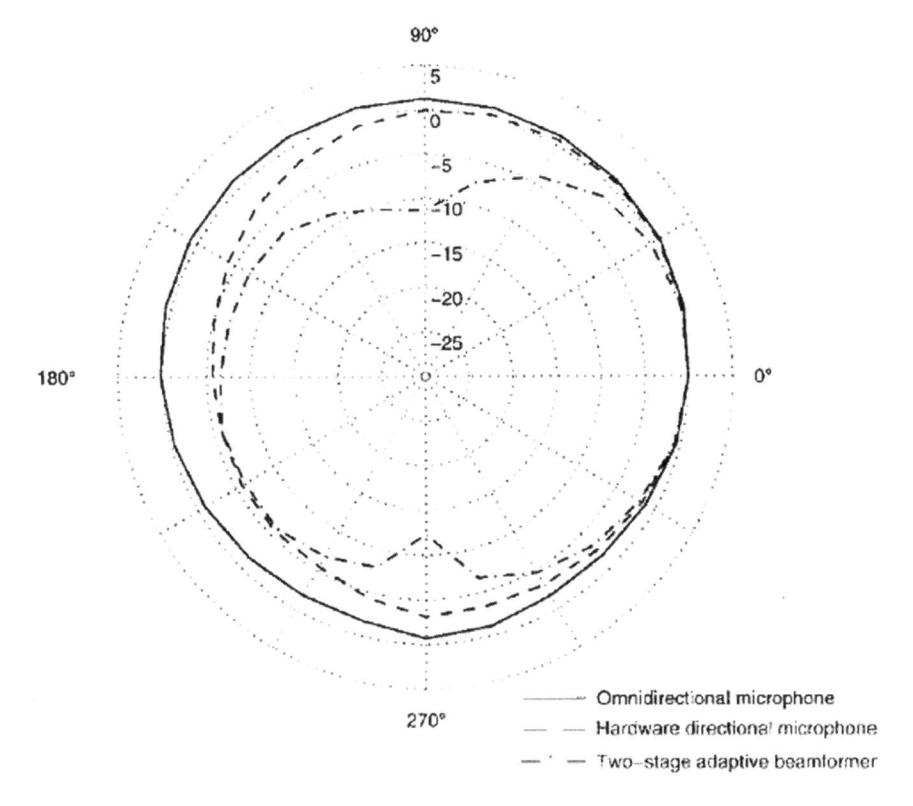

Figure 5-8. AI-weighted directional patterns produced by the two-microphone array of Figure 5-6. The response was measured with the array mounted on a KEMAR manikin under reverberant conditions for a speech source in front of the array (from Maj et al., 2004). The hardware directional microphone had a cardioid polar pattern.

Delay-and-Sum Beam Forming

Most hearing-aid arrays use two microphones due to the limitations on the amount of space available for the microphones in a hearing aid. There are some situations, however, where arrays using more than two microphones are possible. For example, arrays can be mounted across the front or along the temples (side-pieces) of an eyeglass frame. In this section, we consider what happens when the number of microphones in the array is increased. Adaptive processing applied to these larger arrays is then considered in subsequent sections of the chapter.

The microphones in an array can be arranged any way one might want. The array can be in two dimensions or three, be configured as a line or circle or be placed on the surface of a sphere, and can have uniform or nonuniform spacing between the microphones. The simplest geometries are the easiest to analyze, and so this section concentrates on linear arrays having uniform spacing between the microphones. Two basic linear arrangements are commonly used, as shown in Figure 5-9. The axis of an endfire array points toward the desired source of sound, whereas the axis of a broadside array is perpendicular to this direction. Microphones placed along the front of an eyeglass frame would form a broadside array, whereas microphones on the temple would form an endfire array, given a desired source of sound in front of the user.

The signal processing for delay-and-sum beam forming forms a weighted sum of the outputs of the microphones in the array. For an endfire array, the output from each microphone in the array needs to be temporally aligned with the output from the next microphone in the array so that the outputs add in phase. This operation is illustrated in Figure 5-10. The signal from the first microphone in the array is delayed by the length of time it takes for the sound to propagate from the first to the second microphone, and the delayed output from the first microphone is then added to the output from the second microphone. The combined outputs from these two microphones are now in phase and are summed. The combined output is then delayed by the propagation time to the next microphone in the array, and the delayed outputs are again summed. The electronic delays thus duplicate the propagation delays along the entire length of the endfire array. For a broadside array, the signal from the front sound source arrives at all of the microphones at the same time, and the outputs are merely summed.

Two factors are generally of concern in characterizing an antenna array. The first factor is the beamwidth of the array, which is the width of the main lobe of the response pattern and which indicates the ability of the array to attenuate a source of interference close in azimuth to the desired source of sound. The second is the directivity index, which indicates the ability of the array to suppress diffuse interference such as room reverberation, and which was discussed in Chapter 4.

Consider an array consisting of M microphones with a separation d between each microphone. The total array length is then $L = (M - 1)d$. The beamwidth (width of the main lobe) of the array depends on the array length expressed in units of the wavelength of sound at the fre-

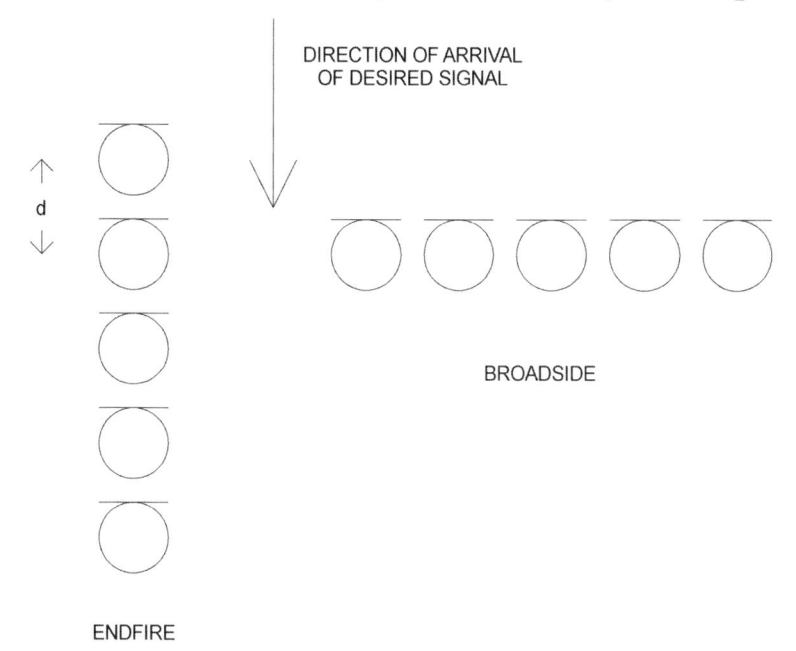

Figure 5-9. Broadside and endfire array geometries.

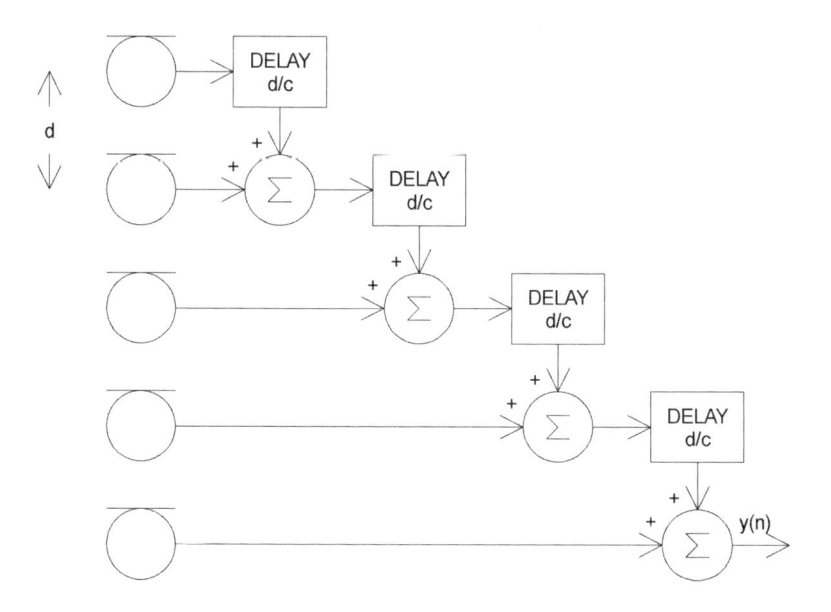

Figure 5-10. Delay-and-sum beam forming for an endfire array.

quency of interest. For a broadside array, the beamwidth from the points where it is 6 dB down from the maximum response level is $BW = 1.21/L$ (Boone, 1987, cited in Soede et al., 1993a), where λ is the wavelength of sound ($\lambda = c/f$ where c is the speed of sound in m/sec and f is the frequency in Hz). The beamwidth thus decreases in inverse proportion to the frequency; doubling the frequency halves the beamwidth. The 6-dB beamwidth for an endfire array is $BW = 1.21(2\lambda/L)^{1/2}$, so for an endfire array doubling the frequency decreases the beamwidth by a factor of $1/\sqrt{2}$. Thus both broadside and endfire arrays become more spatially selective with increasing frequency, but the rate of improvement is more rapid for the broadside array.

Examples of broadside and endfire array patterns are presented in Figure 5-11 for a broadside array and in Figure 5-12 for an endfire array. The arrays in these examples consist of five microphones having a uniform spacing of 2.5 cm between microphones, so each array is 10 cm long. The array response patterns are computed for a frequency of 4 kHz. The beam of the broadside array is formed by summing the outputs of the five microphones, as shown in Figure 5-11A. The response pattern has a narrow main lobe pointing in the forward direction (the z-axis in this figure). Because of the symmetry of the array, the sensitivity is the same for any angle of elevation around the x-axis. Thus, the array has reduced sensitivity to the right (positive x direction) or left (negative x direction), but the sensitivity above (positive y direction), below (negative y direction), or to the rear (negative z direction) is the same as the sensitivity to the front. The broadside array therefore will not attenuate interference coming from directly behind the listener. The three-dimensional response pattern is shown in Figure 5-11C, and the pattern in the x-z plane is shown in Figure 5-11D.

The beam of the endfire array is formed by summing the delayed outputs of the five microphones, as shown in Figure 5-12A and which duplicates the processing diagrammed in Figure 5-10. Again the array has a main lobe pointing in the forward direction indicated by the positive z-axis. Compared to the broadside array, the main lobe of the endfire array is broader. However, the endfire array attenuates sounds coming from the rear because its axis of rotation is the z-axis rather than the x-axis of the broadside array. The delays that temporally align sound waves arriving from in front of the endfire array serve to reduce the temporal alignment of waves coming from the opposite direction, causing partial cancellation of the signal. The DI of the broadside array

(A) Scheme broadside array.

(B) Directivity pattern $Q(k_x, f=4000$ Hz$)$

(C) Three-dimensional diagram

(D) Polar diagram

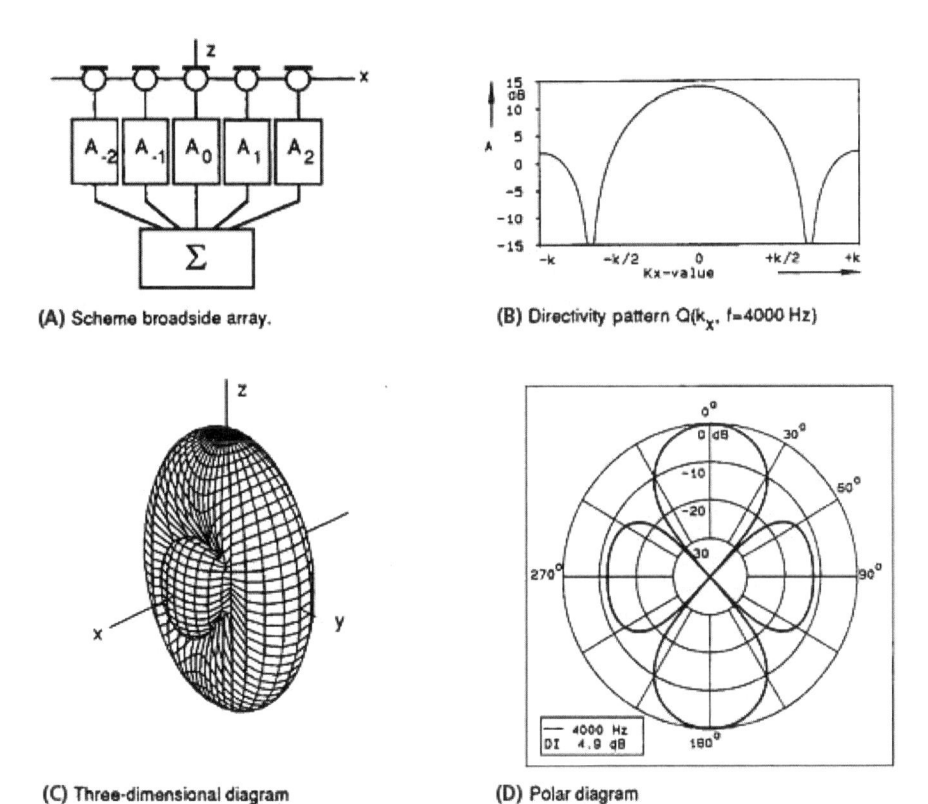

Figure 5-11. Broadside microphone array: **A.** processing block diagram, **B.** directivity pattern as a function of angle from -180 to 180 degree, **C.** three-dimensional polar diagram, and **D.** polar diagram as a function of azimuth (from Soede et al., 1993a). The array consists of five microphones with an overall length of 10 cm, and the analysis frequency is 4 kHz. The z-axis is broadside to the array and the x-axis is parallel to the array, and the polar diagram is in the z-x plane.

at 4 kHz is 4.9 dB, whereas the DI of the endfire array is 7.6 dB. Thus, the broadside array offers a narrower beamwidth, but the endfire array gives better noise attenuation in a diffuse noise field.

A further consideration in the design of a broadside or endfire array is the width of the main directional lobe of the array and the amplitude of the sidelobes. These considerations directly parallel the computation of a DFT. The DFT applies to a signal sampled in time, whereas the microphone array deals with a signal sampled in space. The longer

128 Digital Hearing Aids

(A) Scheme endfire array.

(B) Directivity pattern $Q(k_x, f=4000$ Hz)

(C) Three-dimensional diagram

(D) Polar diagram

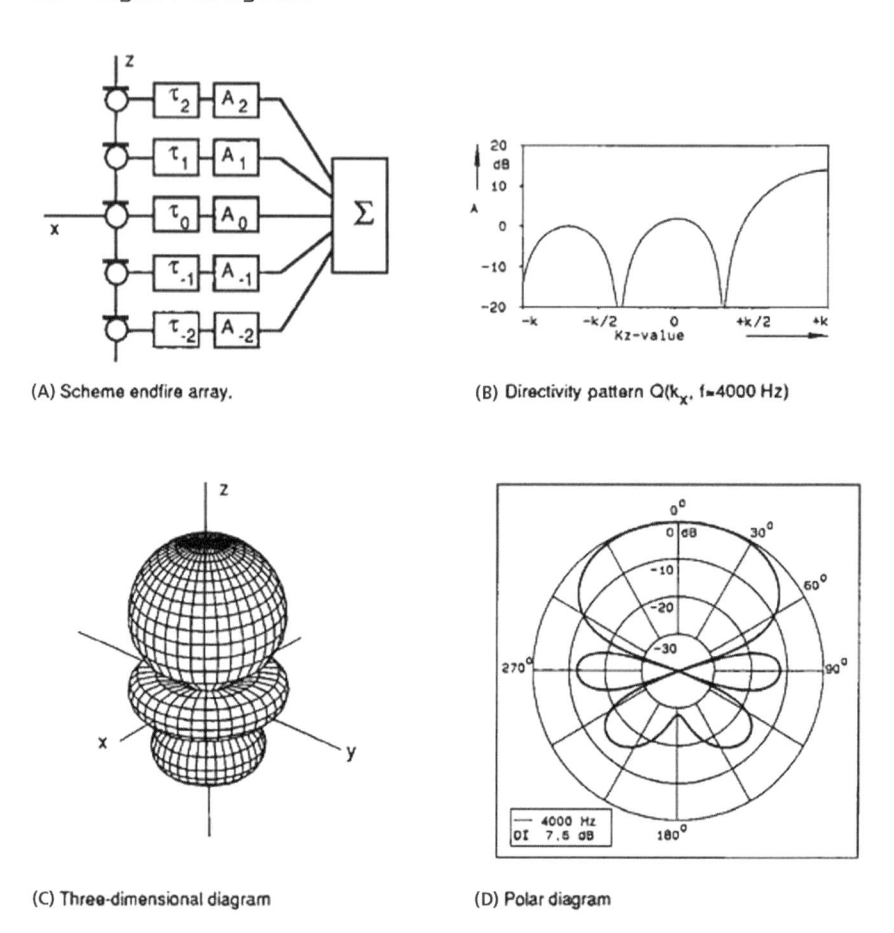

Figure 5-12. Endfire microphone array: **A.** processing block diagram, **B.** directivity pattern as a function of angle from -180 to 180 degrees, **C.** three-dimensional polar diagram, and **D.** polar diagram as a function of azimuth (from Soede et al., 1993a). The array consists of five microphones with a overall length of 10 cm, and the analysis frequency is 4 kHz. The z-axis is endfire to the array and the x-axis is perpendicular to the array, and the polar diagram is in the z-x plane.

the microphone array, the narrower the main lobe. Summing all of the array outputs with equal weights gives the narrowest main lobe width, but also gives the highest sidelobe levels. Applying weights to the array outputs, like applying a raised cosine window to a data sequence before computing its DFT, will increase the width of the main lobe while reducing the amplitude of the sidelobes.

One can also form arrays of directional microphones. If the omnidirectional microphones in an array are replaced by directional microphones, the resultant directional pattern is the product of the gain as a function of angle for the array times the gain as a function of angle for the directional microphone response. The broadside array directional pattern shown in Figure 5-11, for example, would acquire a rear-facing null if the omnidirectional microphones used in that array were replaced by cardioid microphones. But in addition to the improved directional response, the array of cardioid microphones would also acquire the 6 dB/octave frequency-response slope that comes with the directional microphone response.

Adaptive Arrays

Delay-and-sum beam forming combines the microphone outputs to produce a directional pattern having a main lobe pointing in the assumed direction of the desired source of sound. The location of the nulls in the directional pattern is generally not considered when forming the weighted sum of the microphone outputs. In an adaptive array, however, the location of the response nulls is the paramount consideration. The array adapts to position the response nulls in the direction of the strongest sources of interference, and thus maximizes the SNR. So delay-and-sum beam forming is concerned with the characteristics of the main lobe of the response pattern, whereas adaptive array processing is concerned with the nulls and the sidelobes. An array consisting of M microphones can generate $M-1$ nulls in its response pattern, so the adaptive array can suppress $M-1$ separate sources of interference under anechoic conditions. The locations of the nulls are symmetric around the major axis of the array, so there are actually $2(M-1)$ nulls when the mirror images are counted, but only $M-1$ directions can be independently steered. Although an adaptive array can be built using either a broadside or an endfire geometry, an endfire array appears to be more effective in practice (Hoffman et al., 2000).

A block diagram of an adaptive array is presented in Figure 5-13. The output from each microphone feeds an adaptive tapped delay-line filter. The weights from all of the filters are adapted together to optimize the overall array response. A common optimization criterion is to minimize the mean-squared power output by the array, subject to the constraint

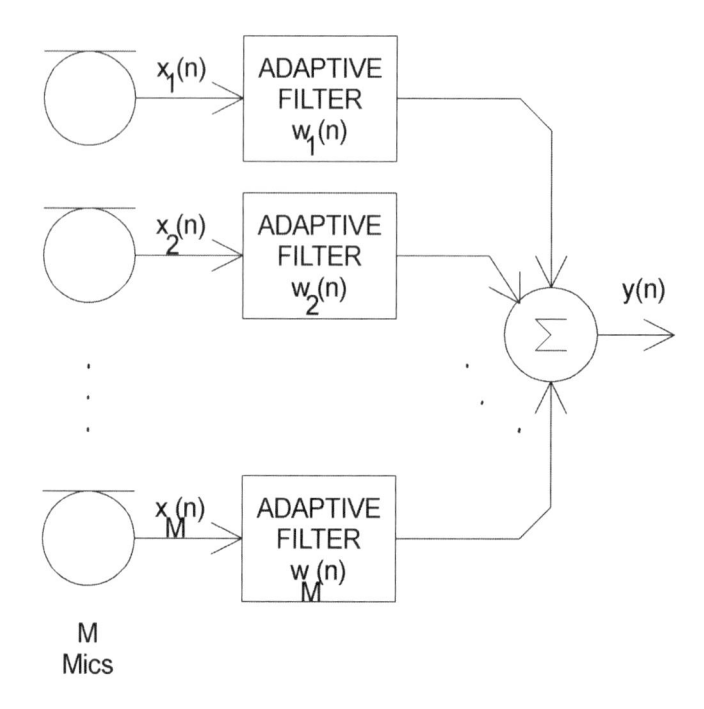

Figure 5-13. Block diagram of an adaptive microphone system.

that a signal coming from directly in front of the array is passed without attenuation (Monzigo & Miller, 1980). The update of the filters uses the correlation between the outputs of the different microphones; the adaptive gain equation of *Eq. (5.2)* is a limiting case where the array consists of two microphones and the adaptive filter consists of just one tap. The adaptive filter update is based on the assumption that the desired signal and the interference are uncorrelated, so the correlations computed between the microphones in the array yield the time delays corresponding to the angles of arrival of each individual sound source at the array. If a strong reflection is present, or if the assumed microphone locations in the array do not match the actual locations, the estimated signal delays will be corrupted and the adaptive system may end up canceling the desired signal instead of the interference (Cox, 1973; McDonough, 1972; Seligson, 1970). Signal cancellation has been observed in arrays designed for hearing-aid applications, with the cancellation caused by strong reflections (Greenberg & Zurek, 1992) or by errors in the assumed microphone locations (Hoffman et al., 1994).

Prevention of signal cancellation can be achieved by applying an additional constraint to the adaptive filter update algorithm. Filters that misadapt and begin to cancel the desired signal tend to show an increase in the magnitudes of the filter coefficients (Cox, 1973). Thus, constraining the magnitude of the adaptive filter coefficients to be less than a preset limit guarantees that the desired signal will never be completely cancelled by the adaptive processing (Cox et al., 1987). This approach, termed the scaled projection algorithm, has been shown to be effective in adaptive hearing-aid arrays used in reverberant rooms (Hoffman et al., 1994; Hoffman et al., 2000; Kates & Weiss, 1996).

Hoffman et al. (1994) simulated head-mounted microphone arrays having from three to seven microphones, with 8- or 16-tap filters at each microphone used to implement an adaptive array incorporating the scaled projection algorithm. The sampling rate was 10.1 kHz. The speech source was in front of the head, and a single noise source was at a 45-degree angle. Reverberant environments were simulated giving direct-to-reverberant power ratios of infinity (anechoic), 6.9, 1.3, and −4.0 dB. The results show that, for the single noise source, increasing the number of microphones in the array had no significant effect on the array performance, whereas the 16-tap filters performed slightly better than the 8-tap filters. The improvement in SNR produced by the array, however, was strongly affected by the direct-to-reverberant ratio, with the array benefit going from about 17 dB at the ratio of infinity (anechoic) to about 3 dB at the ratio of −4.0 dB (e.g., the desired source of sound is beyond the critical distance for the simulated room).

The adaptive array processing can also be implemented in the frequency domain using an FFT approach (Kates & Weiss, 1996). An example of a five-microphone array using block frequency-domain processing is shown in Figure 5-14. The incoming signals at each microphone are read into a buffer, and an FFT is used to transform the signal at each microphone into the frequency domain. The set of weights for each FFT bin is adaptively updated, and the weighted sum at each frequency is then formed. An inverse transform then returns the signal to the time domain where the processed segments are combined using the overlap-add procedure.

Kates and Weiss (1996) investigated the performance of an endfire array 10 cm long composed of five uniformly spaced microphones. The desired signal was a sentence reproduced using a loudspeaker in front

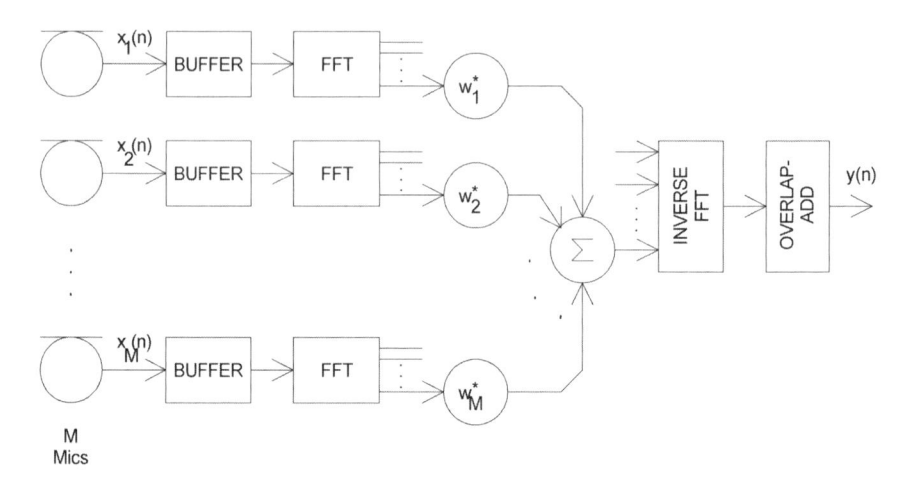

Figure 5-14. Block diagram of a frequency-domain adaptive microphone system.

of the array, and the interference was multitalker babble from a single loudspeaker positioned to one side or behind the array. A diffuse field was also generated by reproducing uncorrelated babble simultaneously from five loudspeakers arranged around the sides and behind the array. Two rooms, an office and a larger conference room, were used for the measurements. For the single source of interference at an input SNR of 0 dB, delay-and-sum beam forming for the array mounted on a microphone stand improved the SNR by an average of 5.3 dB over an omnidirectional microphone, whereas adaptive beam forming gave an average improvement of 11.0 dB. For the diffuse field at an input SNR of 0 dB, delay-and-sum beam forming improved the SNR by an average of 5.1 dB over an omnidirectional microphone, whereas adaptive beam forming gave an average improvement of 10.2 dB. Positioning the array along the side of a dummy head in the location of the left temple of an eyeglass frame reduced the delay-and-sum beam forming performance by about 0.3 dB, and reduced the adaptive processing performance by about 1.0 dB compared to the same array mounted on a microphone stand.

An adaptive array offers substantially better improvements in SNR than delay-and-sum beam forming. But these benefits come at a cost. The adaptive array can partially cancel the desired signal under some conditions, whereas this problem never occurs for delay-and-sum beamforming. The signal processing needed for an adaptive array requires filtering the outputs from each microphone in the array and the mathematical operations needed to update the filter coefficients, and the total computational requirements may be greater than can be realized in a hearing aid while maintaining acceptable battery life.

Superdirective Arrays

Some of the most difficult listening conditions for a hearing-aid user involve multiple sources of interference combined with reverberation, for example, listening to a conversation in a restaurant. Under these conditions the ability of an adaptive array to steer individual nulls in the direction of each interfering sound source is not especially useful because there are many more sources and strong reflections in the room than there are potential nulls in the array directional pattern. Instead of steering nulls, the adaptive array in a diffuse sound field adapts to minimize the total interfering signal power, and this is accomplished by minimizing the levels of the array sidelobes without regard for the null locations. The adaptive array will always converge to the same directional pattern in a completely diffuse noise field. If a diffuse noise field is assumed in advance, one can design a nonadaptive array that gives the same directional pattern as the adaptive system and which optimally improves the SNR. This solution is known as a superdirective array. The superdirective two-microphone array is the hypercardioid response pattern shown in Figure 4-5B.

A superdirective array offers the same performance benefits as an adaptive array in diffuse noise, but the computational demands are greatly reduced as the microphone filters needed for the superdirective array are designed in advance and do not adapt while the array is being used. The response of a superdirective array is not affected by reverberation, and signal cancellation will not occur in the presence of a strong reflection. In an array having M uniformly-spaced microphones, the improvement in SNR for delay-and-sum beam forming is proportional to M. In a superdirective array, the improvement in SNR for external interference is proportional to M^2, and the improvement actually increases as the array dimensions are reduced (Uzkov, 1946).

However, the superdirective array is affected to the same degree as an adaptive array to errors in the assumed microphone locations or to microphone mismatch (Cox et al., 1986). The improvement in the rejection of external interference is obtained by providing large amounts of gain for each microphone in the array and then taking the differences between the outputs of adjacent microphones. The large gains amplify the internal noise of the microphones and the noise adds even when the signal differences are taken. Thus, the greater the rejection of external interference the greater the amplification of the internal noise. Similarly, the large gains combined with the output differences magnify any errors in the assumed amplitude and phase responses of the microphones. Thus, the design of a superdirective array involves a balance between the external interference rejection and the sensitivity to microphone mismatch and internal noise (Cox et al., 1986; Doclo & Moonen, 2003).

Simulation studies for a spherically isotropic noise field (Kates, 1993; Stadler & Rabinowitz, 1993), using endfire array configurations similar to that used by Soede et al. (1993a), show that a superdirective array, constrained to balance the concerns between external interference rejection and sensitivity to microphone mismatch and internal noise, will give a SNR about 5 dB better than that obtained for delay-and-sum beam forming using the same set of microphones. For the broadside array orientation, the superdirective weights average less than 1-dB better SNR than delay-and-sum beam forming. When using omnidirectional microphones, a null at 180 degrees can be imposed on the endfire array beam pattern with only a 0.3-dB penalty in SNR (Kates, 1993), and increasing the number of microphones in the array from five to seven improves the SNR by only about 0.3 dB (Stadler & Rabinowitz, 1993).

Directional patterns for a cardioid microphone, delay-and-sum beam forming, and superdirective processing are presented in Figure 5-15. The endfire microphone array used for parts (B) and (C) of Figure 5-15 consists of five omnidirectional microphones having uniform 2.5-cm spacing, giving a total length of 10 cm. The delay-and-sum directional patterns shown in Figure 5-15B for the array show that this system offers little noise suppression at low frequencies. As the frequency increases the main lobe of the array becomes narrower and the sidelobe level decreases, and both effects lead to increased rejection of off-axis noise. The same general behavior is visible in Figure 5-15C for the superdirective array. However, the superdirective array offers much better directional behavior at all frequencies than is possible with the delay-

Adaptive and Multimicrophone Arrays 135

Figure 5-15. Directional patterns for **A.** cardioid microphone, **B.** five-microphone endfire array using delay-and-sum beam forming, and **C.** five-microphone endfire array using superdirective processing.

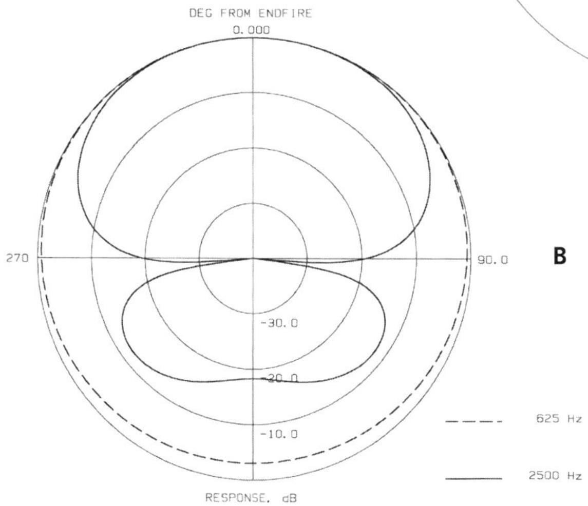

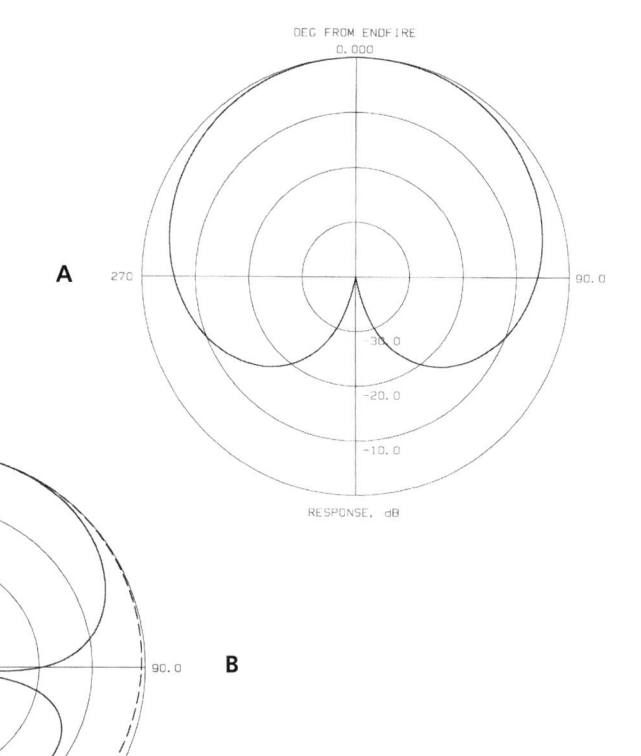

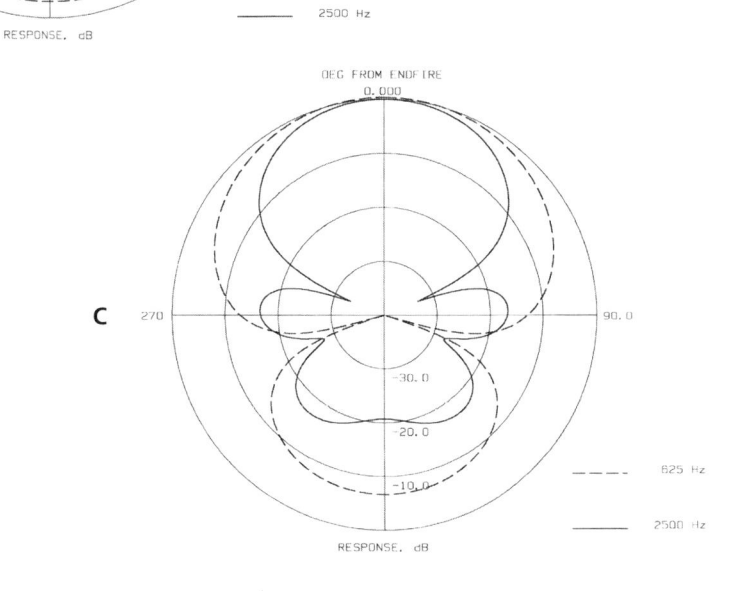

and-sum beamforming. Also, note that the directional response pattern for the superdirective array at 625 Hz is very similar to the hypercardioid directional microphone response shown in Figure 4-5B, so at low frequencies a directional microphone performs almost as well as the endfire array.

One characteristic of delay-and-sum beam forming, adaptive arrays, and superdirective arrays is that the width of the main lobe tends to decrease with increasing frequency, as shown in Figure 5-15C. The frequency response will be flat for a source of sound located at exactly 0 degrees on-axis. But if the desired source of sound shifts around to the side, the changes in the beam patterns at the different frequencies will attenuate the high frequencies more than the low frequencies. This problem can be avoided if the array is designed to have the same mainlobe width at all frequencies. The design procedures to accomplish this end are quite complicated (Doclo & Moonen, 2003; Ward et al., 1995). But like the superdirective array, the design needs to be performed only once, after which fixed filters are used on the output of each microphone in the array.

Widely Spaced Arrays

The arrays considered so far use microphones that are spaced close together, with the expectation that the array would be connected to the input of a hearing aid or would be hand-held. An alternative approach is an array design that places the microphones on opposite sides of the head. The array now spans the head, and the array output is fed into hearing aids at both ears. The array output thus replaces the normal binaural processing with a system that is designed to have better noise-suppression characteristics. An additional concern is that a widely spaced array requires a mechanism for routing the signals from one side of the head to the other in order to perform the beam forming, which means that either a wire or a wireless link is needed. A wire has cosmetic problems, and a wireless link may require more power than can be practically supplied by a hearing-aid battery.

One array design that has been used (Greenberg & Zurek, 1992; Kompis & Dillier, 2001a) is illustrated in Figure 5-16. This design is a Griffiths-Jim adaptive array (Griffiths & Jim, 1982). The array orientation is broadside, and the microphone outputs are combined to form

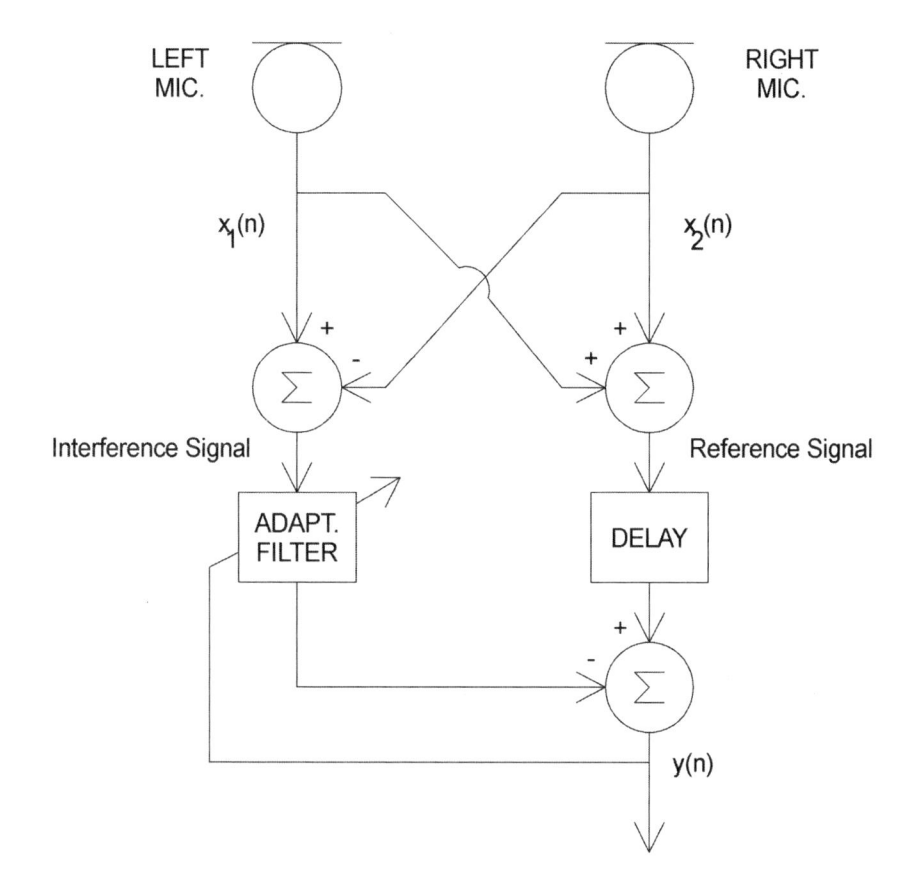

Figure 5-16. Block diagram of a two-microphone array used with the microphones mounted on opposite sides of the head.

reference and interference signals. The reference signal is the delay-and-sum array output formed by summing all of the microphone outputs. Because the array orientation is broadside, the microphone sum gives a main lobe that has its maximum at 0 degrees in front of the array. The interference signal is the difference between the two microphones. For the broadside geometry, the difference of the two microphones gives a cosine directional response that has a null at 0 degrees and peaks to either side. The desired signal is therefore canceled by taking the difference, leaving only the interference.

The interference signal is then adaptively filtered to maximally cancel the interference corrupting the reference signal. As with the adaptive arrays described previously in this chapter, this adaptive system can cancel the desired signal if it is present in both the reference and interference signal outputs; this problem can happen in reverberation where the desired signal originates from the front of the array and is also contained in reflections arriving at the array from azimuths other than 0 degrees. One approach used to prevent signal cancellation is to allow the filter to adapt when only noise is present, and then to freeze the filter coefficients when speech is assumed to be present (Greenberg & Zurek, 1992; Kompis & Dillier, 2001b).

If the adaptive filter in Figure 5-16 is short, the system works to steer nulls in the array directional pattern. For a pair of microphones on opposite sides of the head, the microphone separation is about 15 cm. This distance is half a wavelength at 1100 Hz. For frequencies below 1100 Hz, the adaptive system will create a single null at any given low frequency. At frequencies above 1100 Hz, the adaptive system will generate multiple nulls, one in the direction of the noise source to be canceled and additional nulls as a result of the microphone spacing being greater than half a wavelength.

As the length of the adaptive filter is increased, the system works to model the room impulse response at the microphone locations. During intervals where the desired speech is absent, the adaptive filter minimizes the total power output by the array. If a source of interference is in a room, the output power will be minimized if the sound directly from the source, plus all of the major reflections, in the interference signal are filtered to match the interference components in the reference signal. A filter long enough can include both the direct sound and the reflections, and in theory should do a better job of improving the SNR than a short filter that can just steer a null in the direction of the interfering source and cannot deal with the reflections. The long filter has a problem, however, in that the longer the adaptive filter, the more slowly it adapts. Thus, a filter long enough to model the room reverberation may adapt so slowly that it cannot respond to changes in the arrival times of reflections caused by head motion or which occur as the listener moves about the room.

Experimental and simulation results show that the adaptive array can substantially improve the SNR under some conditions. For a single source of interference and the desired signal absent, Greenberg and Zurek (1992) found that the adaptive array could provide over 50-dB cancellation of the noise under anechoic conditions. However, the benefit compared to delay-and-sum beam forming was reduced to essentially 0 dB in a strongly reverberant environment. Kompis and Dillier (2001b) found a 7-dB improvement compared to delay-and-sum beam forming for the adaptive array in anechoic operation when both a single source of interference and the desired signal were present, but the improvement in SNR was reduced to about 1.5 dB when the reverberation time was increased to 0.8 sec. Kompis and Dillier (2001b) also found that the array performance was reduced as the source of interference was moved away from the array in the test room, and both Greenberg and Zurek (1992) and Kompis and Dillier (2001b) found a strong improvement in the adaptive array performance with increasing adaptive filter length. In both of the cited studies, the adaptive processing was allowed to run until the solutions reached steady state, after which the improvement in SNR was measured; Kompis and Dillier (2001b) made their measurements after 2 sec, whereas Greenberg and Zurek (1992) waited for 13.7 sec.

An alternative approach is to implement the beam forming in the frequency domain (Larson et al., 2004; Lockwood et al., 2004), in a manner similar to that shown in Figure 5-14. The frequency-domain adaptation generates a separate response null at each FFT bin center frequency. This approach has the benefit of rapid adaptation, so movement of the listener should not be a problem. The improvement in SNR for the frequency-domain algorithm is very similar to that produced by the time-domain Griffiths-Jim beam former, with the array benefit decreasing as the room reverberation and the number of interfering sources are increased.

Array Benefits

The results cited thus far indicate that a microphone array can make a substantial improvement in the SNR in a noisy situation. Several studies indicate that improvements in speech intelligibility are directly related to the improvements in SNR. One measure of speech intelligibility is the speech reception threshold (SRT), which gives the SNR at which 50% of the test stimuli are correctly identified (Saunders & Kates, 1997). The more negative the SRT, the worse the SNR at which the listeners can

140 Digital Hearing Aids

Table 5-1. Average Differences in Speech Reception Threshold (SRT) Reported in the Literature for a Selection of Array Designs and Processing Strategies.

Authors	No. of Mics	Array Geom.	Inter-ference	Test Room	Process	Ref. Cond.	ΔSRT Words dB	ΔSRT Sent. dB
Vanden Berghe & Wouters (1998)	2	Omni. Endfire	Single Source 90 deg	Office (RT = .35 s)	Adapt. Filter	Omni. Mic.	-4.7	-5.6
Maj et al. (2004)	2	Omni. Endfire	Single Source 90 deg	Large Room (RT=.76 sec)	Adapt. Filter	Omni. Mic.	-11.2	-11.6
			Diffuse		Adapt. Filter	Omni. Mic.	-2.5	-2.6
Soede et al. (1993b)	5	Card. Broad	Diffuse	Sound-Treated	Delay & Sum	Own Ear	–	-3.3
		Card. Endfire			Delay & Sum		–	-4.1
Hoffman et al. (1994)	3	Omni. Broad	Single Source 45 deg	Simulated Anechoic	Adapt. Array	Omni. Mic.	-15.4	–
	3			Living Rm			-5.1	–
	3			Conf. Rm			-1.4	–
	7			Anechoic			-22.7	–
	7			Living Rm			-10.2	–
	7			Conf. Rm			-3.1	–
Greenberg et al. (2003)	4	Card. Broad	Avg of 1 and 3 Sources	Sound-Treated	Delay & Sum	Bin. Card. Mic		-1.6
					Adaptive		–	-7.0
					Freq Null		–	-9.3
Saunders & Kates (1997)	5	Omni. Endfire	Diffuse	Office (RT = .25 sec)	Cardioid Mic	Omni.	-4.3	-4.0
					Delay & Sum		-1.5	-3.0
					Super		-6.2	-6.3
				Conf Rm (RT = .60 s)	Cardioid Mic		-1.9	-3.0
					Delay & Sum		-0.9	-0.5
					Super		-4.7	-5.1

A negative change in the SRT indicates that the listener could identify the test materials at a poorer SNR. The array geometry is endfire or broadside using either omnidirectional or cardioid microphones. The reverberation time (RT) of the test space is indicated when it was specified by authors. The array processing is either two-microphone using an adaptive filter, delay-and-sum beamforming, an adaptive array, or an adaptive frequency-domain null-steering algorithm.

correctly identify the stimuli and the better their speech-understanding ability. Table 5-1 summarizes the perceptual results from some microphone-array studies that used the SRT to measure speech intelligibility for stimuli consisting of sentences and/or isolated words. The more negative the SRT entry in the table, the greater the benefit from the microphone array. Overall, the studies that use both sentence and isolated words as test materials show similar processing benefits for the two types of stimuli.

The results of Vanden Berghe and Wouters (1998) and Maj et al. (2004) show that a two-microphone array can improve speech intelligibility by up to 11.6 dB when a single source of interference is present, but that the benefit from the processing is reduced to just 2.5 dB for diffuse interference. Soede et al. (1993b) show benefits of 3 to 4 dB for broadside and endfire delay-and-sum arrays comprising five cardioid microphones, but the processing benefit appears to be primarily due to the cardioid microphone response pattern as the results of Saunders and Kates (1997) show a comparable benefit for just a single cardioid microphone.

Hoffman et al. (1994) compared three-microphone and seven-microphone arrays using adaptive processing for a single source of interference. The seven-microphone array gives consistently better speech intelligibility than the three-microphone array. For both arrays, the processing benefit decreases rapidly as the amount of reverberation in the simulated room increases. Note that Hoffman et al. (1994) placed the source of interference at 45 degrees, whereas most of the competing studies place the interference at 90 degrees which is an easier situation for the array processing to handle.

Greenberg et al. (2003) compared speech intelligibility for a four-microphone broadside array to binaural signal presentation. They thus compare the benefit of the array processing, in which the same processed signal is presented to both ears, to the speech intelligibility that would occur in a normal binaural hearing-aid fitting using directional microphones. The single noise source in their experiments was at 90 degrees, whereas the three sources were at 90, 180, and 270 degrees. They show a small benefit using delay-and-sum beam forming, a 7-dB benefit for adaptive array processing using a 285-tap adaptive filter at the 16-kHz sampling rate, and the greatest benefit for a frequency-domain algorithm that steers independent nulls in the direction of the interference in each FFT frequency bin.

Saunders and Kates (1997) compared a cardioid microphone to a five-microphone endfire array using delay-and-sum and superdirective processing. The reference was an omnidirectional microphone. The interference was babble reproduced over five loudspeakers to produce diffuse interference in an office and in a conference room. They found that the delay-and-sum beam forming was less effective than a single cardioid microphone, and that the superdirective processing was the most effective. The array processing benefits were greatly reduced in the room having the greater reverberation time, but even in the worse of the two rooms the superdirective array improved speech intelligibility by 5 dB.

Concluding Remarks

Directional microphones and adaptive microphone arrays represent the only processing techniques that have been consistently shown to improve speech intelligibility in noise. Small arrays, comprising two or three microphones, can be built into a hearing-aid case. An adaptive two-microphone array provides a null in the directional response pattern that can be steered in the direction of a single interfering source of sound. Using an adaptive gain in the two-microphone array forces the null to be in the same direction at all frequencies, whereas using a multitap adaptive filter or frequency-domain processing provides different null directions at different frequencies.

Better performance can be obtained by increasing the number of microphones used in the array. A microphone array using delay-and-sum beam forming offers an improvement over an omnidirectional microphone, but the benefit compared to a directional (e.g., hypercardioid) microphone may be small. The greatest benefit occurs when the microphone array is combined with adaptive or superdirective processing. The adaptive array will be best when there are a small number of interfering sound sources in an environment low in reverberation, whereas the superdirective array is to be preferred in highly reverberant situations as it is immune to the problems of signal cancellation that can occur with an adaptive array.

If microphone arrays are so beneficial, why doesn't everyone use them? The problems are cost and cosmetics. A microphone array requires putting more microphones in the hearing aid and providing more signal processing power in the digital processor, and both of these steps will increase the cost of the hearing aid and reduce battery life. A second concern is cosmetics. A microphone array takes up a lot of space compared to a hearing aid; the five-microphone array used by Kates and Weiss (1996), for example, was 10 cm long, which is the size of a pen or pencil. Much of the work on arrays has concentrated on arrays that can fit along the temple or across the front of a pair of eyeglasses, but this may not be an acceptable solution in a world of fashion-conscious eyewear and contact lenses. So microphone arrays are very effective, but getting people to accept them will be a difficult task.

References

Boone, M. M. (1987). *Design and development of a synthetic acoustic antenna for highly directional sound measurements.* Ph.D. Thesis, Delft University Technology, The Netherlands.

Cox, H. (1973). Resolving power and sensitivity to mismatch of optimum array processors. *Journal of the Acoustical Society of America, 54,* 771–785.

Cox, H., Zeskind, R. M., & Kooij, T. (1986). Practical supergain. *IEEE Transactions on Acoustics, Speech and Signal Processing, 34,* 393–398.

Cox, H., Zeskind, R. M., & Owen, M. M. (1987). Robust adaptive beamforming. *IEEE Transactions on Acoustics, Speech and Signal Processing, 35,* 1365–1376.

Desloge, J., Zimmer, M., & Zurek, P. (2004). Performance benefits of adaptive, multimicrophone, interference-cancelling systems in everyday listening environments. *Journal of the Acoustical Society of America, 115,* 2536.

Doclo, S., & Moonen, M. (2003). Design of broadband beamformers robust against gain and phase errors in the microphone array characteristics. *IEEE Transactions on Signal Processing, 51,* 2511–2526.

Elko, G. W. (2000). *Steerable and variable first-order differential microphone array.* U.S. Patent 6,041,127, issued March 21, 2000.

Greenberg, J. E., Desloge, J. G., & Zurek, P. M. (2003). Evaluation of array-processing algorithms for a headband hearing aid. *Journal of the Acoustical Society of America, 113,* 1646–1657.

Greenberg, J. E., & Zurek, P. M. (1992). Evaluation of an adaptive beamforming method for hearing aids. *Journal of the Acoustical Society of America, 91,* 1662–1676.

Griffiths, L. J., & Jim, C. W. (1982). An alternative approach to linearly constrained adaptive beamforming. *IEEE Transactions on Antennas and Propagation, 30,* 27–34.

Haykin, S. (1996). *Adaptive filter theory.* Englewood Cliffs, NJ: Prentice-Hall.

Hoffman, M. W., Pinkelman, X. F., & Li, Z. (2000). Real-time and off-line comparisons of standard array configurations containing three and four microphones. *Journal of the Acoustical Society of America, 107,* 3560–3563.

Hoffman, M. W., Trine, T. D., Buckley, K. M., & Van Tasell, D. J. (1994). Robust adaptive microphone array processing for hearing aids: Realistic speech enhancement. *Journal of the Acoustical Society of America, 96,* 759–770.

Kates, J. M. (1993). Superdirective arrays for hearing aids. *Journal of the Acoustical Society of America, 94,* 1930–1933.

Kates, J. M., & Weiss, M. R. (1996). A comparison of hearing-aid array-processing techniques. *Journal of the Acoustical Society of America, 99,* 3138–3148.

Kompis, M., & Dillier, N. (2001a). Performance of an adaptive beamforming noise reduction scheme for hearing aid applications. I. Prediction of the signal-to-noise ratio improvement. *Journal of the Acoustical Society of America, 109,* 1123–1133.

Kompis, M., & Dillier, N. (2001b). Performance of an adaptive beamforming noise reduction scheme for hearing aid applications. II. Experimental verification of the predictions. *Journal of the Acoustical Society of America, 109,* 1134–1143.

Larson, J. B., Lansing, C. R., Bilger, R. C., Wheeler, B. C., Phatak, S. A., Lockwood, M. E., et al. (2004). Speech perception in noise with a two-sensor frequency-domain minimum-variance (FMV) beamforming algorithm. *Acoustic Research Letters On-Line, 5,* 100–105.

Lockwood, M. E., Jones, D. L., Bilger, R. C., Lansing, C. R., O'Brien, W. D., Wheeler, B. C., et al (2004). Performance of time- and frequency-domain binaural beamformers based on recorded signals from real rooms. *Journal of the Acoustical Society of America, 115,* 379–391.

Luo, F-L, Yang, J., Pavlovic, C., & Nehorai, A. (2002). Adaptive null-forming scheme in digital hearing aids. *IEEE Transactions on Signal Processing, 50,* 1583–1590.

Maj, J. -B., Wouters, J., & Moonen, M. (2004). Noise reduction results of an adaptive filtering technique for dual-microphone behind-the-ear hearing aids. *Ear and Hearing, 25,* 215–229.

McDonough, R. N. (1972). Degraded performance of nonlinear array processors in the presence of data modeling errors. *Journal of the Acoustical Society of America, 51,* 1186–1193.

McKinney, E. D., & DeBrunner, V. E. (1996). A two-microphone adaptive broadband array for hearing aids. *Proceedings of the IEEE International Conference on Acoustic Speech and Signal Processing*, Atlanta, May 7–10, 1996.

Monzigo, R. A., & Miller, T. W. (1980). *Introduction to adaptive arrays* (pp. 78–105). New York: Wiley.

Saunders, G. H., & Kates, J. M. (1997). Speech intelligibility enhancement using hearing-aid array processing. *Journal of the Acoustical Society of America, 102*, 1827–1837.

Seligson, C. D. (1970). Comment on "High-resolution frequency-wavenumber spectrum analysis." *Proceedings of the IEEE, 58*, 947–949.

Soede, W., Berkhout, A. J., & Bilsen, F. A. (1993a). Development of a directional hearing instrument based on array technology. *Journal of the Acoustical Society of America, 94*, 785–798.

Soede, W., Bilsen, F. A., & Berkhout, A. J. (1993b). Assessment of a directional microphone array for hearing-impaired listeners. *Journal of the Acoustical Society of America, 94*, 799–808.

Stadler, R. W., & Rabinowitz, W. M. (1993). On the potential of fixed arrays for hearing aids. *Journal of the Acoustical Society of America, 94*, 1332–1342.

Uzkov, A. I. (1946). An approach to the problem of optimum directive antennae design. *Comptes Rendus (Doklady) de l'Academie des Sciences de l'URSS, 53*, 35–38.

Vanden Berghe, J., & Wouters, J. (1998). An adaptive noise canceller for hearing aids using two nearby microphones. *Journal of the Acoustical Society of America, 103*, 3621–3626.

Ward, D. B., Kennedy, R. A., & Williamson, R.C. (1995). Theory and design of broadband sensor arrays with frequency invariant far-field beam patterns. *Journal of the Acoustical Society of America, 97*, 1023–1034.

6

Wind Noise

WIND NOISE IS A PROBLEM in many hearing aids. Wind noise is caused by turbulent air flow over the microphone(s) in the hearing aid (Dillon et al., 1999; Wuttke, 1991). Turbulence occurs when air flows around any obstacle, including the head and ear, so it can never be entirely eliminated in a hearing aid placed on the head. Wind noise is often annoying while listening, can overload the microphone preamplifier and generate distortion, and can mask desired speech sounds.

A simple and effective procedure to reduce wind noise is to place a screen over the microphone ports to reduce the turbulence, and many styles of wind screens have been developed for sound-recording microphones (Wuttke, 1991). But a wind screen may not be practical for a hearing aid given constraints on size or appearance, in which case an algorithmic solution is needed to reduce the wind-noise effects. Assuming that the microphone and preamplifier are not overloaded by the wind noise, signal processing can be effective in reducing the annoyance and masking effects. If, however, the major effect of the wind noise is overloading the microphone preamplifier, signal processing that occurs after the preamplifier will not reduce the noise problems.

This chapter discusses the causes and potential solutions for wind noise in hearing aids. The nature of turbulent air flow is reviewed, and this section is followed by measurements of turbulence around the head and its effects on hearing aid output. Turbulence and wind noise are then considered from a signal-processing perspective. Signal characteristics that could be used to design wind-noise reduction algorithms are described, followed by several algorithms that have been proposed to reduce the effects of wind noise in hearing aids.

Turbulence

Wind noise is caused by turbulent airflow. Airflow must change direction when it goes around an obstacle such as the head or the ear, and turbulence will occur when the rate of airflow, relative to the size of the obstacle, exceeds a threshold (Talay, 1975). Once turbulence is established, the changes in particle velocity become large, generating eddies and large spatial pressure differentials. Eddies are generated by the airflow around the head, by the flow over and around the pinna, and by the flow past the tragus and helix. The size and shape of the microphone and hearing aid will also affect the turbulence (Corcos, 1963). In general, the greater the wind velocity or the larger the object, the greater the turbulence.

The flow of air (or any fluid) around an object is laminar at low velocities and turbulent at high velocities. Laminar flow over a flat plate is illustrated in Figure 6-1A. The air moves in straight-line layers along the stream lines from left to right, and no air is exchanged between layers. Laminar flow is also observed along curved surfaces, as shown in Figure 6-1B, in which the flow follows along the shape of the surface. The surface in this illustration is an airplane wing (airfoil), but it could just as easily be the curved surface of the head. In a real fluid, friction between the fluid and the surface slows down the fluid close to the surface as shown in Figure 6-1C, and the closer the air is to the surface the slower it moves. The flow is still laminar, however.

As the fluid velocity increases, it finally exceeds a threshold and the flow becomes turbulent as illustrated in Figure 6-1D. The average velocity of the turbulent flow is given by the wind velocity, but the presence of the eddies causes mixing of the air between layers and destroys the laminar flow. In laminar flow all of the particles within a layer have the same velocity, but in turbulent flow there is a large random component superimposed on the average velocity. The transition from laminar to turbulent flow is illustrated in Figure 6-1E for smoke rising

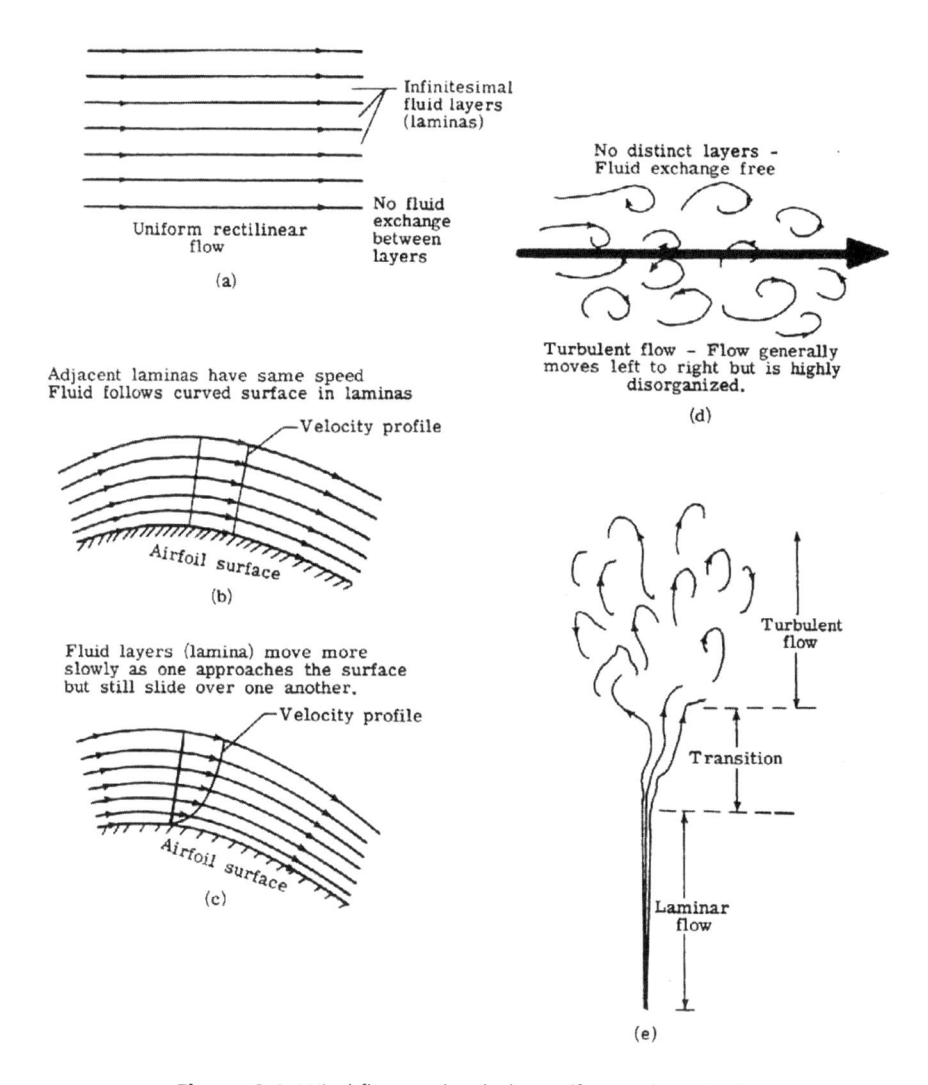

Figure 6-1. Wind flow and turbulence (from Talay, 1975).

from a candle. The smoke initially rises in smooth filaments that result from laminar flow. Sufficiently far from the candle the smoke breaks up into a confusion of eddies that indicate turbulent flow.

Hearing-Aid Measurements

Dillon et al. (1999) undertook a comprehensive set of wind noise measurements, and this section is based on their report. Many of their illustrations and graphs are reproduced in the paper of Thompson and Dillon (2001), which can be accessed on-line. The data presented here were taken in a test chamber at a wind speed of 5 m/sec (18 km/hour, 11 miles/hour). A theoretical analysis shows that the sound pressure level due to the wind is proportional to the square of the wind speed (Strasberg, 1988), so a doubling of the wind speed would be expected to increase the turbulence by a factor of 4 and the resultant wind noise by 12 dB on average. Other factors, including the differences between airflow in a test chamber and flow outdoors, complicate this picture (Morgan & Raspet, 1992), leading to observed increases in outdoor wind noise level that grow somewhat faster with increasing wind velocity.

AIRFLOW AND TURBULENCE

Airflow around the head is illustrated in Figure 6-2 for the KEMAR manikin in a test chamber. The airflow is made visible using a stream of smoke. The flow is laminar as it approaches the head, and the laminar flow is maintained as it intercepts and starts to flow around the head. After the flow passes the head or ear, it becomes turbulent as indicated by a smoke path that has been broadened by the eddies.

The turbulence in the airflow for a completely-in-the-canal (CIC) hearing aid is illustrated in Figure 6-3. The wind originates from 0 degrees (directly in front of the manikin). The x-axis in the figure runs parallel to the side of the head, the z-axis is vertical, and the y-axis extends outward perpendicularly from the side of the head. The turbulence is the root-mean-squared (RMS) sum of the variance in the airflow along the three axes. The CIC hearing aid completely blocks the opening to the ear canal. The greatest amount of turbulence occurs at and immediately behind the upper edge of the pinna, and there is also some turbulence within the concha. The level of turbulence is generally highest following the trailing edge of an obstacle, and the pinna in this case is an obstacle sticking out from the side of the head. The concha diverts some of the airflow downward, which then mixes with the flow coming from in front of the manikin to create strong local eddies.

The turbulence for an in-the-ear (ITE) hearing aid is illustrated in Figure 6-4. The ITE hearing completely fills the concha and presents a

Wind Noise 151

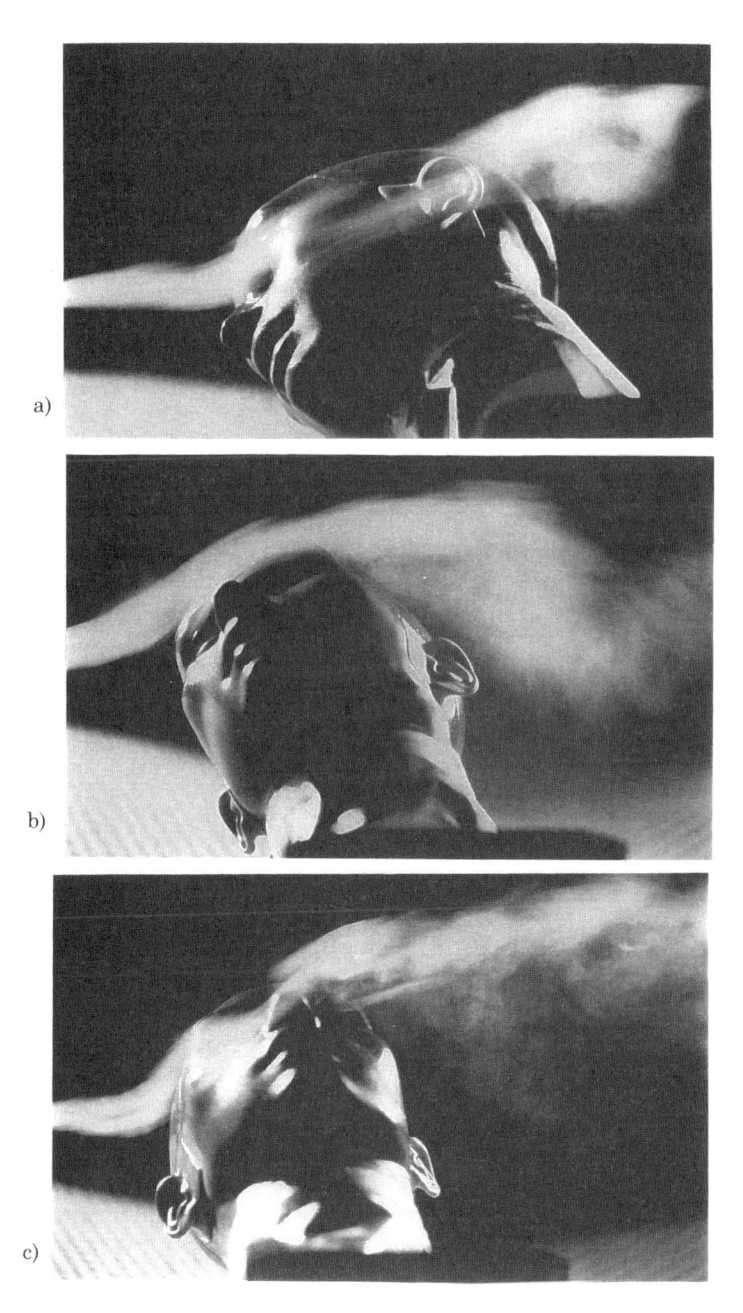

Figure 6-2. Wind flow around the KEMAR manikin made visible using a stream of smoke: **A.** head at 0 degrees, **B.** head at −50 degrees, and **C.** head at −90 degrees. The flow was initially laminar at 5 m/sec (from Dillon et al., 1999).

152 Digital Hearing Aids

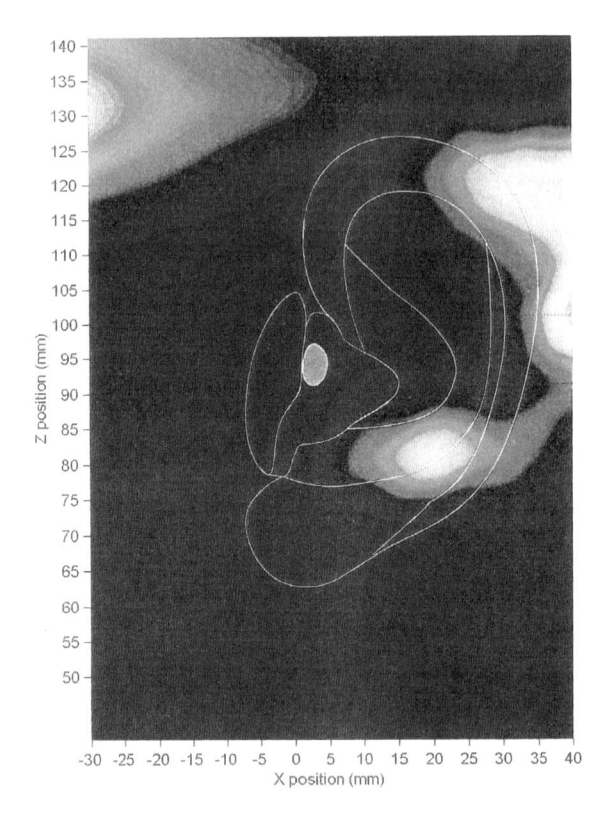

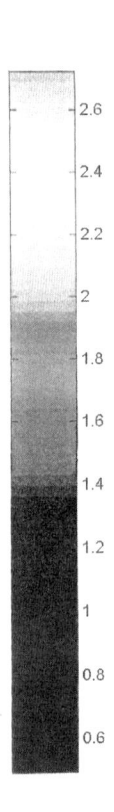

Figure 6-3. Total turbulence velocity around the ear for a CIC hearing aid (from Dillon et al., 1999).

smoother surface to the airflow than the CIC hearing aid. As a result, the eddies within the concha are eliminated, although there is a small amount of turbulence behind the tragus. The turbulence behind the pinna is somewhat greater than observed for the CIC hearing aid.

The turbulence for a behind-the-ear (BTE) hearing aid is illustrated in Figure 6-5. The BTE hearing aid includes the instrument placed behind the pinna as well as the ear hook and tubing that direct the sound into the ear canal. The BTE shows a large amount of turbulence within the upper portion of the pinna and also behind the pinna. The turbulence within the pinna is not seen for the CIC or ITE hearing aids, and is probably due to the ear hook and tubing presenting an obstacle as the airflow approaches the ear. The BTE placement behind the ear also

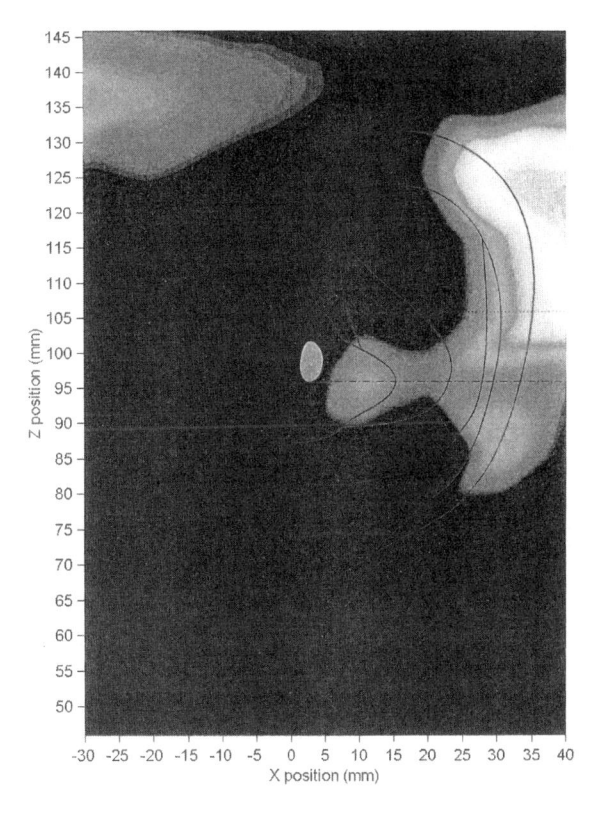

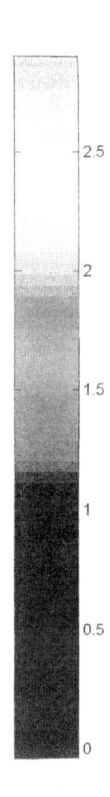

Figure 6-4. Total turbulence velocity around the ear for an ITE hearing aid (from Dillon et al., 1999).

bends the pinna away from the head by a small amount, which may increase the turbulence within as well as behind the pinna. An additional observation is that the microphone in a BTE case, especially the rear microphone in a hearing aid using two microphones, is in a region of greater turbulence than the microphones in CIC or ITE hearing aids.

The turbulence surrounding the ear dissipates rapidly as one moves away from the head. The turbulence for a BTE hearing aid is plotted in Figure 6-6 along the y-axis (perpendicular to the head). BTE location A is above the pinna and approximately 1 cm to the rear of a line projected upward from the tragus. The origin of the y-axis is at the opening to the ear canal and 4 mm from the side of the dummy head. It was not possible to make measurements directly at the surface of the head. The

154 Digital Hearing Aids

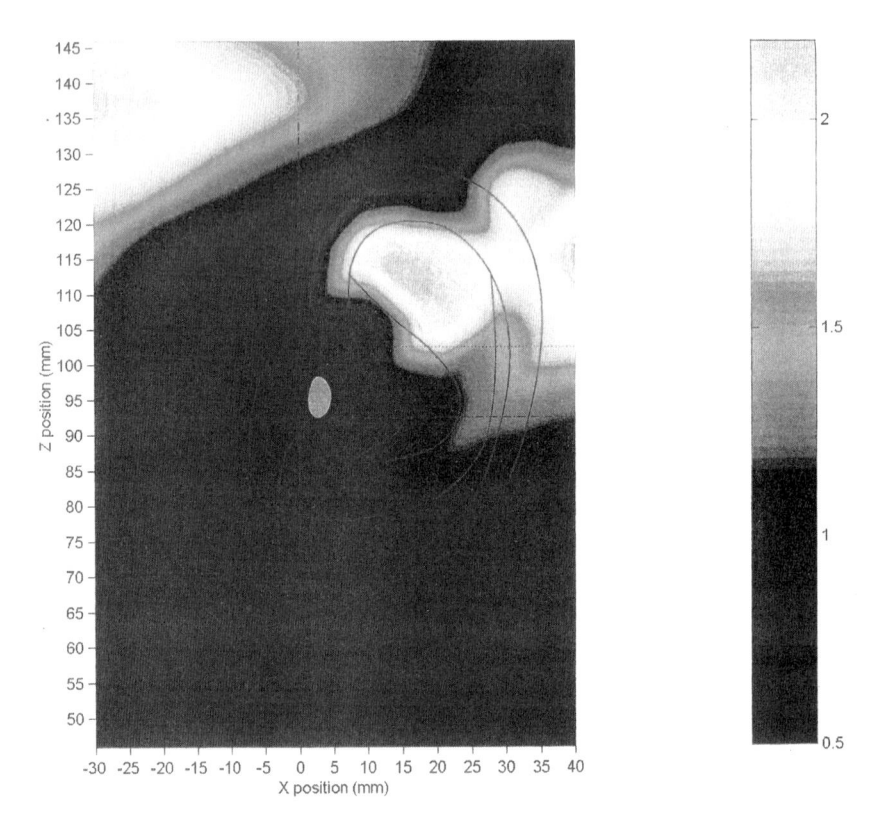

Figure 6-5. Total turbulence velocity around the ear for a BTE hearing aid (from Dillon et al., 1999).

plotted data indicate a maximum in the turbulence at around 7 mm from the head surface, after which it decreases rapidly with increasing distance from the head. Close to the head there is more turbulence when the BTE is present with its earmold, whereas farther from the head there is somewhat greater turbulence when the earmold is absent (BTE still present) and the ear canal is plugged with a CIC instrument. The asymptotes of the curves most likely represent the residual turbulence within the test chamber.

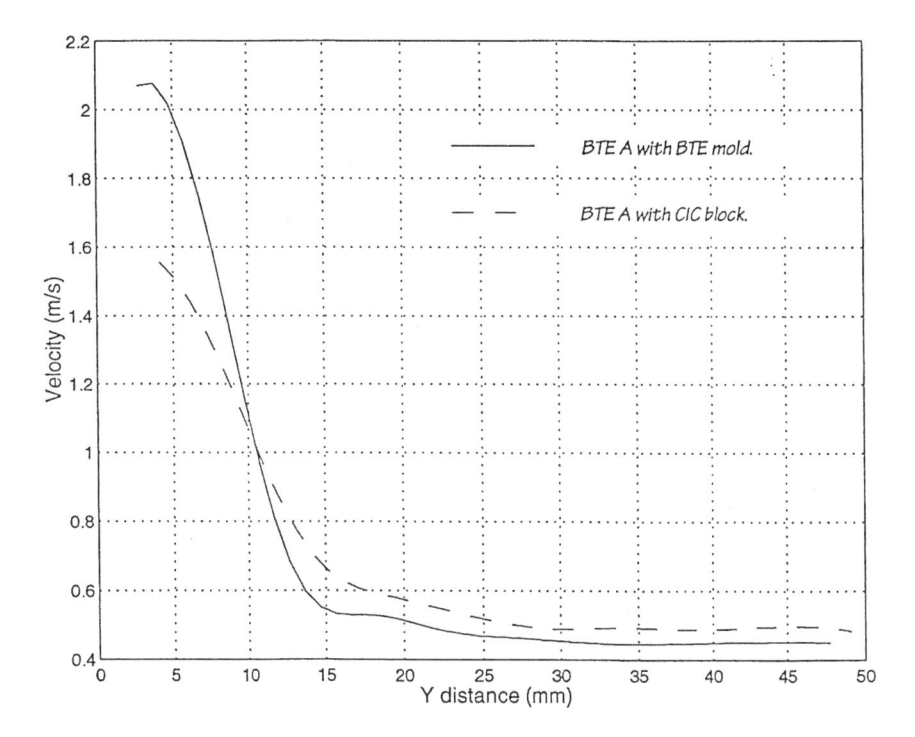

Figure 6-6. Turbulence velocity as a function of the distance perpendicular to the head for a BTE hearing aid with (*solid line*) and without (*dashed line*) the earmold in place (from Dillon et al., 1999).

SOUND PRESSURE

Dillon et al. (1999) also made sound pressure measurements using the same test conditions as were used for the turbulence velocity measurements. The airflow was 5 m/sec (18 km/hour, 11 miles/hour), and the sound pressure was measured using either a hearing-aid microphone or a probe microphone. Measurement were made at various positions corresponding to the microphone inlet ports for CIC, in-the-canal (ITC), ITE, and BTE devices.

Figure 6-7 presents the wind noise measured at BTE position A as the azimuth of the wind moves over a range of 180 degrees An angle of 90 degrees is on the same side of the head as the hearing aid, 0 degrees is directly in front of the manikin, and −90 degrees is on the opposite side

156 Digital Hearing Aids

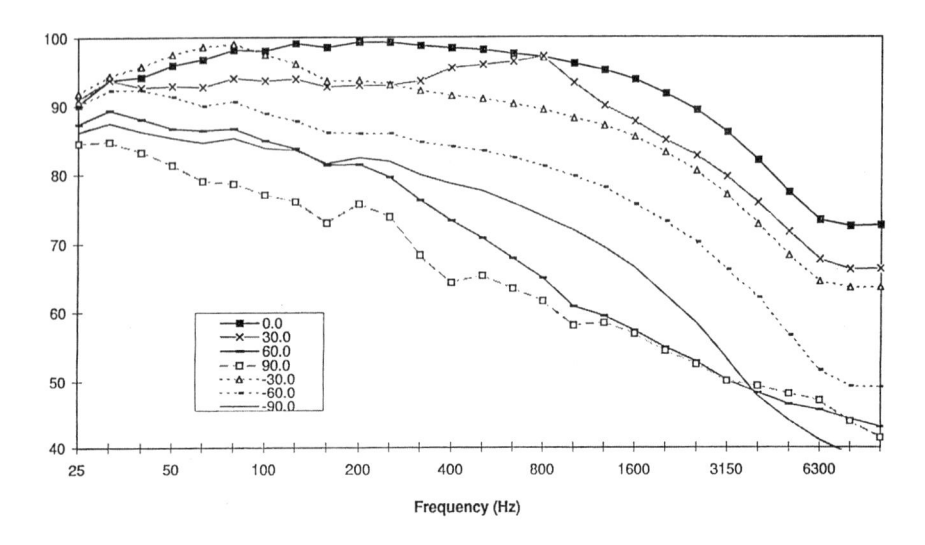

Figure 6-7. Wind noise levels in dB SPL for a BTE hearing aid for different wind directions. A direction of 0 degrees indicates that KEMAR is facing into the wind (from Dillon et al., 1999).

of the head from the ear holding the hearing aid. For wind originating at 0 degrees, the sound spectrum is relatively flat up to about 300 Hz, after which it gradually rolls off. The maximum sound pressure level is nearly 100 dB in the third-octave band centered at 160 Hz, so the total sound pressure level summed across frequency due to the wind at 0 degrees would be in excess of 110 dB SPL. Shifts in the wind direction of 30 degrees to either side reduce the overall sound pressure level by a small amount, but both the 30 and −30-degrees curves have frequency regions where the sound pressure is as high as for 0 degrees.

Shifting the wind direction farther toward the hearing-aid side of the head gives the curves for 60 and 90 degrees, which show a 15- to 20-dB overall reduction in the intensity of the wind noise. Shifting the wind direction farther away from the hearing-aid side of the head gives the curves for −60 and −90 degrees. The wind noise for shifts away from the aided ear is also reduced relative to the level for 0 degrees, but the amount of reduction is not as much as when the hearing aid is facing directly into the wind. One can argue that for a wind direction of 90 degrees, the air flow is still laminar as it moves over the ear, but for −90

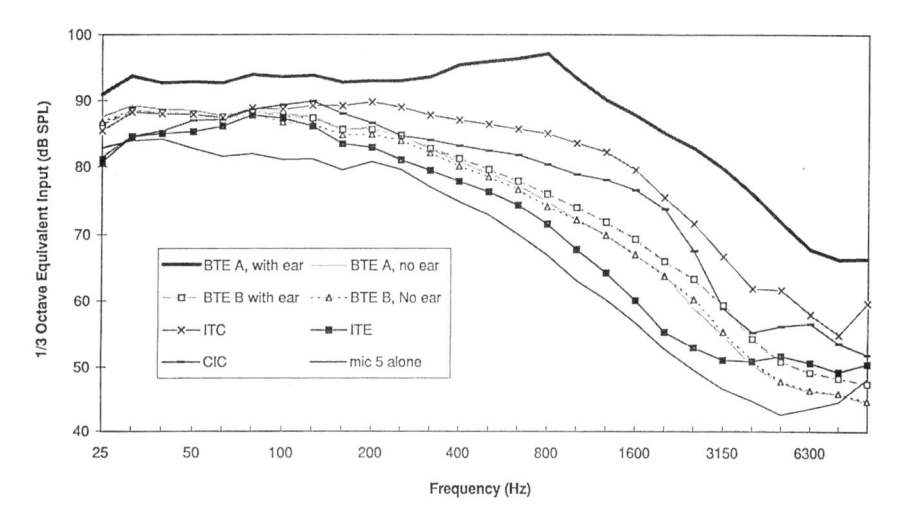

Figure 6-8. Wind noise levels in dB SPL for different hearing aids for the wind coming from an azimuth of 30 degrees (from Dillon et al., 1999).

degrees the hearing aid is in a region of eddies that detach from the flow as with wind moves past the head as shown in Figure 6-2C. The strongest turbulence at the hearing-aid position, however, appears to occur for the wind coming from 0 degrees, which causes strong eddies behind the edge of the pinna, as shown in Figures 6-2A and 6-5.

The wind noise measured for several different hearing aids is plotted in Figure 6-8 for the wind coming from 30 degrees. BTE position B is tucked above the pinna at a spot directly above the tragus, whereas BTE position A is 1 cm to the rear of a line projected upward from the tragus. The BTE sound pressure was measured with the manikin's ear in place, and then repeated with the ear removed from the KEMAR manikin. The greatest amount of wind noise is generated for the BTE in location A, which is consistent with the turbulence plotted in Figure 6-5. Moving the BTE forward by 1 cm to location B greatly reduces the amount of wind noise. Removing the manikin's ear shows that most of the wind noise for the BTE hearing aids is due to the eddies formed as the wind passes over the pinna; removing the pinna removes these eddies and leaves only the noise caused by the wind passing around the head and over the hearing aid case. The ITC and CIC hearing aids have more wind noise than the BTE in position B, and the high amount of wind noise is most likely due to the eddies formed within the concha as shown in Figure 6-3. The ITE, which completely fills the concha, presents the smoothest surface and thus has the fewest eddies in the vicinity of the microphone and the lowest wind noise.

Signal Characteristics

Signal processing to reduce wind noise requires that there be observable differences between the wind noise signal and a signal from a desired source of sound. Wind noise has several characteristics that can potentially be used to distinguish it from other sound sources. Three characteristics, the power spectrum, temporal fluctuations, and spatial correlation, are reviewed in this section.

SPECTRUM

The wind noise spectrum is concentrated at low frequencies (Dillon et al., 1999; Raspet et al., 2006; Wuttke, 1991). The measurements of Wuttke (1991) for a commercial recording microphone show a spectrum that is relatively flat below 100 Hz and with an approximately −12 dB/octave slope above 100 Hz. The measurements of Dillon et al. (1999) for various hearing aids show a wide variation in the wind-noise spectra, but the general behavior is a one-third-octave spectrum that is relatively flat below 300 Hz and inversely proportional to frequency (−6 dB/octave slope) above 300 Hz.

The spectrum of the wind noise also depends on the wind speed. Larsson and Olsson (2004) made recordings of wind noise under a large number of wind conditions using a ReSound Canta 7 BTE attached to a DAT recorder. The sampling rate was 48 kHz with 16-bit quantization. The recordings were made outdoors as they walked around the city of Lund, Sweden. The separate front and rear microphone signals were recorded simultaneously. Average power spectra for the front microphone for classifications of no wind, low wind speed (audible but not annoying), medium wind speed (troublesome), and high wind speed (uncomfortable or painful) are shown in Figure 6-9. Each curve is the average of 10 data files (approximately 3 minutes of data) for each wind-speed classification, and each curve is plotted in dB relative to its maximum intensity. The frequency resolution in Figure 6-9 is 16.25 Hz.

The wind speed spectrum for no wind is limited at high frequencies

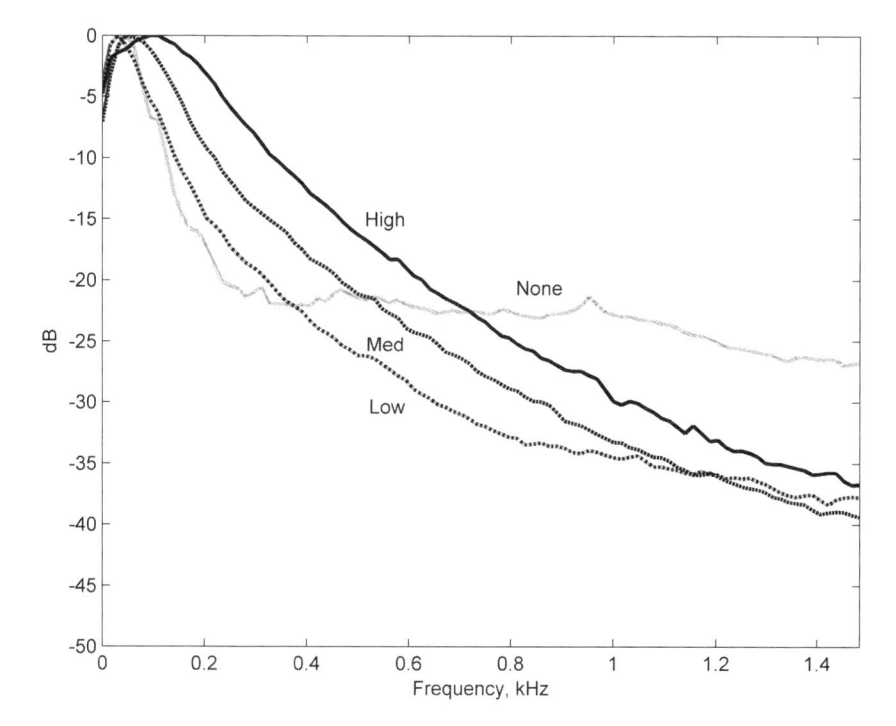

Figure 6-9. Average front-microphone power spectra for different intensities of wind noise from the data of Larsson and Olsson (2004). High intensity is indicated by the solid black line, medium by the dashed line, low by the dot-dash line, and no wind by the dotted line. Ten sound files from recordings made in the city of Lund were averaged for each condition. The average spectra were normalized so that each curve has a peak value of 0 dB.

by the noise floor of the hearing aid and recording apparatus, but some wind noise is apparent even for the no-wind condition where it could not readily be perceived. The low wind speed spectrum has a peak at about 32 Hz, and the peak frequency increases to about 100 Hz as the wind speed increases to high. All three curves for the wind present have a high-frequency slope of about −9 dB/octave. The curves of Figure 6-9 show the peak of the spectrum occurring at a lower frequency than in the data from Dillon et al. (1999) plotted in Figure 6-7. The difference between the two sets of spectra may be due to the Dillon et al. (1999) data being acquired in a test chamber whereas the Larsson and Olsson (2004) data were acquired outdoors where greater fluctuations in the wind velocity would be expected.

TEMPORAL FLUCTUATIONS

The temporal fluctuations of the signal envelope can also be used to separate one type of signal from another if their modulation spectra are sufficiently different. Envelope fluctuations were investigated for speech and wind noise. The spectral analysis used a block size of 24 samples (1.5 msec) at a sampling rate of 16 kHz, with 17 auditory frequency bands realized using digital frequency warping followed by an FFT (Kates & Arehart, 2005). The envelope of each frequency band was computed by sampling the magnitude of the band once per block. The modulation spectrum was then computed from the envelope in each band after the DC component was removed.

The spectra of the envelope fluctuations are plotted in Figure 6-10 for a section of the "Rainbow Passage" spoken by a male talker and in Figure 6-11 for a segment of wind noise having a medium wind speed as characterized by Larsson and Olsson (2004). Both the speech and wind noise modulation spectra are concentrated at frequencies below 5 Hz. The speech has less power at frequencies above 5 Hz than the wind noise, but that would be expected to vary with talker and speech material. Thus, it does not appear that envelope modulation is an effective property for separating speech from wind noise.

CORRELATION

The spatial correlation of the wind noise decreases rapidly with distance (Corcos, 1963, 1964). The wind noise at the two ports of a directional microphone, or at two or more omnidirectional microphones combined to create a directional array, will be uncorrelated despite the microphones being located close to each other. This signal correlation can be used as a test for wind noise. If the signals from the two microphones are correlated, the interference is probably coming from an external source of sound. But if the signals are uncorrelated the interference is most likely wind noise.

Let the signal from the front microphone be given by $x(n)$, and the signal from the rear microphone be given by $y(n)$. The cross-correlation function of the two signals is then, from Eq. (2.12):

$$R_{xy}(j) = \sum_n x(n)y(n+j) \quad \text{Equation (6.1)}$$

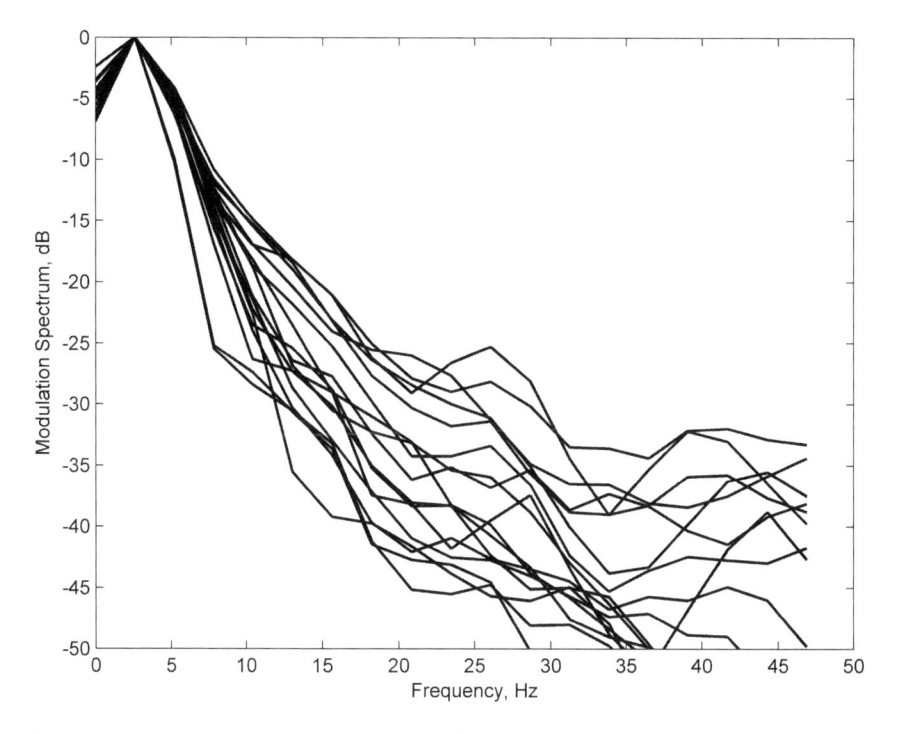

Figure 6-10. Modulation spectra in 17 auditory frequency bands for speech. The stimulus is a segment of the "Rainbow Passage" spoken by a male talker.

For a wave arriving from an external sound source, $x(n)$ and $y(n)$ will differ only by a small time delay. The two signals will therefore be very similar, and the cross-correlation given by Eq. (6.1) will be large for the value of j that corresponds to the delay. In a hearing aid, the value of j will be less than one sample at the sampling rates and microphone separations typically used. Thus, replacing j by 0 leads to only a very small error at the low frequencies where wind noise has its greatest intensity.

For wind noise, the signals $x(n)$ and $y(n)$ have independent fluctuations and the sum of their product will tend toward zero. One can thus form a wind-noise detection statistic:

$$\Gamma = \frac{\sum_n x(n)y(n)}{\sum_n x^2(n)} \qquad \text{Equation (6.2)}$$

162 Digital Hearing Aids

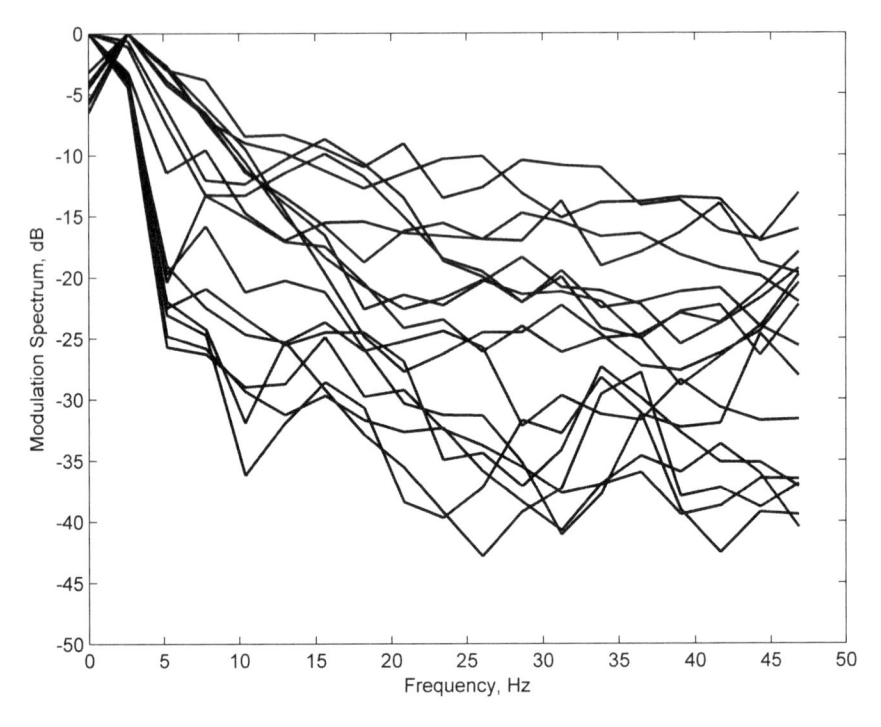

Figure 6-11. Modulation spectra in 17 auditory frequency bands for wind noise. The stimulus is a segment of wind noise having a medium wind speed.

The quantity Γ will approach 1 for sound from an external source, and will tend toward 0 for wind noise.

A statistic related to Eq. (6.2) is to use the difference between the front and rear microphone signals instead of their correlation (Elko, 2003; Petersen et al., 2004). If $x(n)$ and $y(n)$ are similar, as would occur for an external sound source, then their difference will tend toward zero. If $x(n)$ and $y(n)$ are predominantly wind noise, their difference or sum will form a new random variable with twice the power of either signal alone. The difference/sum noise-detection statistic (Elko, 2003) is then:

$$\Delta = \frac{\sum_n |x(n) - y(n)|^2}{\sum_n |x(n) + y(n)|^2} \qquad \text{Equation (6.3)}$$

The quantity Δ will approach 0 for sound from an external source, and will tend toward 1 for wind noise.

Wind-Noise Reduction

The techniques available for reducing wind noise can be divided into two general categories: acoustic and algorithmic. Acoustic wind noise reduction involves modifying the microphone environment to reduce the amount of turbulence at the microphone. An acoustic solution, such as a wind screen, can reduce the wind noise with little effect on the response to the desired signal. In many situations a wind screen is not practical due to size or cosmetic concerns (in other words, a wind screen tends to be big and ugly), in which case the preferred solution is an algorithm that will reduce the sound intensity at those frequencies that are dominated by wind noise or which will switch from directional to omnidirectional microphone mode in a two-microphone array. Many patent applications have been filed on algorithms for wind-noise suppression, and some recent applications are cited in this section.

DIRECTIONAL MICROPHONES

A consequence of the lack of spatial correlation of the wind noise is that the wind noise power for a directional microphone, assuming an equalized low-frequency response, will always be greater than for an omnidirectional microphone. A directional microphone works by subtracting the signal at the rear microphone or port from the signal at the front. The desired signal is correlated at the two locations and the subtraction partially cancels the low frequencies of the desired signal, giving a frequency-response slope of 6 dB/octave The low frequencies are usually restored by providing a low-frequency boost to the directional microphone output.

However, the wind noise at the two microphone locations is uncorrelated and is increased by combining the two signals. Combining uncorrelated signals always increases the signal power independent of the relative phase of the signals; adding the signals or subtracting the signals will both increase the total power of the uncorrelated components. Equalization to give a flat low-frequency response in a directional microphone restores the low frequencies of the desired signal, but it amplifies the uncorrelated wind noise. The resultant increase in wind noise power can become uncomfortably loud. Switching to omnidirectional mode in the wind removes the equalization and can greatly reduce the annoyance from the wind noise.

WIND SCREENS

Wind screens reduce wind noise by reducing the turbulence at the sensing surface of the microphone. A wind screen is thus an acoustic rather than a signal-processing solution to the problem of wind noise, and is the only solution that will prevent overloading the microphone preamplifier or the analog-to-digital (A/D) converter at high wind velocities. Wind screens for recording microphones are typically baskets of metal mesh or open-cell foam (Wuttke, 1991). For a pressure (omnidirectional) microphone, a wind screen made of open-cell foam can be effective. The foam attenuates the wind fluctuations around the microphone and can reduce the A-weighted wind noise by approximately 40 dB, although the cell spacing and porosity of a foam windscreen often causes a small roll-off in the microphone frequency response above 10 kHz.

A metal basket works best with a pressure-gradient (directional) type of microphone. The basket encloses a small volume of air, and the pressure becomes uniform within the enclosed space as long as the dimensions of the space are small compared with the wavelength of sound. If both ports of the directional microphone are within the basket, then the instantaneous pressure at the two microphone ports will be the same at low frequencies. Thus, the pressure at the two ports is equalized, the diaphragm displacement eliminated, and the wind noise is reduced. However, equalizing the pressure can also reduce the low-frequency response of the microphone and will compromise the low-frequency directivity. At high frequencies, the dimensions of the volume are comparable to the acoustic wavelengths, and standing waves within the basket can adversely affect the microphone frequency response and directivity.

A foam windscreen is somewhat less effective for a directional microphone. It can reduce the wind noise by about 30 dB for a cardioid microphone, whereas a mesh basket windscreen can reduce the wind noise by about 40 dB for the same sensor (Wuttke, 1991). However, although the foam windscreen is not as effective in reducing wind noise, it also has a much smaller effect in reducing the microphone directivity index at low frequencies. For example, the front-to-back ratio of a Schoeps MK 4 cardioid microphone is about 15 dB at 100 Hz. A foam windscreen reduces the front-to-back ratio to about 10 dB, whereas a basket-type windscreen reduces the front-to-back ratio to about 0 dB.

SPECTRUM ALGORITHMS

One of the characteristics of wind noise, as shown above, is that the spectrum is concentrated at low frequencies. In a hearing aid using a single microphone the spatial correlation is not available as a test for wind noise, so the spectral shape or the low-frequency sound intensity are the most useful available indicators. One approach (Kates, 2007) is illustrated in Figure 6-12. The shape of the long-term spectrum is monitored, and the fraction of the total signal power that is found at low frequencies is used to indicate the presence of wind noise. If this fraction exceeds a preset threshold, the low-frequency gain of the hearing aid is reduced.

This approach to wind-noise suppression can be very useful in a BTE using a directional microphone and designed for an open fitting. This type of hearing aid, because of the open fitting, provides very little amplification in the ear canal for frequencies below 800 Hz. However, the equalization used to compensate for the 6 dB/octave slope of the microphone response provides a large amount of low-frequency boost. The low frequencies provide little benefit for speech intelligibility due to the open fitting, but the instrument can still have a large amount of wind noise when used outdoors. The low-frequency attenuation provided by the algorithm of Figure 6-12 will greatly reduce the intensity of the wind noise, but will have only a minimal effect on speech intelligibility as most of the speech low frequencies enter the ear canal directly and are not affected by the reduction in the hearing aid amplification.

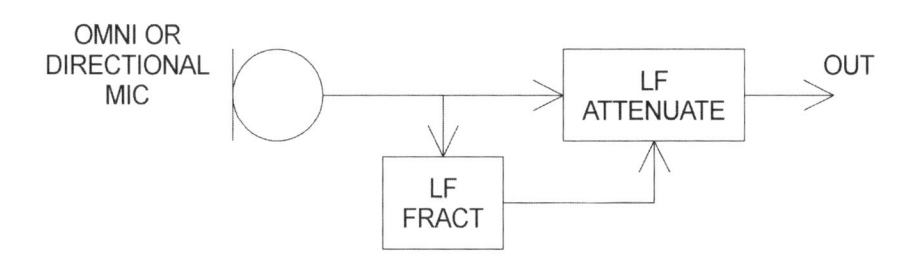

Figure 6-12. Block diagram of a single-microphone wind noise suppression system.

Another spectral-based approach, proposed by Luo (2005), exploits the fact that wind noise tends to be much more intense than speech at low frequencies. The wind-noise detector in this patent application uses a set of frequency bands. A low-frequency band is selected as the "master" band, and the signal level in this band is compared to an absolute threshold. The signal levels in the other frequency bands are also compared to absolute thresholds in each respective band. The signal level in each band is then attenuated based on the fraction of the time the master band is above its threshold combined with the fraction of the time the signal in the given frequency band is above threshold. The wind-noise detector can also extended to a two-microphone array and used to switch the hearing-aid microphone between omnidirectional and directional modes.

CORRELATION ALGORITHMS

The amount of correlation between the front and rear microphone signals forms a reliable wind-noise detection statistic. Petersen et al. (2004), for example, propose low-pass filtering of front and rear microphone signals to emphasize the low frequencies where wind noise is the strongest. They then form the cross-correlation statistic Γ given by *Eq. (6.2)*. Dickel and Knapp (2002) prefer to use the absolute value of the difference between the front and rear microphone signals, and compare the difference against an absolute threshold to detect wind noise. This latter approach combines into a single statistic the high sound pressure levels induced by the wind and the loss of correlation between the front and rear microphone signals.

Figure 6-13 shows a wind noise reduction system that combines the correlation detection of Petersen *et al.* (2004) with the microphone mode switching proposed by Dickel and Knapp (2002). If the normalized cross-correlation Γ given by *Eq. (6.2)* is high, the hearing aid connects the rear microphone and operates in the directional microphone mode. If Γ approaches 0, the wind-noise detector indicates that wind noise is present and the rear microphone is disconnected, thus switching the hearing aid into an omnidirectional mode that uses just the front microphone.

The correlation detection for wind noise can also be performed in the frequency domain. An example of such a system (Elko, 2003) is shown in Figure 6-14, which implements a frequency-domain version of the correlation-based wind-noise detection given by *Eq. (6.2)*. The

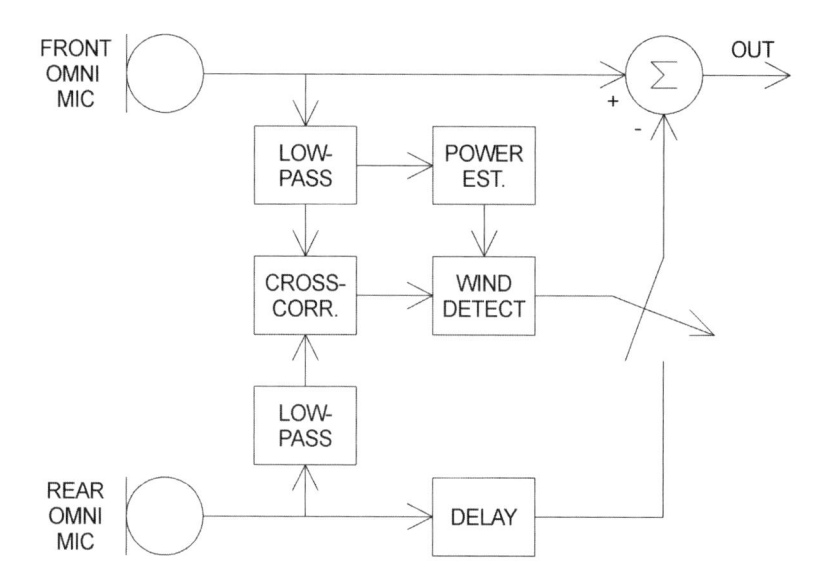

Figure 6-13. Block diagram of a two-microphone wind noise suppression system in which the microphone cross-correlation controls a switch between directional and omnidirectional operation.

signals from the front and rear microphones are divided into overlapping blocks, and each block is transformed into the frequency domain using the FFT. A directional microphone response is implemented in the frequency domain in this example by taking the difference between the FFT of the front microphone signal and the FFT of a delayed version of the rear microphone signal. The cross-correlation is then performed in the frequency domain by averaging the product of the front- and rear-microphone FFTs in each FFT frequency bin. The normalization is provided by averaging the power in each frequency bin for the front-microphone signal and dividing the front-rear cross-correlation in that bin by the front-microphone power. If the normalized cross-correlation is high in a given frequency bin, the gain for that bin is set close to 1. If the normalized cross-correlation is low in a given frequency bin, the gain for that bin is set close to 0. The gains are then applied to the spectrum of the directional microphone response. The filtered spectrum is transformed into the time domain via an inverse FFT, and the signal blocks combined using the overlap-add procedure.

168 Digital Hearing Aids

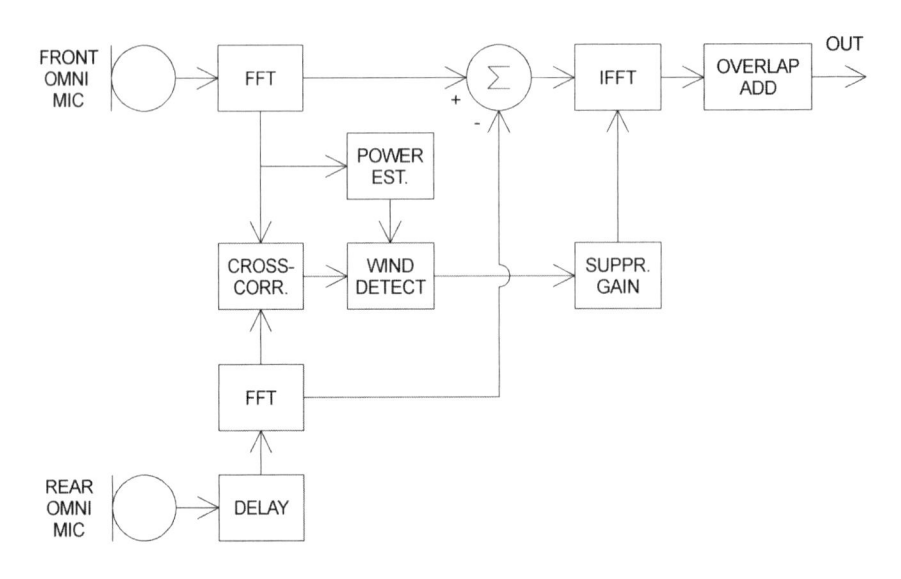

Figure 6-14. /Block diagram of a two-microphone wind noise suppression system implemented in the frequency domain and using the cross-correlation between the front and rear microphones to adjust the suppression gain.

A frequency-domain version (Elko, 2003) of the difference/sum wind-noise detection system of Eq. (6.3) is presented in Figure 6-15. The operation is similar to that shown in Figure 6-14. The numerator of the detection statistic in each FFT bin is formed from the difference of the FFTs of the front and rear microphone signals, and the denominator is formed from their sum. If the difference/sum ratio is low the signal in that FFT bin is assumed to be from an external source, and the gain is set high. If the difference/sum ratio is high, the signal in the FFT bin is assumed to be wind noise and the gain is set low.

A comparison of the wind-noise detection behavior for the frequency-domain correlation and difference/sum approaches is plotted in Figure 6-16. The test signal is a segment of continuous discourse spoken by a male talker and presented in wind noise at a 0-dB SNR. The value of the normalized cross-correlation is very low for the first three frequency bands, which span 0 to 270 Hz and where the wind noise is more intense than the speech. The normalized cross-correlation then climbs rapidly, approaching 1 at about 420 Hz, and remains close to 1 throughout the frequency region where the speech is more intense than

Wind Noise 169

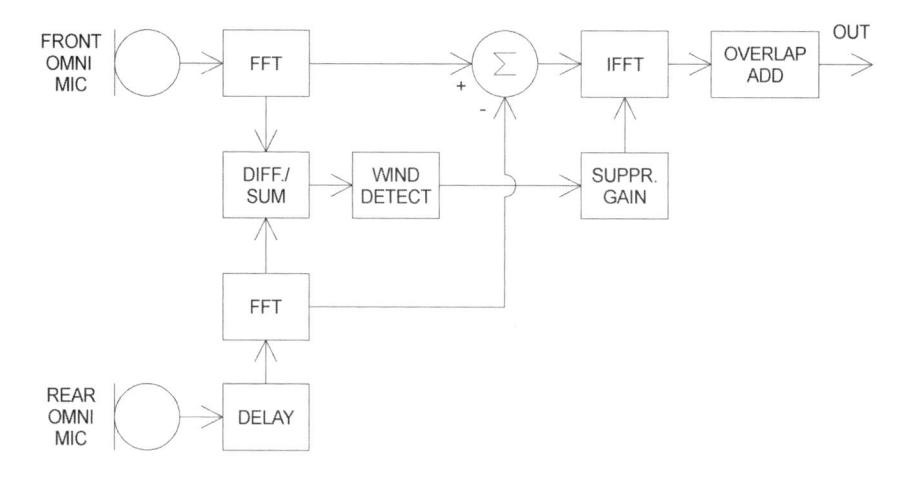

Figure 6-15. Block diagram of a two-microphone wind noise suppression system in which the cross-correlation is replaced by taking the difference between the signals at the two microphones.

the wind noise. At frequencies above 3.7 kHz the normalized cross-correlation falls off due to the reduction in power in the speech signal at high frequencies. The difference/sum starts out at a relatively high value for the first two frequency bands (0 and 135 Hz), and then drops rapidly toward 0 as the speech signal power exceeds that of the wind noise. The difference/sum value then starts to climb slowly with increasing frequency, as opposed to the normalized cross-correlation which remains at a relatively constant value. The problems associated with wind noise are most severe below 1 kHz, however, and in this low-frequency region both wind-noise detection approaches appear to be accurate.

ADAPTIVE ARRAYS

Depending on the array design, the processing in an adaptive array can also offer some reduction of wind noise. Arrays that configure the microphones into directional response patterns before processing, such as the ones shown in Figures 5-2 through 5-4, will have a problem with wind noise. The adaptive processing in these arrays steers a null toward the assumed external source of interference, but the array frequency response always has a rising 6-dB/octave slope and the response equalization will always amplify the wind noise at low frequencies.

170 Digital Hearing Aids

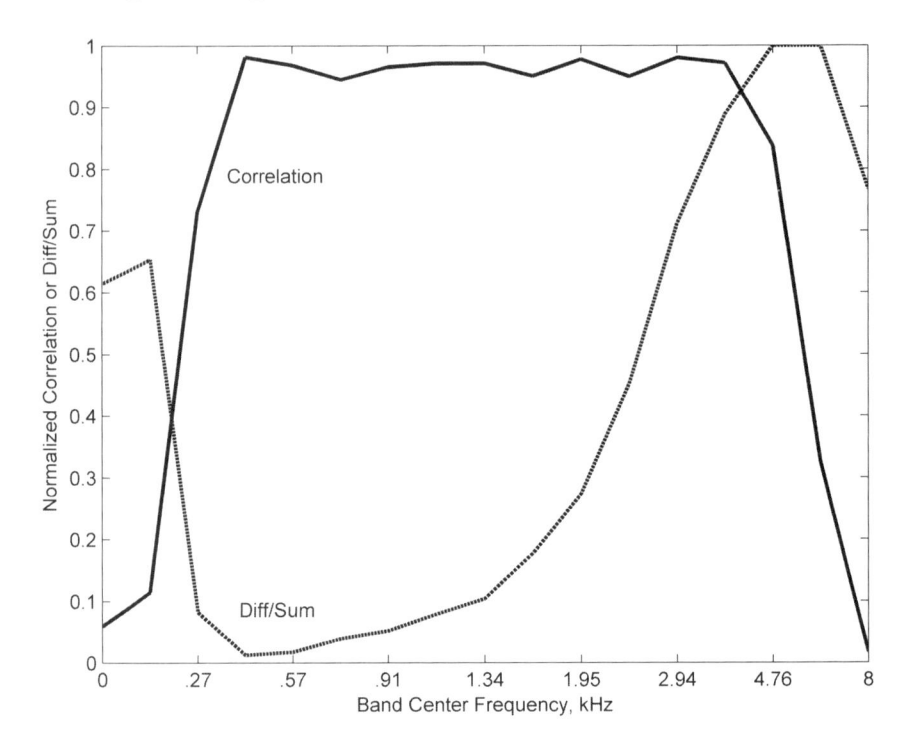

Figure 6-16. The normalized cross-correlation wind-noise detection statistic given by Eq. (6.2) and the difference/sum statistic given by *Eq. (6.3)* plotted as a function of frequency for a 17-band auditory frequency analysis system. The stimulus is a portion of the "Rainbow Passage" spoken by a male talker in wind noise at a 0-dB SNR.

A more general array design that combines the outputs from multiple omnidirectional microphones, as shown in Figure 5-13, has a response behavior that also adapts to the source of the interference and which can adapt to wind noise. If the interference is due to an external source of sound, the array will adapt to steer a null in the direction of the source. However, if the interference is dominated by wind noise, the array will adapt to minimize the wind noise instead of creating and steering a null.

The wind noise is uncorrelated from one microphone to the next, which is the same mathematically as the interference being a more intense version the random noise produced by each microphone. For this situation, the adaptive processing will adjust the array to reduce the internal rather than the external noise. The internal noise, and hence the wind noise, is minimized by averaging the signals across the microphones in the array, which results in the array processing converging to delay-and-sum beam forming. The change from directional nulls for external sources of interference to delay-and-sum beam forming for wind noise is equivalent to switching from a directional microphone with an equalized low-frequency response to an omnidirectional microphone with a flat-frequency response. The wind noise is reduced by a comparable amount.

Furthermore, for delay-and-sum beam forming the wind noise components at each microphone sum in random phase whereas the desired signal components sum in phase. The result is an additional reduction in the wind noise power of 3 dB relative to the desired signal power for each doubling of the number of microphones in the array.

Concluding Remarks

Wind noise is caused by turbulent airflow past the microphone ports of a hearing aid. The turbulence is produced by the head and by the pinna, concha, and tragus of the ear. Wind noise levels up to 110 dB SPL have been measured for a BTE in wind at 5 m/sec. The amount of wind noise depends on the square of the wind velocity, so velocities greater than the 5 m/sec will result in greatly increased amounts of wind noise. The amount of wind noise also depends on the type of hearing aid, with BTE hearing aids generally having highest wind noise and ITE hearing aids having the lowest. Finally, the amount of wind noise depends on the orientation of the hearing aid with respect to the wind direction, with the greatest amount of wind noise for the user facing directly into the wind and the lowest amount for the user at 90 degrees to the wind.

Wind noise can be reduced using acoustic means and through signal processing. A wind screen smoothes the airflow over the hearing aid, and wind screens can be very effective in reducing wind noise. However, wind screens for hearing aids face problems due to the size and appearance of the screen, and a wind screen can interfere with the frequency response and directional characteristics of a directional microphone.

Signal processing to reduce wind noise needs to be able to detect wind noise in the presence of other acoustic signals. The important signal characteristics of wind noise are that it is concentrated at low frequencies and that the wind noise is uncorrelated when the signals at different microphone locations are compared. Both the frequency and correlation properties of wind noise have been used to design effective detection strategies. The wind noise intensity can be reduced, once it is detected, by reducing the low-frequency gain of the hearing aid.

A directional microphone has an inherent 6-dB/octave frequency-response slope, and a directional microphone requires a low-frequency boost to restore a flat-frequency response. This low-frequency boost also amplifies the wind noise, so directional microphones have much more severe wind noise problems than omnidirectional microphones. One solution, in a hearing aid that uses two microphones to provide directional behavior, is to select the directional mode when the wind noise is low and to switch to omnidirectional mode when high levels of wind noise are detected. The adaptive processing in some microphone arrays essentially provides this kind of switching behavior by smoothly changing from adaptive directional nulls when an external source of interference is dominant to summing the microphone outputs when wind noise is dominant.

References

Corcos, G. M. (1963). Resolution of pressure in turbulence. *Journal of the Acoustical Society of America, 35*, 192–199.

Corcos, G. M. (1964). The structure of the turbulent pressure field in boundary layer flows. *Journal of Fluid Mechanics, 18*, 353–378.

Dickel, T., & Knapp, B. (2002). *Method for operating a hearing aid or hearing aid system, and a hearing aid and hearing aid system.* U.S. Patent Application No. US 2002/0037088 A1, Published March 28, 2002.

Dillon, H., Roe, I., & Katch, R. (1999). *Wind noise in hearing aids: Mechanisms and measurements.* National Acoustic Labs Australia: Report to Danavox, Phonak, Oticon, and Widex, January 13, 1999.

Elko, G. (2003). *Reducing noise in audio systems.* U.S. Patent Application No. US 2003/0147538 A1, Published August 7, 2003.

Kates, J. M. (2007). *A hearing aid with suppression of wind noise.* U.S. Patent Application No. 20070030989, issued February 8, 2007.

Kates, J. M., & Arehart, K. H. (2005). Multi-channel dynamic-range compression using digital frequency warping. *EURASIP Journal of Applied Signal Processing, 2005*, 3003–3014.

Larsson, P., & Olsson, P. (2004). *Detection of wind noise in hearing aids*. Masters Thesis, Department of Electroscience, Lund Institute of Technology, March, 2004.

Luo, H. (2005). *Method and device for processing an acoustic signal*. Euro. Patent Application No. EP 1 519 626 A2, Published March 30, 2005.

Morgan, S., & Raspet, R. (1992). Investigation of the mechanisms of low-frequency wind noise generation outdoors. *Journal of the Acoustical Society of America, 92*, 1180–1183.

Petersen, K. S., Boganson, G., Kjems, U., & Nielsen, T. B. (2004). *Device and method for detecting wind noise*. U.S. Patent Application No. US 2004/0161120 A1, Published Aug. 19, 2004.

Raspet, R., Webster, J., & Dillion, K. (2006). Framework for wind noise studies. *Journal of the Acoustical Society of America, 119*, 834–843.

Strasberg, M. (1988). Dimensional analysis of windscreen noise. *Journal of the Acoustical Society of America, 83*, 544–548.

Talay, T. A. (1975). *Introduction to the aerodynamics of flight*. Report SP-367. Scientific and Technical Information Office, NASA, Washington, D.C. (available at http://history.nasa.gov/SP-367/cover367.htm).

Thompson, S. C., & Dillon, H. (2001). Wind noise in hearing aids. Presented at the 13th Annual Convention of the American Academy of Audiology, San Diego, April 21, 2001. (available at http://www.knowleselectronics.com/engineering/publications/general.asp).

Wuttke, J. (1991). Microphones and the wind. *Journal of the Audio Engineering Society, 40*, 809–817.

7
Feedback Cancellation

IN A SYSTEM WITH FEEDBACK, a fraction of the system output gets added back into the input. In most hearing aids, the mechanical and acoustic feedback limits the maximum gain that can be achieved by the instrument. The feedback path includes effects of the hearing-aid microphone, amplifier, receiver, as well as the vent acoustics described in Chapter 3 or acoustic leaks that may occur in the fit of the earmold or shell within the ear canal. In Chapter 3 it was also pointed out that external acoustic factors, such as a telephone handset or hat, will also contribute to the feedback path. System instability caused by feedback is sometimes audible as a continuous high-frequency tone or whistle emanating from the hearing aid, and momentary instabilities in a hearing aid can result in short chirps, ringing that persists after an input sound stops, or other audible artifacts. In most instruments, venting the earmold used with a BTE or venting the shell of an ITE or CIC hearing aid establishes an acoustic feedback path that limits the maximum possible gain to less than 40 dB for a small vent and even less for a large vent (Kates, 1988).

The goal in most hearing aid fittings is to achieve the target frequency response chosen for a given hearing loss. If feedback is present in the hearing aid, however, it may not be possible to get high enough amplification, and speech intelligibility may suffer. In designing signal processing to reduce the effects of feedback, the objective is to achieve as much gain as possible over a wide frequency range while minimizing whistles, chirps, ringing, and other processing artifacts. And one has to be careful that the cure is not worse than the disease—the signal processing used to compensate for the feedback should not introduce its own processing artifacts that could degrade the output signal from the hearing aid.

Several approaches have been tried to reduce the effects of feedback in hearing aids. The simplest is to reduce the gain in the frequency region where feedback peaks are expected to occur, and many hearing aids use this approach. A notch filter adjusted during the hearing-aid fitting can be used to reduce the gain in the selected narrow frequency region. The system is made more stable, reducing the potential for whistling, but the gain reduction may also reduce intelligibility. A more complex approach is to mathematically model the feedback path and to subtract the model output from the microphone signal. In the best of all possible worlds the model will completely cancel the feedback signal at the hearing-aid input, leading to increased gain with no deleterious changes in the hearing-aid frequency response. However, the feedback path model is often imperfect, and the mismatch between the modeled and real feedback path responses can lead to instability in the hearing aid and a recurrence of the whistles and chirps that we are trying to eliminate.

In this chapter, we consider the effects of feedback in hearing aids and the signal-processing approaches that have been proposed to reduce these effects. The first question addressed is what feedback does to the response of a hearing aid that does not have any feedback reduction. The acoustics of the vent and the resultant feedback path are described, and the hearing-aid transfer function including feedback is discussed. Simple solutions to feedback, such as notch filters, are discussed next. The bulk of the chapter is dedicated to adaptive feedback cancellation algorithms as these have the greatest potential for reducing feedback effects in hearing aids. The chapter concludes with a discussion of some of the limitations on feedback cancellation, including room reverberation and nonlinear distortion.

The Feedback System

The existence of feedback in a hearing aid modifies the response of the entire system. The degree to which the system response is changed depends on the interaction of the hearing aid processing with the feedback path. Processing to reduce feedback effects then modifies this system to produce a new system that has even more complicated behavior. Before proceeding to the proposed solutions for feedback, it is therefore worthwhile to study the behavior of a hearing aid without any feedback reduction as many of the limitations of the solutions are directly related to the behavior of this basic system.

SYSTEM EQUATIONS

A block diagram of a hearing aid is shown in Figure 7-1. It assumed that the hearing aid uses a vent, and that the vent provides the major feedback path. Mechanical feedback can be caused by the vibrations of the receiver diaphragm being transmitted back to the microphone diaphragm through contact with the hearing-aid shell, and the mechanical feedback will be subsumed as part of the overall acoustic feedback path. The hearing aid processing is represented by $H(f)$, and the microphone, amplifier, and receiver responses are represented by $M(f)$, $A(f)$, and $R(f)$, respectively. If there were no feedback and no vent, then the hearing aid frequency response would be given by

$$Y(f) = X(f)[M(f)H(f)A(f)R(f)] \quad Equation\ (7.1)$$

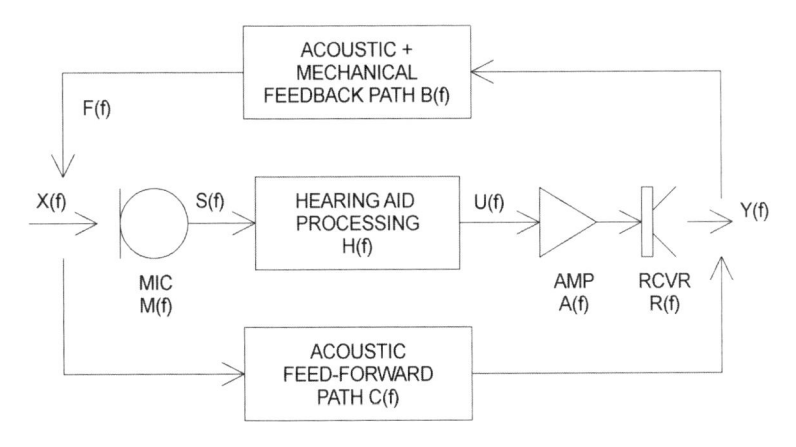

Figure 7-1. Block diagram showing a hearing aid with the feedback and acoustic feed-forward signal paths.

where $X(f)$ is the input signal and the product of the transfer functions in the square brackets is the total processing effect of all of the elements that make up the hearing aid.

Now consider the hearing aid with a vent. The vent provides a feedback path, represented by $B(f)$, that leads from the ear canal back to the microphone. The vent also provides an unamplified feed-forward path $C(f)$ from the opening of the vent in the outer ear (near the microphone in an ITE) directly into the ear canal. The pressure at the microphone is therefore the sum of the signal arriving from the external source and the feedback from the ear canal, and the pressure in the ear canal is the sum of the amplified hearing-aid signal plus the unamplified signal that comes directly through the vent. Combining all of these signals leads to the transfer function for the hearing aid (Kates, 1999; Rafaely & Hayes, 2001):

$$Y = X \frac{C + H[MAR]}{[1 - BC] - H[MARB]} \quad \text{Equation (7.2)}$$

The terms in Eq. (7.2) are all functions of frequency, but the frequency variable f has been suppressed to make the equation more concise.

It will be shown a little later in this section that the product $B(f)C(f) \ll 1$. Given the assumption that $B(f)C(f) \ll 1$, Eq. (7.2) reduces to the simpler form

$$Y = X \frac{C + H[MAR]}{1 - H[MARB]} \quad \text{Equation (7.3)}$$

Assume that there is no feedback, in which case $B(f) = 0$. The denominator of Eq. (7.3) then reduces to 1, and the hearing-aid response is the desired response given by Eq. (7.1) combined with the vent feed-forward path. Note that it is very difficult to design a physical system in which a vent allows sound propagation in one direction (feed-forward) but not the other (feedback), but in the world of mathematical simulations this is easily done and can be quite useful for understanding the system behavior.

When feedback is present, $B(f) \neq 0$ and the denominator of Eq. (7.3) is no longer exactly 1. As the denominator deviates from 1, the system transfer function deviates from the desired response. The danger occurs for a denominator close to zero at some frequency; if the denominator actually reaches zero, the transfer function for $Y(f)$ involves a division by zero which indicates infinite output amplitude. A stable system is one in which a finite input yields a finite output, so the system becomes unstable. In practice an infinite output level cannot be achieved given the finite power stored in the hearing-aid battery, but the system tries its best to reinforce the output at the frequency at which the gain is infinite, resulting in a continuous whistle output by the hearing aid.

The goal is to guarantee that the hearing aid is always stable. If there is no feedback reduction, as in this example, then the only option is to turn down the gain. A mathematical statement is that stability is ensured if the hearing-aid gain $H(f)$ is selected so that (Egolf, 1982; Kates, 1999):

$$|H[MARB]| < 1 \quad \text{Equation (7.4)}$$

If Eq. (7.4) is satisfied, then the denominator of Eq. (7.3) will always be greater than zero and the hearing aid will be stable.

SYSTEM RESPONSE

Most hearing aids are vented or use vented earmolds, so the behavior of the vent will dominate that of feedback path. The vent can be modeled as an acoustic tube (Egolf et al., 1985; Kates, 1988), with the length of the tube determining its resonance frequency and radius of the tube determining the amount of signal attenuation. This model behavior is plotted in Figure 7-2 for a tube 2.2 cm long and with a radius varying from 0.05 to 0.20 cm. As the vent radius is increased the amplitude of the feedback path transfer function increases, and the vent transfer function has a sharp peak at about 7 kHz due to the tube resonance. Acoustic modifications to the vent (Lybarger, 1982; Macrae, 1983) can provide some benefit by reducing the magnitude of the response at high frequencies.

The feedback transfer function for the vent is compared to the feedforward transfer function in Figure 7-3. The transfer functions for the two directions are very different despite it being the same vent. The difference is due to the radiation properties at the end of the vent. For the feedback path response, the vent is terminated at the side of the head, so a simple model of the acoustic load is the radiation impedance of a

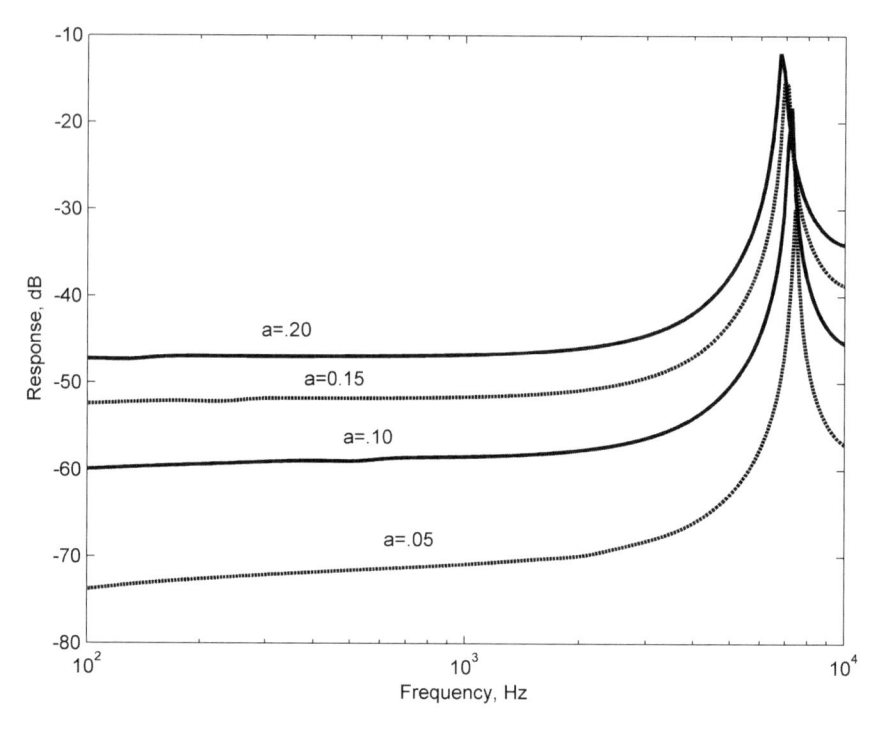

Figure 7-2. Feedback path magnitude transfer functions for a vent in a simulated ITE hearing aid as a function of the vent radius a. The vent length is 2.2 cm.

piston in an infinite baffle. For the feed-forward path response, the vent is terminated by the acoustic volume of the ear canal in parallel with the impedance of the ossicles and tympanic membrane. As a result of these differences in the terminating impedance, the feedback path response is that of an acoustic resonator, whereas the feed-forward response is a low-pass filter that also has a resonance peak at high frequencies.

Note that the gain of the feedback path is very low at low frequencies where the response of the feed-forward path is at its peak. Also note that the resonance peaks in the vicinity of 7 to 8 kHz in the feedback and feed-forward path responses are at different frequencies and that both are very sharp. Thus the assumption that $B(f)C(f) \ll 1$ that was made in going from Eq. (7.2) to Eq. (7.3) is valid for this simulation.

An ITE hearing aid was simulated (Kates, 1988) using the vent responses shown in Figure 7-3. The gain of the hearing aid was set to 45 dB

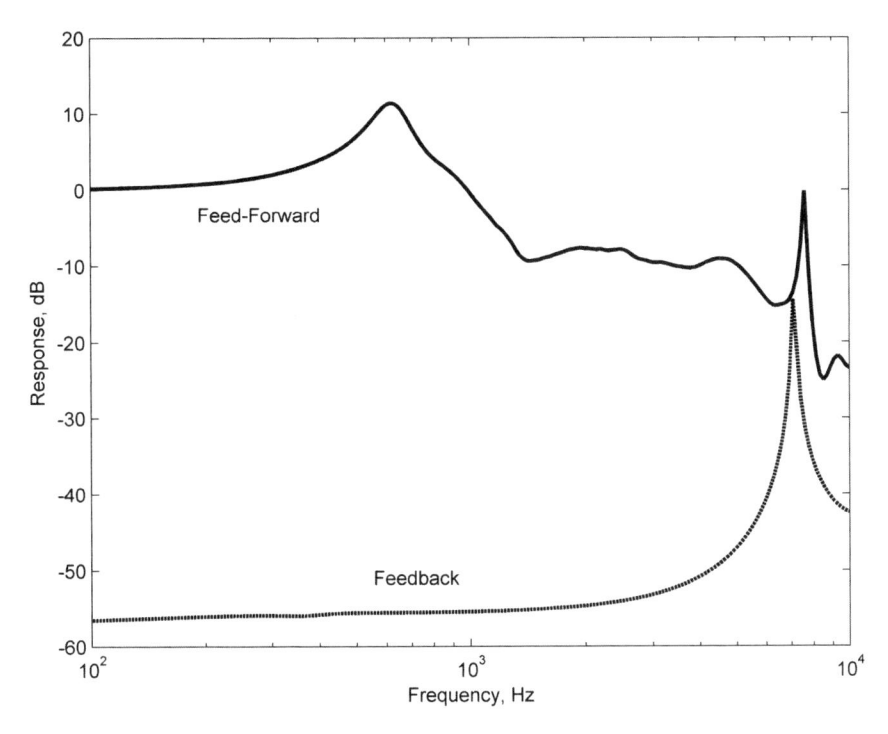

Figure 7-3. Vent feedback and feed-forward magnitude transfer functions in a simulated ITE hearing aid. The vent length is 2.2 cm and the radius a = 0.12 cm.

in order to push it close to instability. The simulation results are plotted in Figure 7-4. The hearing aid response was calculated using *Eq.* (7.2) for the complete system (solid line), and for the system with the feedback response $B(f)$ set to zero while keeping the feed-forward response $C(f)$ as calculated (dashed line). A naïve consideration of the feedback path plotted in Figure 7-2 would lead one to expect that the hearing aid would approach instability at the frequency corresponding to the peak of the feedback path response at approximately 7 kHz. Instead, the hearing aid shows a large increase in system output at about 5.5 kHz, with a reduction in output at 2.5 kHz and an increase at 1.8 kHz. One factor is the decrease in the magnitude of the receiver and microphone responses above 5 kHz, which decreases the overall magnitude of the transfer function $H[MARB]$. One must also remember that the denominator of *Eq.* (7.3) approaches zero when the magnitude of the term $H[MARB]$ approaches

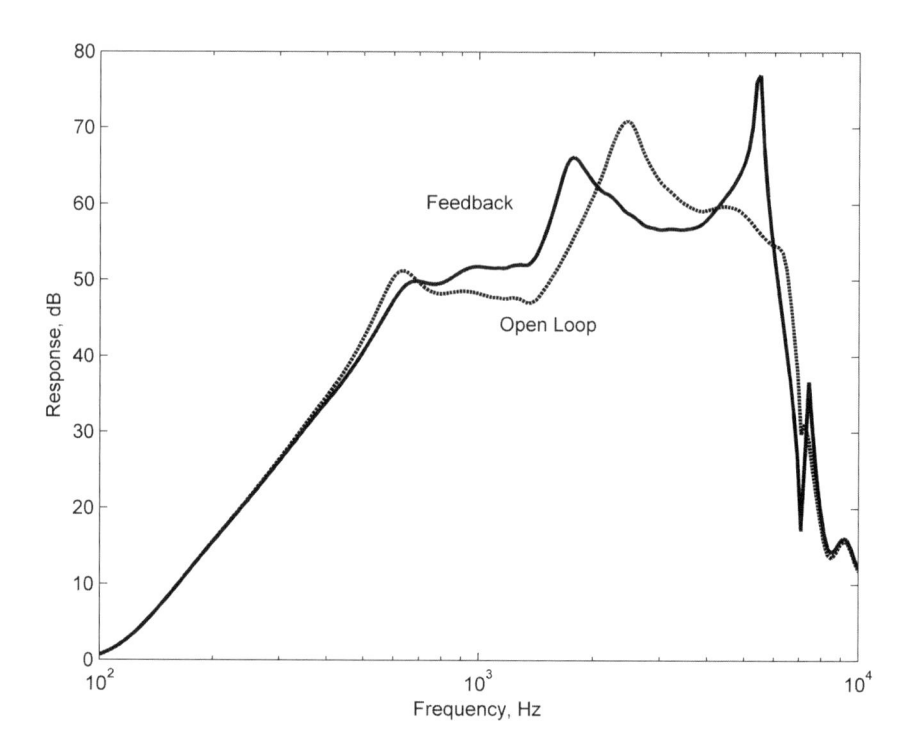

Figure 7-4. Magnitude frequency response for a simulated ITE hearing aid with an amplifier gain of 45 dB. The solid line shows the system response with the feedback and feed-forward paths through the vent. The dashed line shows the system response with the vent feed-forward path present but the feedback path removed.

1 and its phase is 0 degrees. Instability requires both an amplitude and a phase match, and the phase effects are not obvious when just considering the magnitude frequency response of the feedback path. Thus, the effects of the feedback on the overall system response are surprisingly complicated, and small changes in the feedback path may lead to large and unexpected changes in the system response.

The behavior of real feedback paths is much more complicated than the simple simulation results shown in Figure 7-2. Three feedback path responses are plotted in Figure 7-5 for measurements from a BTE mounted on a dummy head (Kates, 1999). The magnitude of the feedback paths measured on the dummy head has been empirically observed to be about 10 dB greater than those on a real person, but has the same general shape to the response. The earmold for BTE was unvented

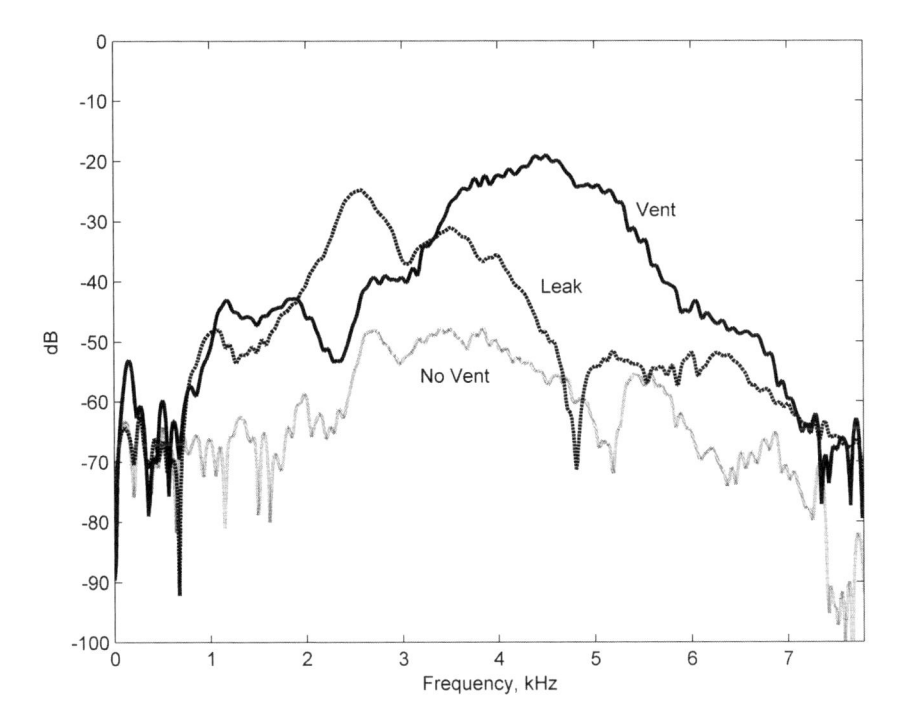

Figure 7-5. Feedback path magnitude frequency response measured on a dummy head for a BTE hearing aid. The earmold had no vent (*dotted line*), no vent but fitted loosely to ensure an acoustic leak (*dashed line*), or was vented (*solid line*).

(dotted line), unvented but shifted in the ear canal to give a leaky loose fit (dashed line), or vented (solid line). The fit of the unvented earmold in the ear canal of the dummy head was very tight, and the feedback path response shows 50 dB or greater attenuation. Introducing a leak into the earmold fitting causes a large change in the feedback path response, with a peak occurring at about 2.6 kHz. The vented earmold has a feedback path response with a large peak at about 4.5 kHz. Thus, changing the vent configuration can have a large effect on the behavior of the feedback path.

The measurements were repeated for the same hearing and earmold configurations, but with a telephone handset positioned close to the pinna of the dummy head. These handset measurements are plotted in Figure 7-6. The overall shape of the measurements for the handset

184 Digital Hearing Aids

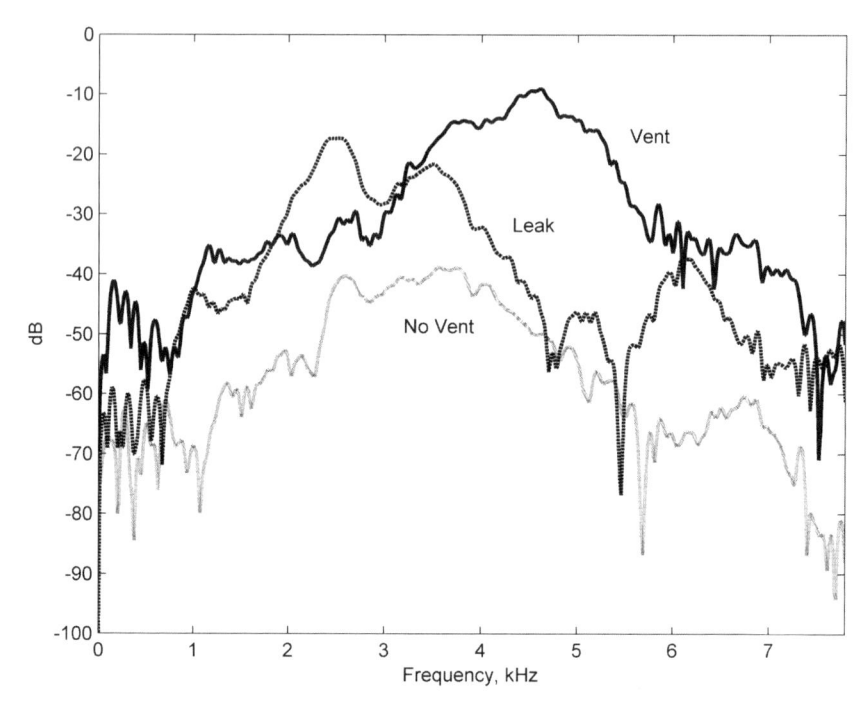

Figure 7-6. Feedback path magnitude frequency response measured on a dummy head for a BTE hearing aid. A telephone handset was positioned next to the pinna of the head. The earmold had no vent (*dotted line*), no vent but fitted loosely to ensure an acoustic leak (*dashed line*), or was vented (*solid line*).

close to the pinna are similar to those for the unoccluded pinna, but the curves all lie about 10 dB higher. Thus, a hearing aid that was stable for normal use may become unstable when the user uses the telephone, puts on a hat, or stands close to a wall. Other feedback path measurements (Hellgren et al., 1999; Stinson & Daigle, 2004) have shown similar changes in the feedback path response as external objects such as a telephone handset, hand, or hat are moved closer to the hearing aid, with the proximity of a reflecting surface causing increases in the feedback path response of 10 to 20 dB.

Gain-Reduction Solutions

The simplest solution to reduce the occurrence of feedback problems is to reduce the gain in order to satisfy Eq. (7.4). But the gain does not need to be reduced everywhere; it only needs to be reduced in the frequency region where feedback problems are expected to occur. Improving the system stability by reducing the gain in selected frequency regions is a technique that has been used for many years in public address (PA) systems, and has also found application in hearing aids.

One approach is to insert a notch filter in the amplified signal path (Boner & Boner, 1965). A notch filter attenuates the system response over a narrow frequency region. A block diagram of a hearing aid using a notch filter is presented in Figure 7-7. The approximate transfer function for this system is given by:

$$Y = X \frac{C + HN[MAR]}{1 - HN[MARB]} \quad \text{Equation (7.5)}$$

Imagine that the hearing aid is unstable without the notch filter, that is $|H[MARB]| > 1$ over a narrow frequency region. The notch filter $N(f)$ can then be designed so that it attenuates the system response across the unstable frequency region. The result is that $|HN[MARB]| < 1$ and the system is now stable. However, the notch filter also reduces the system

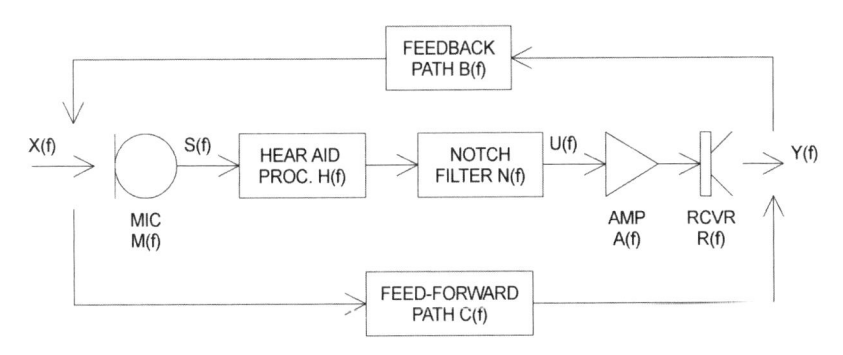

Figure 7-7. Block diagram of a hearing aid using a notch filter for feedback reduction.

gain over the selected frequency region, and the resultant reduction in amplification could reduce speech intelligibility. If the frequency region over which the hearing aid is unstable is small, say less than half an octave, then the loss in intelligibility would be small as well. In some multichannel hearing aids the gain reduction is provided by attenuating one or more of the frequency bands, thus saving on computation but attenuating the signal over a wider bandwidth.

Using this approach requires that the peaks of the system response be identified in advance and an appropriate notch filter inserted into the system. The measurement of the hearing-aid magnitude frequency response in the ear canal can be performed during the hearing-aid fitting, but this measurement represents only one of many possible listening situations where the hearing aid could become unstable. A change in the feedback path, such as that caused by bringing a telephone handset close to the ear, could still drive the system unstable.

A more elegant solution is to reduce the gain only when oscillation caused by feedback is detected, and to limit the gain reduction to the frequency region where the feedback has rendered the system unstable. One approach is to monitor the input signal $X(f)$. If $X(f)$ is a tone indicative of oscillation caused by an unstable system, a notch filter $N(f)$ can be inserted into the signal path at the frequency of the tone.

Patronis (1978) proposed correlating the input signal with a delayed version of itself to detect whistling in a PA system. If whistling is present, the signal at the microphone will be nearly a sinusoid. If the delay is an integral number of periods of the sinusoid, then the delayed waveform will perfectly overlap the undelayed input and the correlation will be very high. Voiced speech is also periodic, so the delay must be longer than the typical duration of syllables (200 to 300 msec) in speech. If a high degree of correlation between the direct and delayed input signal is detected, the gain of the hearing aid is reduced using a notch filter or by attenuating one or more of the frequency bands in a multiband system. Kaelin et al. (1998) proposed a similar idea, but used a frequency-domain analysis to detect high degrees of correlation in individual frequency bands and reduce the gain in those bands. Music may still present a problem to the correlation detection, however, so such a system would need to be turned off in a "music" mode.

Adaptive Feedback Cancellation

The approaches to improving the hearing-aid stability discussed so far are based on reducing the gain of the hearing aid. Ideally, one would like to improve the system stability without any gain reduction. Adaptive feedback cancellation techniques mathematically model the feedback path response and subtract the modeled response from the signal input to the hearing aid. A perfect match would mean that the feedback signal at the microphone would be completely canceled by the modeled signal, and the system would be completely stable for any amount of amplification. In practice, feedback-cancellation systems typically permit 10 to 15 dB additional gain in a hearing aid before the systems become unstable (Dyrlund et al., 1994; Greenberg et al., 2000; Hellgren, 2002; Kates, 2001; Maxwell & Zurek, 1995), although the system benefit is often less for tonal inputs or for large changes in the feedback path.

The limitation on feedback cancellation is the accuracy to which the feedback path can be modeled. The feedback path can change, as illustrated in Figures 7-5 and 7-6, and the model needs to be able to track these changes in the feedback path response. Furthermore, the model and the procedures used to estimate the feedback path response should not cause any degradation in the hearing-aid output. Some early algorithms, for example, proposed injecting a continuous low-level noise signal into the hearing-aid signal path to assist in measuring the feedback path response (Dyrlund & Bisgaard 1991; Dyrlund et al., 1994; Engebretson & French-St. George, 1993; Engebretson et al., 1990). However, the injected noise needs to be at a relatively high intensity to be of any use and would be audible to most listeners (Odelius, 2003). Another proposal (Kates, 1991) was to turn off the hearing-aid amplification when instability due to feedback was detected, measure the feedback path response, and then turn the hearing-aid amplification back on. The advantage of this approach is that the measurement of the hearing-aid feedback path response is very accurate (Maxwell & Zurek, 1995), but there is the obvious disadvantage of interrupting the desired signal.

The algorithms used in hearing aids today attempt to measure the feedback path response while the hearing aid is in use for any possible listening condition or input signal. These requirements make feedback cancellation a very difficult problem to solve. In the remainder of this section, we describe the approaches being used for feedback cancellation in hearing aids and the techniques that are used to improve algorithm behavior under difficult conditions such as when tonal inputs are present.

System Equations

A block diagram of a hearing aid incorporating feedback cancellation is presented in Figure 7-8. In some systems the feedback path is modeled by a single filter $W(f)$ but in this example the filter is separated into three components (Kates, 1999): a delay, a fixed (nonadaptive) filter, and an adaptive FIR filter $G(f)$. The delay and the fixed filter represent aspects of the physical feedback path, such as the microphone and receiver responses, that are expected to change very slowly over time. The adaptive filter then models those parts of the feedback path, such as the vent and associated external acoustic effects, that would be expected to change rapidly (e.g., putting on a hat). The objective of the adaptive filter is to match the output of the feedback path model $V(f)$ as closely as possible to the actual feedback signal as received by the microphone, given by $F(f)M(f)$. The error signal $E(f) = S(f) - V(f)$ is used to control the adaptation of the filter modeling the feedback path.

The transfer function of the hearing aid given in Eq. (7.2) is modified by the presence of the feedback-cancellation filter. The resultant system transfer function is given by (Kates, 1999):

$$Y = X \frac{C + H[WC + MAR]}{[1 - BC] - H\{MARB - W[1 - BC]\}} \quad \text{Equation (7.6)}$$

Invoking the assumption $B(f)C(f) \ll 1$ leads to the simplified equation

$$Y = X \frac{C + H[WC + MAR]}{1 - H[MARB - W]} \quad \text{Equation (7.7)}$$

The condition for stability then becomes:

$$|H[MARB - W]| < 1 \quad \text{Equation (7.8)}$$

Feedback Cancellation

[Figure 7-8 block diagram]

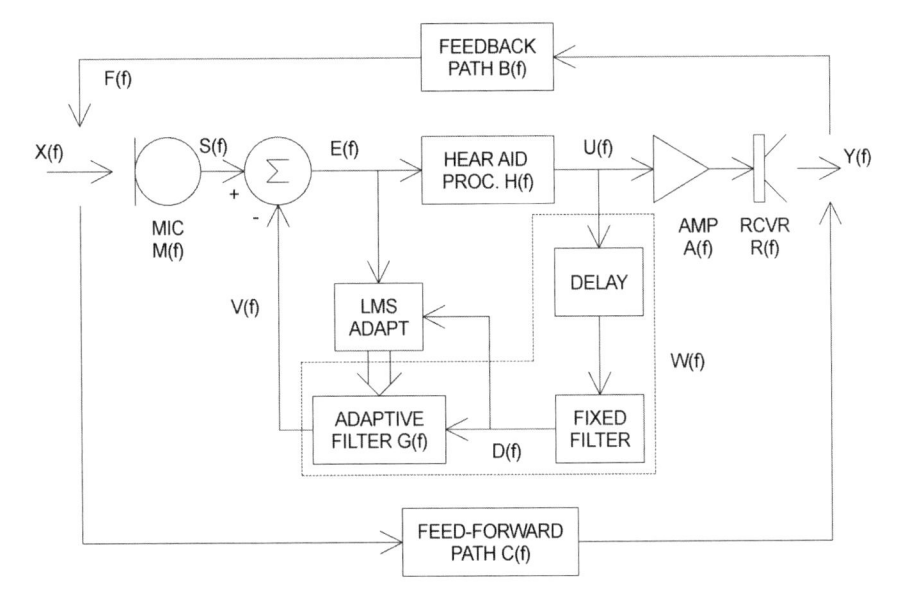

Figure 7-8. Block diagram of an adaptive feedback cancellation system.

The stability criterion for the hearing aid without feedback cancellation was given by Eq. (7.4), which showed that the instrument will be stable if the gain H(f) is chosen so that

$$|H| < \frac{1}{|MARB|} \quad \text{Equation (7.9)}$$

With feedback cancellation, the hearing aid will be stable if the gain H(f) satisfies

$$|H| < \frac{1}{|MARB - W|} \quad \text{Equation (7.10)}$$

If W(f) is a good model of the actual feedback path MARB, then the denominator of Eq. (7.10) will be smaller than the denominator of Eq. (7.9), and H(f) can be made correspondingly larger. The difference in the maximum stable gains possible between Eqs. (7.9) and (7.10) in the hearing aid is often used as a criterion in determining the effectiveness of the feedback cancellation. The limitation to the maximum possible increase in gain is thus the accuracy of the feedback path model.

LMS ADAPTATION

The procedure for updating the adaptive filter $G(f)$ operates in the time domain. The error signal in the time domain $e(n)$ is compared to the output $d(n)$ of the fixed portion of the feedback path model. The adaptive FIR filter coefficients $\{g_k(n)\}$ are then adapted using a power-normalized version of the LMS algorithm (Haykin, 1996; Widrow et al., 1976) to minimize the average power in the error signal $e(n)$, where the error power is given by:

$$\varepsilon(n) = e^2(n) \quad \text{Equation (7.11)}$$

The adaptation algorithm uses the correlation between $e(n)$ and $d(n)$ to update $g_k(n)$:

$$g_k(n+1) = g_k(n) + \frac{2\mu}{\sigma_d^2} e(n)d(n-k) \quad \text{Equation (7.12)}$$

where the subscript k is the index for the filter coefficients. The factor μ controls the rate of adaptation; increasing the value of μ gives faster adaptation to changes in the feedback path, but also increases the expected error in the feedback-path model. The value of μ is generally small, so the update of each filter coefficient represents an average over many data samples. The factor σ_d^2 is the power in the signal $d(n)$; this term normalizes the rate of adaptation so that the system responds just as quickly at low signal levels as at high signal levels.

The update for the kth filter coefficient uses the cross-correlation between the sequence $e(n)$ and the sequence $d(n)$ delayed by k samples. If the error signal and the delayed input to the correlation move in the same direction and at the same frequency, then the corresponding coefficient of the adaptive filter will be incremented. If the fluctuations in $e(n)$ and $d(n)$ are independent of each other, then the changes in $g_k(n)$ will average out to zero and the filter coefficient will remain unchanged.

The adaptive filter update works best when the input signal $x(n)$ is white Gaussian noise. White noise has the property that the correlation of the signal with itself for any non-zero time delay is zero. That is, the average of $x(n)x(n-k)$ is zero for $k \neq 0$, and gives the signal power for $k = 0$. Now imagine that the hearing aid processing $H(f)$ is just an amplifier having a gain of 0 dB along with a microphone and receiver also having ideal flat responses, and that the feedback path $B(f)$ is a pure time delay of L samples. The filter update given by Eq. (7.12) will be zero for every filter coefficient $k \neq L$, and will converge to the amplitude of the delayed feedback signal for $k = L$. In the case of a more general feedback path response, the correlation of $e(n)$ and $d(n)$ will yield the impulse response of the feedback path and the model will be exact.

Now consider a sinusoid as the input $x(n)$. The sinusoid will be present at the input $x(n)$ and also in the error signal $e(n)$. The sinusoid will be amplified by the hearing aid processing, so an amplified and delayed version of the sinusoid will also appear in the hearing-aid output $y(n)$ and in the input to the adaptive filter $d(n)$. Because $e(n)$ and $d(n)$ are both sinusoids at the same frequency, they will be highly correlated, and the correlation between the two sinusoids will be much greater than any signal correlations related to the feedback path transfer function. Because the adaptive filter coefficient update is driven to minimize the error signal, the filter will adapt by shifting the amplitude and phase of $d(n)$ so that the filtered signal $v(n)$ cancels the sinusoid at the microphone output $s(n)$. The result is that for a sinusoidal input signal, adaptive feedback cancellation stops modeling the feedback path and instead adapts to cancel the input signal.

CONSTRAINED ADAPTATION

A challenge in designing an adaptive feedback-cancellation system is to ensure that the system accurately models the feedback path while never canceling a sinusoid or tonal input signal. To achieve this end, the behavior of the LMS adaptation needs to be modified. One approach, constrained adaptation (Kates, 1999), lets the adaptation proceed normally as long as the adaptive filter remains close to an assumed "correct" reference filter, and prevents the adaptive filter coefficients from drifting too far from this presumed correct solution. The constraints prevent the system from canceling a sinusoidal input, but may also prevent the system from adapting fully to a large change in the feedback path.

Adaptation Equations

Two types of constraints were proposed by Kates (1999). The first is a clamp on the distance that the filter coefficients are allowed to deviate from the reference. Let the input to the hearing aid be a sinusoid. As explained above, this input will drive the adaptive feedback cancellation filter away from the desired model of the feedback path. Assume that we have made an initial model of the feedback path $W(f,0) \approx MARB$ when the hearing aid was fit to the user. It is now some time later and the feedback path model is given by $W(f,m)$ for processing block m. The stability criterion given by Eq. (7.10) is $|H\|MARB - W(f,m)| < 1$. The actual feedback path transfer function $MARB$ is not available, but the initial measurement of the feedback path is. The stability criterion can then be approximated by $|H\|W(f,0) - W(f,m)| < 1$, assuming that the feedback path has not changed substantially. Stability for a sinusoidal input will be maintained as long as the feedback path model stays close to the initial measurement.

The frequency-domain constraint using the initial feedback path measurement can be translated into the time domain. Let $g_k(0)$ represent the adaptive feedback path filter coefficients established when the instrument was fit to the user. The clamp constraint limits the maximum deviation of the adaptive filter from this initial setting:

$$\frac{\sum_{k=0}^{K-1}|g_k(n) - g_k(0)|}{\sum_{k=0}^{K-1}|g_k(0)|} < \gamma, \quad \gamma \approx 2 \quad \text{Equation (7.13)}$$

The clamp works like keeping a dog in a fenced yard; the filter coefficients (the dog) can move around freely within the area established by the constraint (the fence), but are prevented from moving outside the fence.

The second constraint modifies the error given by Eq. (7.11) that is used to guide the coefficient adaptation. The modification is a cost constraint that penalizes deviations of the adaptive filter coefficients if they move away from the initial values. The modified error contains a penalty for large filter coefficients:

$$\varepsilon(n) = e^2(n) + \beta \sum_{k=0}^{K-1} [g_k(n) - g_k(0)]^2 \quad \text{Equation (7.14)}$$

The LMS adaptive filter coefficient update equation then becomes:

$$g_k(n+1) = g_k(n) - 2\mu\beta[g_k(n) - g_k(0)] + \frac{2\mu}{\sigma_d^2} e(n)d(n-k)$$

Equation (7.15)

If the filter coefficients are close to the initial values, the standard LMS update term from Eq. (7.12) dominates the adaptation. However, if the filter coefficients move away from the initial values, the β term grows in magnitude and pulls the coefficients back toward the initial values. The cost constraint works like an elastic band; for small deviations from the initial values the restoring force is small, but for large deviations the restoring force is large and quickly pulls the coefficients back toward the initial values.

Initialization

The constrained adaptation requires a reference filter $\{g_k(0)\}$ that is normally set during the initial fitting of the hearing aid to the user. A block diagram of an initialization procedure (Kates, 2002) is presented in Figure 7-9. A periodic excitation sequence is used to measure the feedback path response of the hearing aid inserted in the user's ear. The normal hearing-aid processing is disabled during the initialization, so the system measures the feedback path response in situ, and produces an accurate estimate of the overall transfer function *MARB*. A noiselike stimulus having a flat power spectrum is desirable, and a maximum length sequence (Rife & Vanderkooy, 1989; Schneider & Jamieson, 1993; Vanderkooy, 1994) has proven effective in practice. A response is collected for each period of the excitation, and the responses are averaged together to suppress the effects of external noise sources. Because the excitation is periodic, it creates a buzzing sound in the listener's ear while the initialization is performed.

The impulse response of the feedback path is extracted by cross-correlating the averaged outputs with one period of the excitation se-

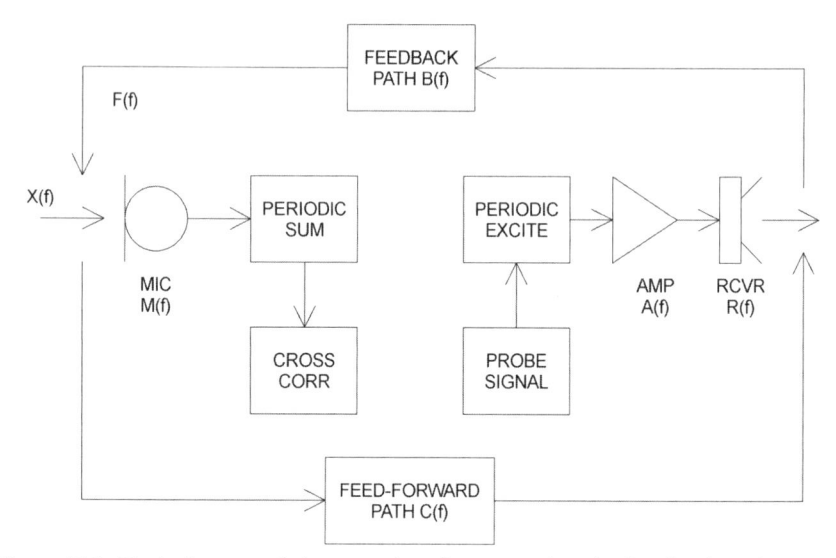

Figure 7-9. Block diagram of the procedure for measuring the feedback path response during initialization.

quence. System identification techniques (Ljung, 1987) are then used to compute a minimum mean-squared error model fit to the observed impulse response. The Kates (2002) model incorporates three pieces as shown in Figure 7-8: a fixed delay, a short recursive (IIR) filter that represents the slowly varying portion of the feedback path (microphone, amplifier, and receiver), and the initial coefficients for the adaptive FIR filter that represents the rapidly varying portion of the feedback path (vent plus external acoustics and acoustic leaks). Splitting the feedback path model into three pieces creates a model that is short and computationally efficient, but which still accurately represents the major characteristics of the feedback path.

Simulation Results

The feedback-cancellation system of Figure 7-8 was simulated in MATLAB. A BTE hearing aid was used, and the feedback path was the vented earmold response shown in Figure 7-5. The feedback path model consisted of a delay, a fixed 5-pole IIR filter, and an adaptive FIR filter having 8 taps. The fit of the initial feedback path model to the actual feedback path measurement is shown in Figure 7-10. The model does a

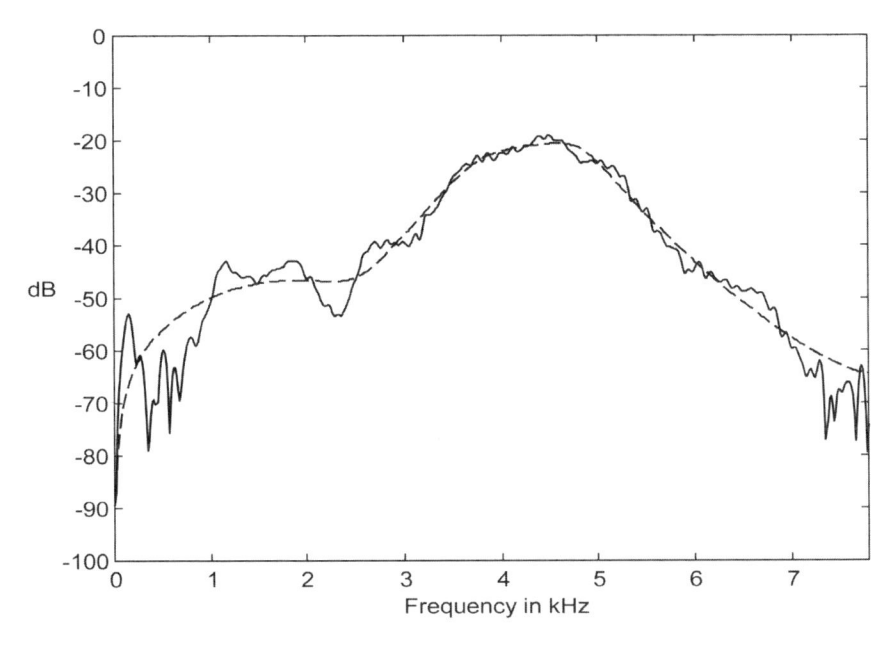

Figure 7-10. Magnitude frequency response for the measured hearing aid vent (*solid line*) and the 5-pole 8-tap FIR model (*dashed line*) fit by the initial parameter estimation.

good job of reproducing the overall shape of the feedback path magnitude frequency response, but does not have enough degrees of freedom to reproduce the fine structure of the feedback path (we return to the question of model accuracy in the section on processing limitations).

The simulated hearing aid was then excited with a 2-kHz sinusoid and the feedback-cancellation system was allowed to adapt for 10 sec. As the unconstrained feedback cancellation system adapts in the presence of the sinusoid, it will adjust the adaptive filter to cancel the signal. If the sinusoid had an initial amplitude of 1 V at the output of the hearing aid, then the signal amplitude will decrease as the system adapts. This behavior is plotted in Figure 7-11. The envelope of the sinusoid at the output of the hearing aid decreases exponentially for the unconstrained adaptation. With the clamp constraint, the envelope starts to decay. The adaptive filter coefficients then reach the limit imposed by the clamp at about 4 sec, after which the envelope remains at a constant amplitude. With the cost function constraint, the envelope shows a slower initial

196 Digital Hearing Aids

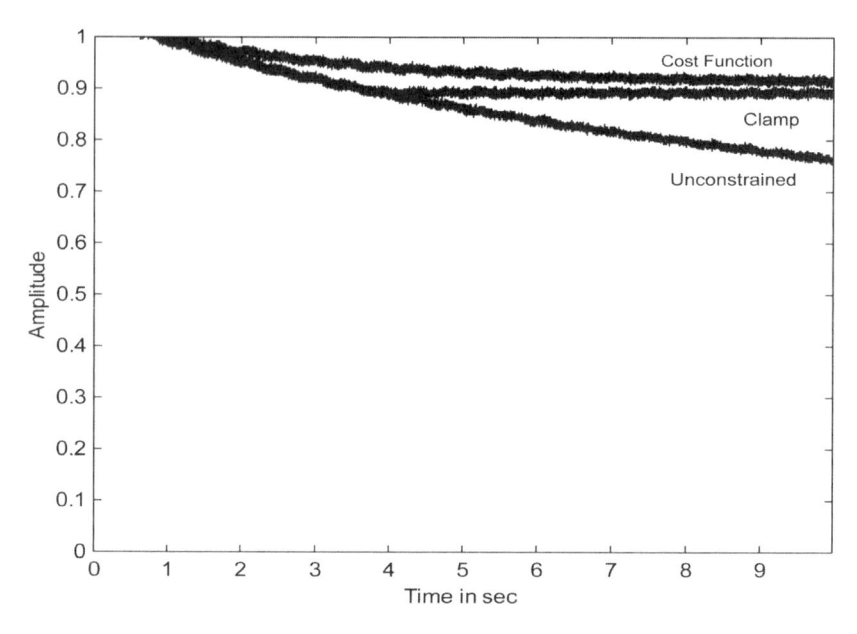

Figure 7-11. Envelope of the hearing-aid output signal for the 2-kHz sinusoid using unconstrained adaptation, clamped adaptation, and adaptation with the coefficient cost function.

rate of decay, and proceeds toward an asymptote that is similar to the signal attenuation limit of the clamp.

An alternative way of visualizing the effects of the filter adaptation is to plot the relative error between the actual and modeled feedback path responses. The initial fit of the model to the feedback path will have a small error, but as the filter adapts to cancel the sinusoid, the filter coefficients will drift away from the correct values and the error will increase. This behavior is plotted in Figure 7-12. The error for the unconstrained adaptation appears to grow without limit. With clamp constraint, the error starts to grow just as for the unconstrained adaptation, but then the error reaches the limit allowed by the algorithm and the error is prevented from growing any further. With the cost function constraint, the error grows more slowly as the constraint constantly pushes the filter coefficients back toward the initial values, and the error appears to be heading toward an asymptote similar to the maximum error allowed by the clamp.

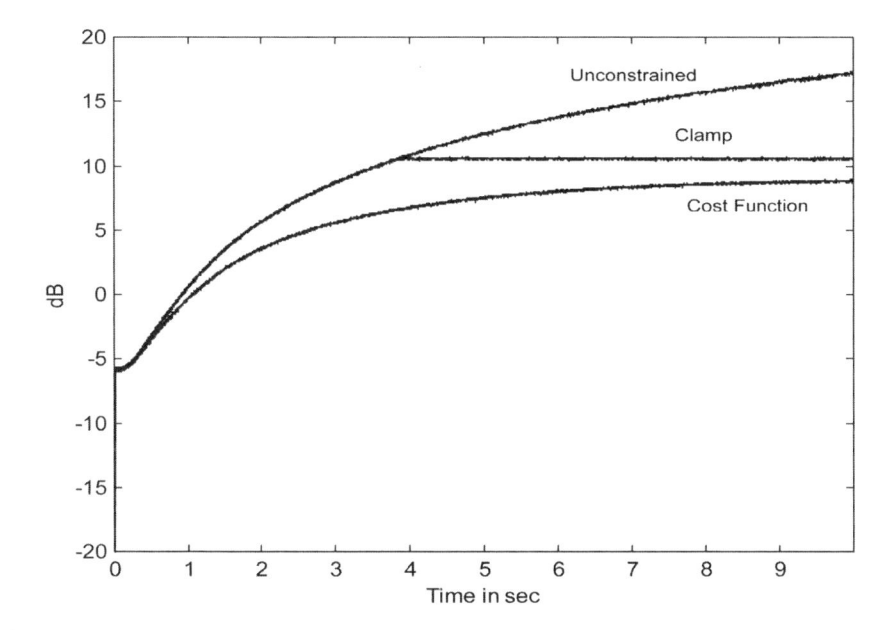

Figure 7-12. Normalized signal for the difference between the feedback path model and the measured feedback path for the 2-kHz sinusoid using unconstrained adaptation, clamped adaptation, and adaptation with the coefficient cost function.

The magnitude frequency responses of the adaptive FIR filter in cascade with the fixed IIR filter at the end of the 10-sec adaptation are plotted in Figure 7-13 for the three adaptation conditions. All of the adaptive filters drift away from the correct response. The adaptation for the sinusoidal input does not model the feedback path, but rather adjusts the gain and phase at 2 kHz to cancel the input signal. What happens to the filter response at other frequencies is not controlled by the LMS adaptation, and any filter shape is possible. So in Figure 7-13, the filter response for the unconstrained adaptation has moved substantially away from the initial filter response at all frequencies. With the clamp and cost function constraints, the filter has moved a large distance in the vicinity of 2 kHz, but has not drifted as far from the true response at frequencies above 4 kHz.

The constrained adaptation prevents cancellation of a sinusoidal input signal. However, the constraints may also prevent complete adapta-

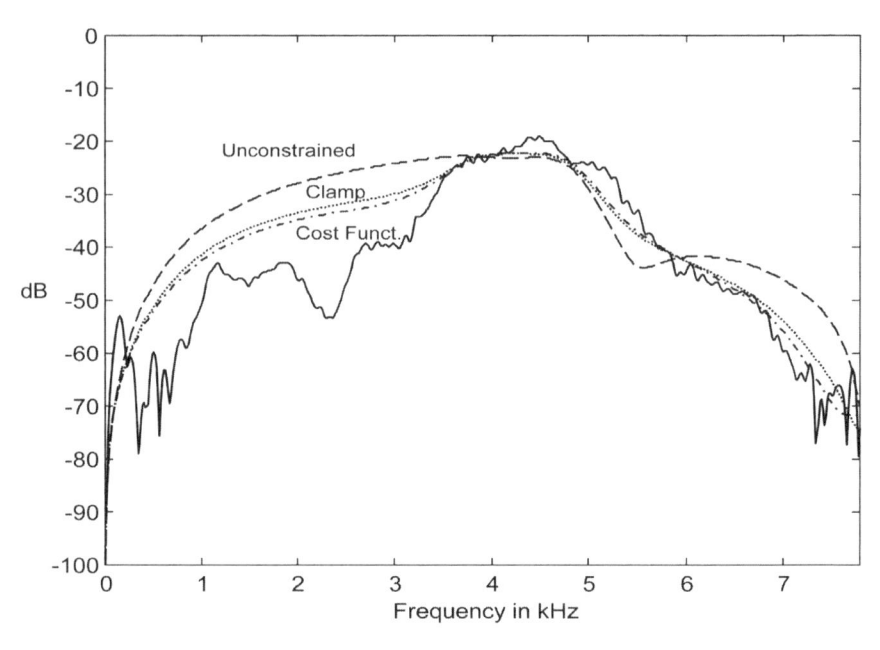

Figure 7-13. Magnitude frequency response for the vented BTE hearing aid feedback path (*solid line*), and the 5-pole 8-tap FIR model after adapting for 10 sec. The response for the unconstrained adaptation is given by the dashed line, the response for the clamped adaptation by the dotted line, and the response for the coefficient cost function by the dot-dash line.

tion to the new feedback path when there is a large change, as would occur when the user places a telephone handset close to the aided ear. Constrained adaptation is therefore a useful but imperfect solution to the complex problem of adaptive feedback cancellation.

DECORRELATION TECHNIQUES

The situations that have been considered so far are a white noise input, in which case the adaptive filter worked perfectly because its inputs were uncorrelated, and a sinusoidal input, in which case the adaptive filter failed unless the adaptation was constrained because its inputs were highly correlated. An alternative to constrained adaptation is to ensure that the signals $e(n)$ and $d(n)$ used for the LMS coefficient adaptation in Eq. (7.12) are as uncorrelated with each other as possible.

Interrupted Adaptation

A simple approach would be to let the adaptation proceed if $e(n)$ and $d(n)$ are uncorrelated (noiselike), but stop the adaptation and freeze the filter coefficients if $e(n)$ and $d(n)$ are sufficiently correlated (tonal or periodic). But this simple approach has a problem. Imagine that a hearing-aid user answers the telephone and her hearing aid starts to whistle. If the adaptation stops, the system will never adjust to the new feedback path and the hearing aid will whistle until the handset is removed.

Delay

A second approach is to insert a delay into the feedback path model or into the hearing aid processing $H(f)$. Many signals are correlated with each other for short time delays, but become increasingly uncorrelated as the time separation increases. Bustamante et al. (1989) proposed placing a delay in the feedback path to reduce the correlation between $e(n)$ and $d(n)$. Siqueira and Alwan (2000) showed that for a colored noise input the LMS adaptive filter of Eq. (7.12) had a large error in modeling the feedback path. Inserting a delay in the hearing-aid processing greatly improved the model accuracy, whereas a delay in the feedback model signal path provided a smaller improvement. However, there will still be some situations, such as the whistle example in the paragraph above, in which no amount of delay will remove the signal correlation and the system will fail to adapt to the correct model of the feedback path.

Filtered-X Algorithm

A more effective solution is to provide filters that modify $e(n)$ and $d(n)$ prior to the LMS adaptive filter update. A block diagram of this approach, termed the Filtered-X algorithm, is presented in Figure 7-14. A filter $P(f)$ operates on $E(f)$ and an identical filter operates on $D(f)$ to provide modified inputs to the LMS adaptation (Chi et al., 2003; Hellgren, 2002). The effect of the filter $P(f)$ is related to the concept of group delay discussed in Chapter 2. If a filter has a high narrow peak it will have a large group delay because the phase response of the filter response changes rapidly over the frequency interval containing the steep filter slopes. Similarly, if a signal spectrum has a high narrow peak, the correlation between the signal and delayed versions of itself will be high over a long period of time proportional to the group delay of the equivalent filter. The pair of filters $P(f)$ are designed to flatten the spectrum of the signals and thus reduce the time interval over which their correlations are high. The shorter the correlation distance, the better the adaptive filter will behave.

The system shown in Figure 7-14 uses a pair of fixed filters to modify the inputs to the LMS cross-correlation. The inputs are given by:

$$Q(f) = E(f)P(f)$$
$$Z(f) = D(f)P(f)$$
Equation (7.16)

The adaptive filter coefficient update then proceeds as presented in Eq. (7.12), except that the modified inputs are used:

$$g_k(n+1) = g_k(n) + \frac{2\mu}{\sigma_d^2} q(n)z(n-k)$$ Equation (7.17)

Speech is often the input signal of interest, and Hellgren (2002) proposed setting $P(f)$ to compensate for the long-term average spectrum of speech. As speech has most of its power at low frequencies, the filter $P(f)$ would be a high-pass filter. Kates (2002) also proposed using a high-pass filter for $P(f)$.

One way of considering the effects of the high-pass filter is that, for low frequencies, the filter reduces the amplitude of the signals being correlated. The reduced amplitude of signals $q(n)$ and $z(n)$ in Eq. (7.17) is equivalent to keeping the signal amplitudes at their original levels and instead reducing the value of μ at low frequencies. Thus, the effect of the high-pass filter is to reduce the rate of adaptation at low frequencies while maintaining a high rate of adaptation at high frequencies. If the hearing aid whistles at a high frequency, the system will adapt to cancel the whistle. If the input is a low-frequency tonal signal, such as voiced speech or music, the rate of adaptation will be much slower and the feedback path model will only shift a small amount from the correct model and the signal will not be substantially modified.

As an example of the frequency-dependent rate of adaptation, consider the hearing aid and feedback cancellation system simulated in a previous section. In addition, use a high-pass filter $P(f)$ given by a simple first-difference operation:

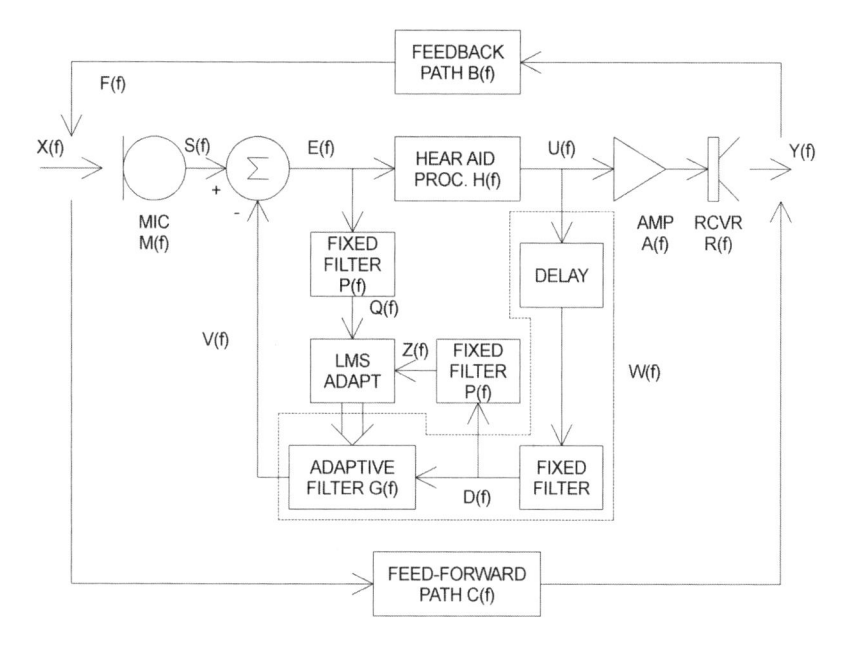

Figure 7-14. Block diagram for the filtered-X feedback cancellation algorithm.

$$q(n) = e(n) - e(n-1)$$
$$z(n) = d(n) - d(n-1)$$

Equation (7.18)

at a 16-kHz sampling rate. This filter will attenuate signals below 4 kHz and will pass signals above 4 kHz, and is an approximate inverse filter for the long-term spectrum of speech. A tone at 1 kHz was used to test the susceptibility of the feedback cancellation to speech or music, whereas a tone at 4 kHz was used to test the ability of the system to cancel whistling. Given a long enough observation time, all of the systems will cancel either sinusoid. However, the rate of signal attenuation in dB/sec depends strongly on the design of the adaptive system as shown in the first two rows of Table 7-1. The conventional LMS system rapidly cancels both sinusoids, whereas the filtered-X system using the high-pass filter cancels the 1-kHz tone much more slowly than the 4-kHz tone.

The use of a fixed filter in the filtered-X algorithm assumes that the characteristics of the input signal are relatively constant. However, in the real world the input signal is constantly changing. To get accurate

TABLE 7-1. Rate of Cancellation of a Sinusoid in dB/sec for the Conventional Adaptive Feedback Cancellation, for the Filtered-X Algorithm Using a Fixed High-Pass Filter for $P(f)$, and for the Filtered-X Algorithm Using an Adaptive Notch Filter for $P(f)$

Adaptation Algorithm	Rate of Sinusoid Cancellation, dB/sec	
	1 kHz	4 kHz
Conventional LMS	9.1	5.2
Filtered-X: 1st-order Diff.	0.3	2.8
Filtered-X: Adaptive Notch	0.006	3.3

feedback-path models for all possible input signals, the filter $P(f)$ should change dynamically to whiten any input to the cross-correlation operation. Thus, the fixed filter $P(f)$ should be replaced by an adaptive filter, as shown in Figure 7-15.

If the expected deviation from a flat input signal spectrum is primarily peaks due to the presence of tones, then a notch filter can be used to remove the tones while leaving the remainder of the background noise. Kates (2004) proposed using an adaptive notch filter to remove a tone at an arbitrary low frequency in the input signal. The notch filter is attractive as it can be implemented using only a few mathematical operations. Because the notch adapts, it can shift its center frequency to remove any tone within a desired frequency range, say below 4 kHz in an ITE, and multiple notches can be used in cascade to flatten the spectrum of more complex periodic inputs. Consider the example from the paragraph above, but use a single adaptive notch filter to cancel the 1-kHz sinusoid prior to the LMS adaptation. The results are presented in the bottom row of Table 7-1. The adaptive notch filter is very effective in preventing the cancellation of the 1-kHz sinusoid, and constraining the notch to lie below 4 kHz still allows the system to cancel the assumed whistle at 4 kHz.

A more general approach is to use an adaptive filter that can whiten an arbitrary input spectrum (Kates, 2004; Rafaely et al., 2003; Spriet et al., 2005) and not just remove spectral peaks. Spriet et al. (2005) show that for speech and music inputs, the use of an adaptive filter $P(f)$ greatly improves the accuracy of the feedback path model over that produced by the filtered-X algorithm using a fixed filter. Their simulation results suggest that the adaptive filter would allow up to 10 dB additional hearing-aid gain over the use of a fixed filter.

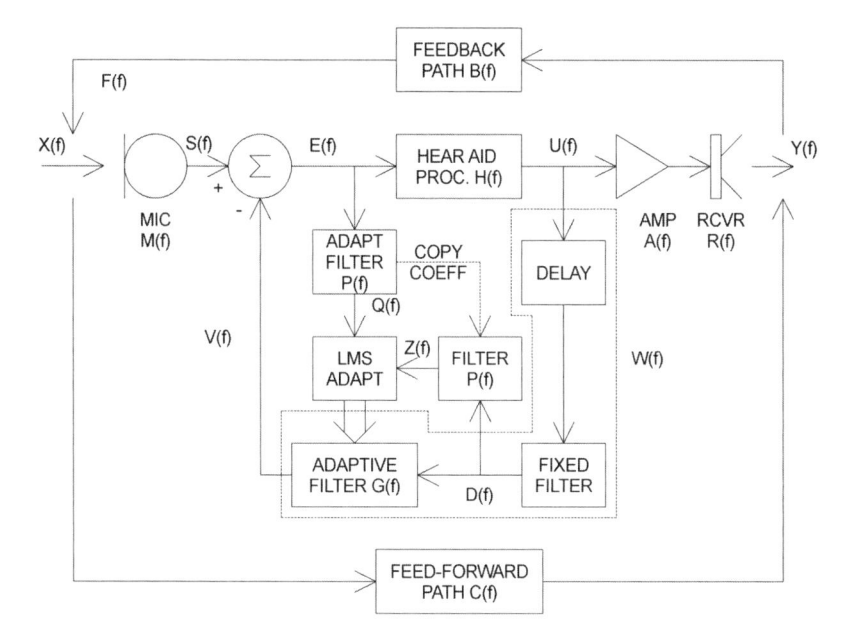

Figure 7-15. Block diagram for the filtered-X algorithm using adaptive filters to pre-whiten the input to the coefficient update.

FREQUENCY-DOMAIN ADAPTATION

The feedback-cancellation algorithms considered thus far operate in the time domain. It is also possible to implement feedback cancellation in the frequency domain. A frequency-domain system uses a filter bank or the FFT to separate the feedback path model into a group of models, each model representing the feedback behavior in a different frequency band. The adaptive filter in each band is represented by a single weight (having both a gain and a phase shift) within each frequency band. The equivalent time-domain feedback-cancellation filter is given by the inverse FFT of the frequency-domain filter described by the set of weights.

An example of a frequency-domain system (Kaelin et al., 1998; Kuo & Voepel, 1993; Wyrsch & Kaelin, 1999) is presented in Figure 7-16. This system performs all of the hearing-aid processing in the frequency domain. It uses an FFT at the input to the processing to transform the signal into the frequency domain, and an inverse FFT at the system output to return to the time domain. The adaptive feedback cancellation in one of the FFT bins is illustrated in the figure; identical processing is implemented for each of the other FFT bins. The error signal $E(k)$ is

204 Digital Hearing Aids

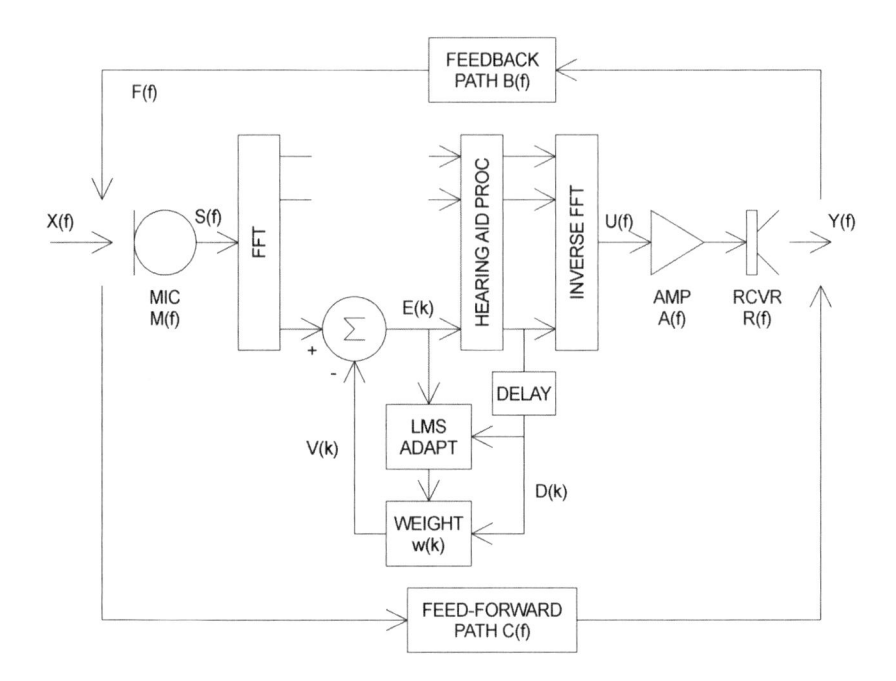

7-16. Block diagram for a frequency-domain adaptive feedback-cancellation system where the entire hearing-aid processing is implemented in the frequency domain. The feedback cancellation is shown for one of the FFT bins.

computed in the kth FFT bin, and this is cross-correlated with the delayed hearing-aid output $D(k)$ in the same frequency band to update the adaptive filter coefficient $w(k)$. The normalized LMS algorithm as given by Eq. (7.12) is typically used. The feedback path model is then $V(k) = w(k)D(k)$, which is subtracted from the input to produce the signal in the frequency band with the feedback removed.

It is also possible to update the feedback-cancellation filter in the frequency domain while the rest of the hearing-aid processing is performed in the time domain. On example of this processing strategy (Morgan & Thi, 1995) is illustrated in Figure 7-17. The adaptive feedback cancellation in one of the FFT bins is illustrated; identical processing is implemented for each of the other FFT bins. The error signal and the delayed hearing-aid output are both transformed into the frequency domain using the FFT. The outputs in each FFT bin are cross-correlated and the normalized LMS algorithm is used to update the adaptive filter coefficient $w(k)$. The feedback-cancellation filter frequency response (magnitude and phase) is completely described by the set of filter coefficients. The time-domain filter is then produced using the inverse FFT of the filter coefficients.

One advantage of frequency-domain adaptive filtering is that each filter coefficient is adapted independently of the others. In particular, the normalized LMS algorithm divides the cross-correlation in each frequency band by the power in that band, thus equalizing the signal power across the spectrum prior to updating the adaptive filter coefficients. This power normalization is equivalent to the spectral whitening provided by the filtered-X algorithm, and has the same advantage of reducing the adaptation problems caused by sinusoidal input signals.

The disadvantage of frequency-domain adaptation is the increased computational load. Division operations in digital signal processing use a lot of battery power. The normalized LMS algorithm in the time domain uses a single division to normalize the cross-correlation by the total signal power, whereas normalized LMS in the frequency domain requires a division in each frequency band. The FFT operations shown in Figure 7-17 require additional signal processing over a time-domain system as well, and will also impact the battery drain.

In summary, excellent adaptive feedback-cancellation performance can be achieved either in the time domain or in the frequency domain. The selection of one approach over the other will depend more on the practical considerations of power consumption, data memory requirements, and whether the other algorithms in the hearing aid already use FFT processing.

Processing Limitations

The progress being made in developing feedback-cancellation algorithms would lead one to believe that we will soon have hearing aids with arbitrarily large amounts of amplification, perfect fidelity, and never a feedback whistle. The real world is not quite so accommodating. Even with the filtered-X approach, there are limitations on the algorithms that will limit the amount of additional gain that can be realized in a hearing aid. Two limitations are considered in this section. One is the effect of the room in which the hearing-aid user is listening, and the other is the effect of nonlinear distortion.

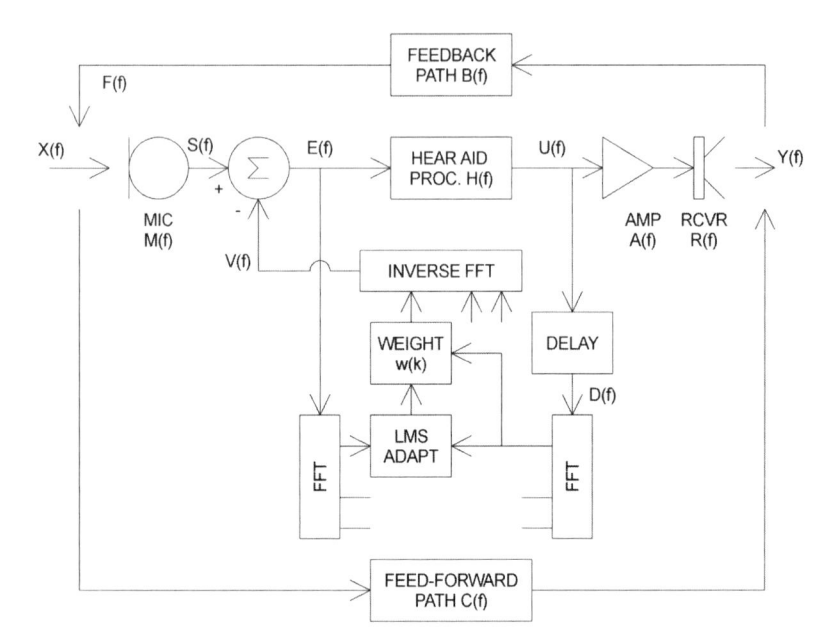

Figure 7-17. Block diagram for a frequency-domain adaptive feedback-cancellation system where only the feedback-cancellation processing is implemented in the frequency domain. The feedback cancellation is shown for one of the FFT bins.

ROOM REFLECTIONS

Measurements of feedback cancellation made in rooms, as opposed to anechoic chambers or treated test booths, generally show a maximum increase in hearing-aid gain of 10 to 15 dB. The amount of additional gain is essentially independent of the adaptive filter length for FIR filters having from 16 to 190 taps (Greenberg et al., 2000; Kates, 2001). One cause for this limitation in the benefit of the adaptive feedback cancellation is the acoustic reflections that occur in the room.

Reverberation in a room typically persists for a much longer time than the impulse responses of the electromechanical components in the hearing aid or the direct acoustic path from receiver to microphone. A short adaptive filter used to model the components and the acoustic environment in the ear canal and the local vicinity of the head will not be long enough to model the room reverberation. Changes in the reverberation as the user moves about the room will change the feedback path, but the feedback cancellation filter will not be able to model these changes. Increasing the length of the adaptive filter may not improve performance if the filter is not long enough to include the time delays corresponding to the major room reflections. Reverberation therefore becomes an important limitation to the effectiveness of feedback cancellation in hearing aids (Kates, 2001).

Measurement Procedure

The effects of reverberation on feedback cancellation were studied for feedback path measurements made in an office. A behind-the-ear (BTE) hearing aid was mounted on the right ear of an acoustic manikin. An open fitting, in which the earmold was replaced by the receiver tubing held in place with an annular support, was used to get the greatest possible intensity for the feedback path signal. The hearing aid was

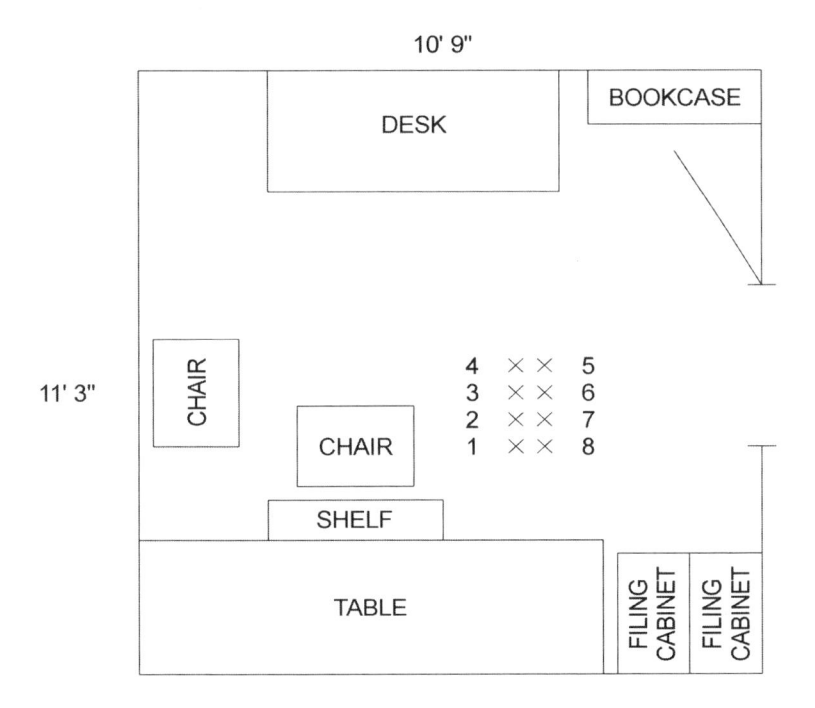

Figure 7-18. Office used for the room feedback path measurements. The measurement locations, numbered from 1 through 8, are on a grid with a 6-inch (15-cm) spacing.

connected via a cable to a real-time digital processing system, and the sampling rate was 15.625 kHz. The feedback path response was measured for the dummy head placed at eight locations in an office representative of a small room. The office floor plan is shown in Figure 7-18. The eight measurement positions are indicated by the crosses in the figure, numbered from 1 through 8, and the manikin always faced away from the office door. The measurement locations are on a grid with 6-inch (15-cm) spacing. The time delays for early reflections from the walls to either side of the manikin will shift by about 1 msec as it is moved from one location to the next, and this will shift the locations of the peaks and valleys in the feedback path frequency response perturbations caused by the reflections.

The feedback model initialization described previously was performed for each of the eight locations. The feedback path impulse response was obtained by the circular convolution of the MLS sequence with the summed response to the periodic 255-sample MLS excitation. A total of 10 sec of data was acquired at each of the eight locations in the room. The hearing aid was left in place on the dummy head as it was moved from one location to the next to determine the effects of changing position within the room. The initial feedback path model was a cascade of a delay, a fixed 5-pole IIR filter, and an adaptive FIR filter having either 8, 16, or 32 taps.

Measurement Results

The model fit to the measurement made at location 1 is presented in Figure 7-19. The actual response is given by the solid line, whereas the model is indicated by the dashed line. The model does a good job of fitting the peaks at 2.8 and 3.7 kHz, and is less accurate in fitting the magnitude frequency response at the lower levels occurring at lower and higher frequencies. However, the feedback reduction will depend primarily on the fit of the model to the actual feedback path in the vicinity of the peaks, and the errors in fitting the low-level portions of the feedback path response will have little effect on the system stability.

The measured impulse responses determined using the MLS procedure are plotted in Figure 7-20 for the eight separate room locations. It is apparent from the overlaid responses in the figure that there is very little variation during samples 100 to 150 of the impulse response as the room location is changed. This is the time interval where the ringing of the receiver resonances and the immediate acoustic effects of the ear ca-

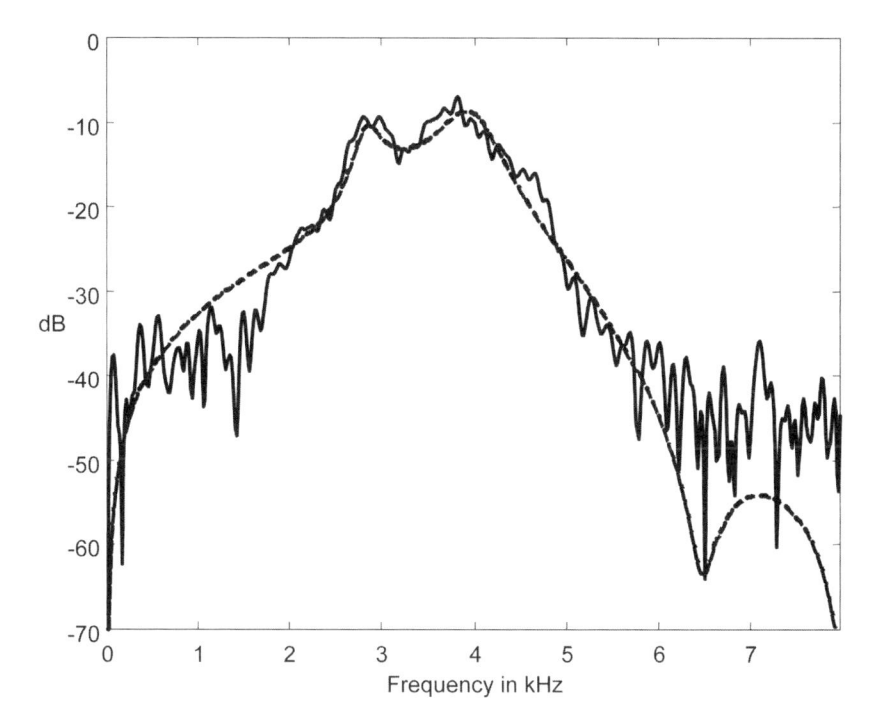

Figure 7-19. Fit of the feedback path model to the measured response at location 1 in the room.

nal and pinna would be expected to dominate, followed by the shoulder bounce (mounting board for the dummy head) approximately 20 to 25 samples later. These acoustic factors would not be expected to depend on the location within the room.

The first room reflection appears at about sample 160 in Figure 7-20. This signal is probably due to a reflection from the opened office door, as measurements made with the door closed did not show this reflection. However, substantial variation is seen in the interval between 180 and 250 samples. As the manikin is moved within the room, there will be shifts in the distance from the hearing aid to the walls near the table and desk, as shown in Figure 7-18. Thus, the reflections from these two walls will arrive at different times, creating the apparent randomness in the overlaid impulse responses. There is another strong reflection with very little variance at about 340 samples, indicating a reflection path such as a ceiling reflection that would not depend strongly on the location of the manikin in the room.

210 Digital Hearing Aids

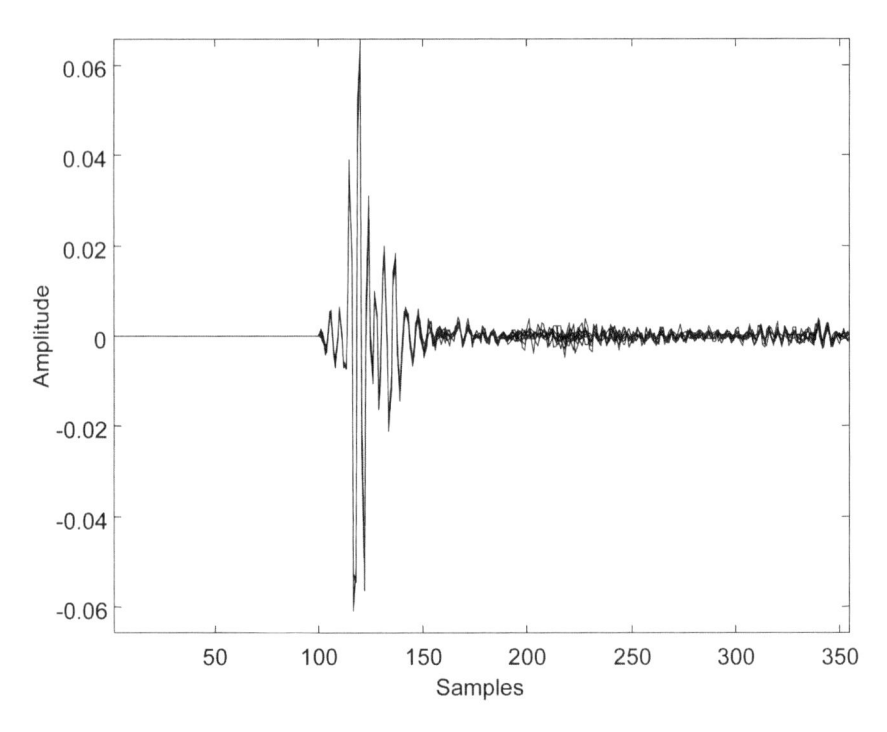

Figure 7-20. Eight feedback-path impulse responses comprising one response from each of the eight room measurement locations.

The magnitude frequency responses computed from the feedback path impulse responses of Figure 7-20 are plotted in Figure 7-21. The variation in the impulse responses translates into a corresponding variation in the frequency responses. The greatest variation in dB is at the low and high frequencies where the signal is weakest and the measurement would be most strongly affected by background noise, and the least variation occurs at the frequency response peaks. The signal will not be affected by noise in the vicinity of the peaks at 2.8 and 3.7 kHz, but the overlaid frequency response plots still span a 2-dB range around these peaks. This response variation is thus due to the changes of position of the manikin in the room, and indicate that even small displacements within the room can result in noticeable differences in the feedback path responses.

If the variation in the peaks of the feedback path frequency responses are caused by room reflections, then removing the reflections should

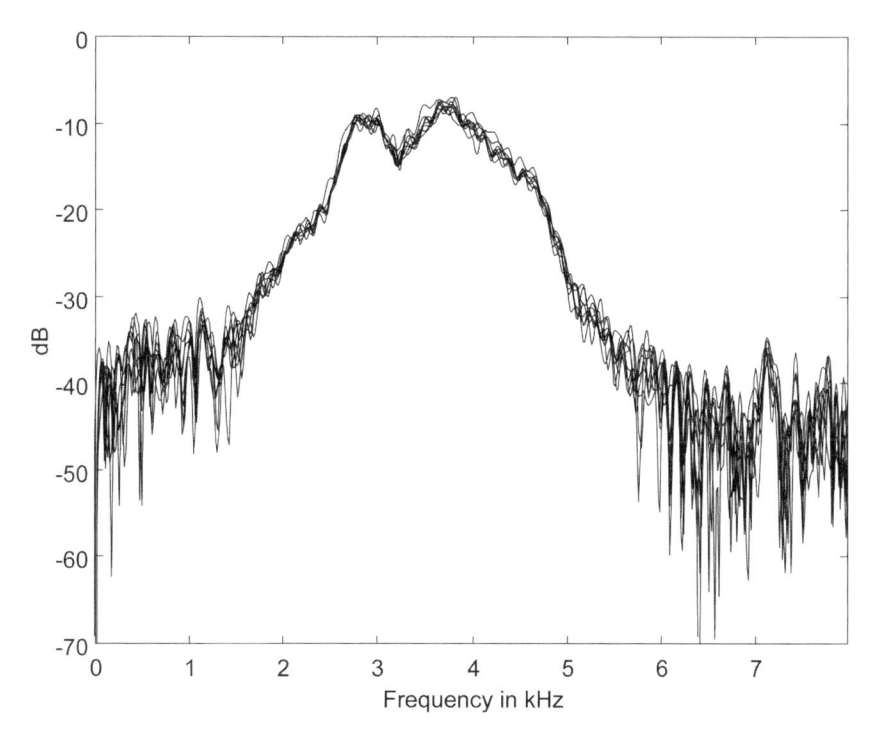

Figure 7-21. Magnitude frequency responses obtained from the eight impulse responses shown in Figure 7-18.

reduce the variation. The early part of the impulse responses is assumed to be due to the hearing aid, vent and ear acoustics, and the shoulder bounce, whereas the later part is assumed to be predominantly room reverberation. Thus windowing the impulse responses of Figure 7-20 to keep the early part of the responses while attenuating the later portion will preserve the head-level effects while suppressing the room. The result of the windowing is shown in Figure 7-22. It is clear that the superimposed frequency responses in the vicinity of the peaks in Figure 7-22 show much less variability than the corresponding curves in Figure 7-21, thus reinforcing the interpretation that the variation in the room reflection pattern from one measurement location to the next is a major factor in the feedback path.

Digital Hearing Aids

TABLE 7-2. Maximum Stable Gain (MSG) in dB for the Initial Feedback Cancellation Poles and Zeroes.

Room Location	No FB Can.	8-Tap FIR	16-Tap FIR	32-Tap FIR
1	7.0	17.1	20.4	22.1
2	7.5	18.1	18.1	21.2
3	7.6	15.7	20.5	19.2
4	7.8	15.5	19.7	19.1
5	8.0	15.3	18.6	17.4
6	7.6	15.9	21.0	21.7
7	8.1	17.4	19.7	23.4
8	8.1	16.3	21.2	21.5
Avg.	7.7	16.4	19.9	20.7

The test conditions are no feedback cancellation, an 8-tap FIR filter, a 16-tap filter, and a 32-tap filter. No filter adaptation has taken place.

Maximum Stable Gain

An important question is whether the differences in the measured feedback paths cause differences in the expected feedback cancellation performance. The results are shown in Table 7-2. The maximum stable gain (MSG) without feedback cancellation averages 7.7 dB, whereas that for the 8-tap FIR filter gives 16.4 dB, the 16-tap FIR filter gives an average of 19.9 dB, and the 32-tap FIR filter gives an average of 20.7 dB. Thus, the feedback cancellation using the 8-tap FIR filter results in a 8.7-dB improvement in the expected maximum gain over no feedback cancellation. Increasing the FIR filter length to 16 taps improves the expected performance by just 3.5 dB, and doubling the length again to 32 taps adds only an additional 0.8 dB. The 32-tap filter should be long enough to model the shoulder bounce, but this increased filter length did not make a significant improvement in feedback cancellation performance because the increased filter length is still insufficient to model the room reflections. Successfully modeling the reverberation within a room requires a much longer filter; acoustic echo cancellation, for example, can require an FIR filter of up to 4000 taps at an 8-kHz sampling rate to model the room reverberation (Haneda et al., 1994).

Even though the benefit of a longer FIR filter is limited by the presence of room reverberation, there may be some conditions where increasing the filter length will lead to measurable improvements in feedback

TABLE 7-3. Maximum Stable Gain (MSG) in dB for the Initial Feedback Cancellation Poles and Zeroes Computed for the Windowed Impulse Responses.

Room	MSG, dB			
Location	No FB Can.	8-Tap FIR	16-Tap FIR	32-Tap FIR
1	8.3	19.8	23.8	27.8
2	8.1	20.8	22.4	31.4
3	8.0	19.1	23.0	27.4
4	8.3	19.6	21.8	26.1
5	8.5	19.2	22.4	28.7
6	8.4	19.2	23.7	30.0
7	8.9	19.8	21.8	29.4
8	8.5	19.4	23.6	29.2
Avg.	8.4	19.6	22.8	28.8

The window consisted of a 10-sample linearly rising portion to the peak of the impulse response, a flat portion of 40 samples, and a linearly decreasing portion of 25 samples. The test conditions are no feedback cancellation, an 8-tap FIR filter, a 16-tap filter, and a 32-tap filter. No filter adaptation has taken place.

cancellation performance. In situations where reverberation is minimal, such as walking outdoors, the degrees of freedom in the longer filter will not be wasted trying to model the reverberation but will instead be available to model the feedback path in the vicinity of the head.

Reduced reverberation was simulated by windowing the measured impulse response. The window was the same as used for the magnitude frequency response curves of Figure 7-22. For each of the eight locations, the MSG without feedback cancellation, and the MSG with feedback cancellation using 8-tap, 16-tap, and 32-tap FIR filters were computed for the windowed impulse response data. The results are shown in Table 7-3. The MSG without feedback cancellation averages 8.4 dB, whereas that for the 8-tap FIR filter gives 19.6 dB, the 16-tap FIR filter gives an average of 22.8 dB, and the 32-tap FIR filter gives an average of 28.8 dB. Thus, the feedback cancellation using the 8-tap FIR filter results in a 11.2 dB improvement in the expected maximum gain over no feedback cancellation. Increasing the FIR filter length to 16 taps improves the expected performance by only 3.2 dB, and doubling the length again to 32 taps adds a further 6.0 dB.

These results confirm the supposition that the benefit of longer filters depends on the amount of reverberation. Increasing the number of taps in the filter allows a better model of either the reverberation or

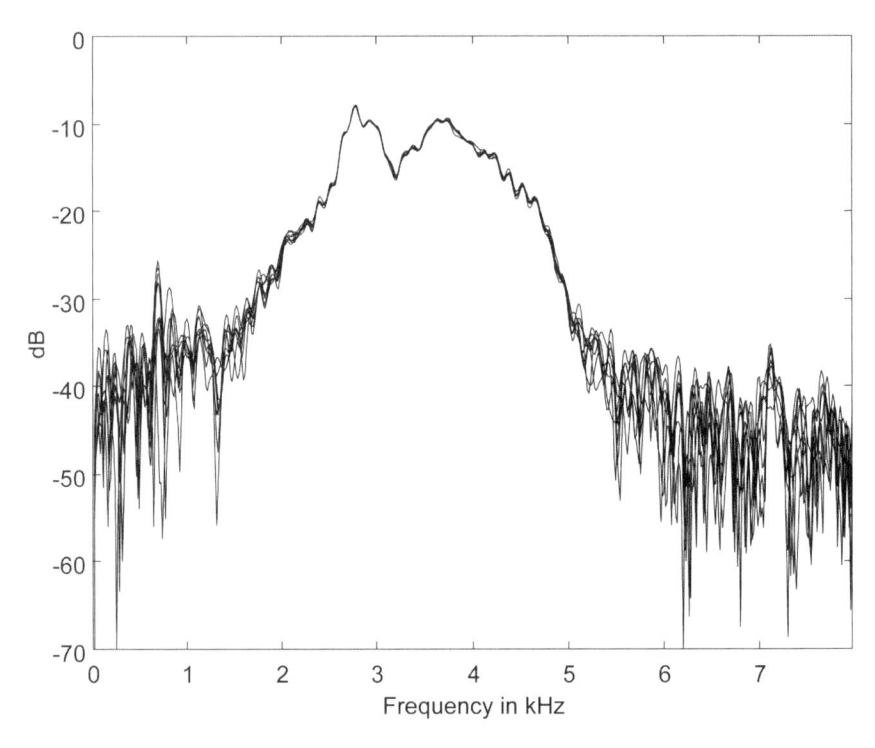

Figure 7-22. Magnitude frequency responses obtained from the eight impulse responses shown in Figure 7-18 after the reverberant tail was removed by windowing.

the residual error in the ear-level feedback path, depending on which is greater. Increasing the FIR filter length from 8 to 16 taps yielded similar results for the full-length and windowed impulse responses, which indicates that the 16-tap filter is still modeling the ear-level feedback path and not the room. The 32-tap FIR filter gave a much bigger improvement for the windowed impulse response than for the full-length response, which indicates a much better model of the ear-level response than for the shorter filters in the absence of reverberation. When reverberation is present, however, the 32-tap filter tries to model the reverberation ripples because these ripples in the frequency response are greater in magnitude than the residual errors in modeling the ear-level feedback path.

Room reverberation causes perturbations in the feedback path response that depend on the location within the room. A short feedback-cancellation filter will fit a smooth curve through the measured data, and THUS will give an average improvement that will be similar everywhere in the room because the reverberation is essentially ignored in the feedback path model. The stronger the reverberation, the less the benefit because the errors between the actual feedback path and the model will be greater. A longer filter in the absence of reverberation, as simulated by the windowed response, will do a better job of modeling the ear-level feedback path and will give additional headroom. However, the longer filter will try to model the reverberation when it is present, and very little benefit will result from the increased filter length unless the filter is long enough to substantially encompass the early reflections in the room.

NONLINEAR DISTORTION

There is an assumption hidden in the feedback cancellation algorithms. The assumption is that the hearing aid is a linear system. The feedback path model includes the microphone, hearing-aid processing, amplifier, and receiver. The model assumes that each of these components is a linear system, although the adaptive filter in the model allows for some temporal variation of the system transfer functions as long as that variation is slow. However, the amplifier and receiver in the hearing aid can produce large amounts of nonlinear distortion under some operating conditions. In a power aid, for example, the designers might choose to drive the receiver beyond the linear limits of the diaphragm suspension or magnetic circuit (Warren, 2000) in order to get sufficient output for a profound hearing loss, and the power amplifier might be driven into saturation as well. The linear model used in the feedback cancellation cannot reproduce these amplifier and receiver nonlinearities, and the presence of nonlinear distortion will limit the accuracy of the feedback path model.

As an example, consider the hearing-aid receiver. At low signal levels the receiver output can be modeled as a linear function of the input. At high signal levels, however, the diaphragm suspension runs of travel, and eventually the diaphragm will reach its maximum possible displacement. It won't be able to move any further no matter how much additional force is applied. In an ideal receiver the output could be represented a scaled version of the input:

$$y(n) = ax(n) \quad \text{Equation (7.19)}$$

In a system with nonlinear distortion, the receiver output can be modeled as a power series:

$$y(n) = \sum_{p=1}^{P} a_p x^p(n) \quad \text{Equation (7.20)}$$

One approach to feedback cancellation would therefore be to add a nonlinear power series model of the amplifier and receiver behavior to the feedback path, with the adaptive filter modeling the remaining linear acoustic behavior. A more general approach is to use a separate adaptive filter for each term in the power series expansion and then sum the outputs (Küch et al., 2005). The potential benefits of nonlinear feedback cancellation will probably only be achieved in devices, such as power aids, that operate at high levels of nonlinear distortion; for most hearing aids the limitations imposed by reverberation will most likely be reached before the limitations due to distortion.

Concluding Remarks

Feedback in a hearing aid limits the maximum gain that can be achieved in the device. The solutions to feedback fall into two broad categories: (1) gain reduction, and (2) feedback cancellation in which the feedback path is modeled mathematically and subtracted from the microphone signal. Gain reduction is a simple solution that always works if the gain is reduced sufficiently, but the loss of amplification may also reduce the audibility of speech. Feedback cancellation can improve the stability of the hearing aid and allow for up to 10 to 15 dB additional gain over an instrument that does not use feedback cancellation, and promises no detrimental modifications of the hearing-aid response.

Feedback cancellation appears to be the perfect solution, except that it has its own problems. An adaptive feedback-cancellation filter is needed to model the dynamic changes in the feedback path. However, the basic adaptive filter algorithm is sensitive to tonal input signals, and adapts to cancel the tone rather than model the feedback path. Improved algorithms, such as the filtered-X algorithm, can greatly reduce the sensitivity of the system to tonal inputs without imposing an undue computational burden. But even if the problems concerning tonal inputs can be solved, there are additional limitations caused by room reflections and nonlinear distortion. A substantial amount of progress has been made in feedback cancellation, but there is still a need for additional research.

References

Boner, C. P., & Boner, C. R. (1965). Minimizing feedback in sound systems and room ring modes with passive networks. *Journal of the Acoustical Society of America*, 37, 131–135.

Bustamante, D. K., Worrell, T. L., & Williamson, M. J. (1989). Measurement of adaptive suppression of acoustic feedback in hearing aids. *Proceedings of the 1989 International Conference on Acoustic Speech and Signal Processing*, Glasgow (pp. 2017–2020).

Chi, H. -F., Gao, S., Soli, S. D., & Alwan, A. (2003). Band-limited feedback cancellation with a modified filtered-X LMS algorithm for hearing aids. *Speech Communication*, 39, 147–161.

Dyrlund, O., & Bisgaard, N. (1991). Acoustic feedback margin improvements in hearing instruments using a prototype DFS (digital feedback suppression) system. *Scandinavian Audiology*, 20, 49–53.

Dyrlund, O., Henningsen, L. B., Bisgaard, N., & Jensen, J. H. (1994). Digital feedback suppression (DFS): Characterization of feedback-margin improvements in a DFS hearing instrument. *Scandinavian Audiology*, 23, 135–138.

Egolf, D. (1982). Review of the acoustic feedback literature from a control systems point of view. G. A. Studebaker & F. H. Bess, (Eds.) In *The Vanderbilt Hearing-Aid Report*, (pp. 87–90), Upper Darby, PA: Monographs in Contemporary Audiology.

Egolf, D., Howell, H., Weaver, K., & Barker, S. (1985). The hearing aid feedback path: Mathematical simulation and experimental verification. *Journal of the Acoustical Society of America*, 78, 1578–1587.

Engebretson, A. M., & French-St. George, M. (1993). Properties of an adaptive feedback equalization algorithm. *Journal of Rehabilitation Research and Developments*, 30, 8–16.

Engebretson, A. M., O'Connell, M. P., & Gong, F. (1990). An adaptive feedback equalization algorithm for the CID digital hearing aid. *Proceedings of the 12th Annual International Conference of the IEEE Engineering in Medicine and Biology Society*, Part 5, (pp. 2286–2287), Philadelphia.

Greenberg, J. E., Zurek, P. M., & Brantley, M. (2000). Evaluation of feedback-reduction algorithms for hearing aids. *Journal of the Acoustical Society of America*, 108, 2366–2376.

Haneda, Y., Makino, S., & Kaneda, Y. (1994). Common acoustical pole and zero modeling of room transfer functions. *IEEE Transactions on Speech and Audio Processing, 2*, 320–328.

Haykin, S. (1996). *Adaptive filter theory* (3rd ed.). Upper Saddle River, NJ: Prentice-Hall.

Hellgren, J. (2002). Analysis of feedback cancellation in hearing aids with Filtered-X LMS and the direct method of closed loop identification. *IEEE Transactions on Speech and Audio Processing, 10*, 119–131.

Hellgren, J., Lunner, T., & Arlinger, S. (1999). System identification of feedback in hearing aids. *Journal of the Acoustical Society of America, 105*, 3481–3496.

Kaelin, A., Lindgren, A., & Wyrsch, S. (1998). A digital frequency-domain implementation of a very high gain hearing aid with compensation for recruitment of loudness and acoustic echo cancellation. *Signal Processing, 64*, 71–85.

Kates, J. M. (1988). A computer simulation of hearing aid response and the effects of ear canal size. *Journal of the Acoustical Society of America, 83*, 1952–1963.

Kates, J. M. (1991). Feedback cancellation in hearing aids: Results from a computer simulation. *IEEE Transactions on Signal Processing, 39*, 553–562.

Kates, J. M. (1999). Constrained adaptation for feedback cancellation in hearing aids. *Journal of the Acoustical Society of America, 106*, 1010–1019.

Kates, J. M. (2001). Room reverberation effects in hearing aid feedback cancellation. *Journal of the Acoustical Society of America, 109*, 367–378.

Kates, J. M. (2002). Adaptive feedback cancellation in hearing aids. In J. Benesty & Y. Huang (Eds.), *Adaptive signal processing* (pp. 23–57). New York: Springer.

Kates, J. M. (2004). *Feedback cancellation in a hearing aid with reduced sensitivity to low-frequency inputs.* U.S. Patent 6,831,986, issued December 14, 2004.

Küch, F., Mitnacht, A., & Kellermann, W. (2005). Nonlinear acoustic echo cancellation using adaptive orthogonalized power filters. *Proceedings of the International Conference on Acoustic and Signal Processing, 2005*, Philadelphia.

Kuo, S. M., & Voepel, S. (1993). Digital hearing aid with the lapped transform. *Digital Signal Processing, 3*, 228–239.

Ljung, L. (1987). *System identification: Theory for the user.* Englewood Cliffs, NJ: Prentice-Hall.

Lybarger, S. F. (1982). In G. A. Studebaker & F. H. Bess, (Eds.), *The Vanderbilt Hearing-Aid Report* (pp. 87–90). Acoustic feedback control. Upper Darby, PA: Monographs in Contemporary Audiology.

Macrae, J. (1983, January). Vents for high-powered hearing aids. *Hearing Journal*, pp. 13–16.

Maxwell, J. A., & Zurek, P. M. (1995). Reducing acoustic feedback in hearing aids. *IEEE Transactions on Speech and Audio Processing, 3*, 304–313.

Morgan, D. R. & Thi, J. C. (1995). A delayless subband adaptive filter architecture. *IEEE Transactions on Signal Processing, 43*, 1819–1830.

Odelius, J. (2003). *Generation of probe signal for feedback cancellation systems*. Masters Thesis Reg nr: LiTH-ISY-EX-3449, Linköpings Universitet, Linköpings, Sweden.

Patronis, E. T. (1978). Electronic detection of acoustic feedback and automatic sound system gain control. *Journal of the Audio Engineering Society, 26*, 323–326.

Rafaely, B., & Hayes, J. L. (2001). On the modeling of the vent path in hearing aid systems. *Journal of the Acoustical Society of America, 109*, 1747–1749.

Rafaely, B., Shusina, N. A., & Hayes, J. L. (2003). Robust compensation with adaptive feedback cancellation in hearing aids. *Speech Communication, 39*, 163–170.

Rife, D. D., & Vanderkooy, J. (1989). Transfer-function measurement with maximum-length sequences. *Journal of the Audio Engineering Society, 37*, 419–444.

Schneider, T., & Jamieson, D. G. (1993). A dual-channel MLS-based test system for hearing-aid characterization. *Journal of the Audio Engineering Society, 41*, 583–594.

Siqueira, M. G., & Alwan, A. (2000). Steady-state analysis of continuous adaptation in acoustic feedback reduction systems for hearing aids. *IEEE Transactions on Speech and Audio Processing, 8*, 443–453.

Spriet, A., Proudler, I., Moonen, M., & Wouters, J. (2005). Adaptive feedback cancellation in hearing aids with linear prediction of the desired signal. *IEEE Transactions on Signal Processing, 53*, 3749–3763.

Stinson, M. R., & Daigle, G. A. (2004). Effect of handset proximity on hearing aid feedback. *Journal of the Acoustical Society of America, 115*, 1147–1156.

Vanderkooy, J. (1994). Aspects of MLS measuring systems. *Journal of the Audio Engineering Society, 42*, 219–231.

Warren, D. M. (2000). *Differential-algebraic equations governing nonlinear transducer networks*. Preprint 5223, 109th Audio Engineering Society Convention, Los Angeles, August, 2000.

Widrow, B., McCool, J. M., Larimore, M. G., & Johnson, C. R., Jr. (1976). Stationary and nonstationary learning characteristics of the LMS adaptive filter. *Proceedings of the IEEE, 64*, 1151–1162.

Wyrsch, S., & Kaelin, A. (1999). Adaptive feedback cancellation in subbands for hearing aids. *Proceedings of the International Conference on Acoustic Speech and Signal Processing, 2*, (pp. 921–924), Phoenix, AZ, March 15–19, 1999.

8

Dynamic-Range Compression

THIS CHAPTER PROVIDES AN OVERVIEW of dynamic-range compression in digital hearing aids. The focus of the chapter is on the technology used to build digital compression systems. The rationale for compression is to compensate for the reduced dynamic range found in the impaired ear and the increased growth of loudness (recruitment) that accompanies hearing loss. Several survey papers (Braida et al., 1979; Dillon, 1996; Souza, 2002) have presented overviews of compression algorithms and their effectiveness from an audiologic perspective. The results have been mixed; nonetheless, multichannel compression is implemented in the vast majority of digital hearing aids. There is also an on-going argument as to whether compression time constants should be fast (syllabic) to render audible all portions of the speech signal (Villchur, 1973), or slow to preserve the speech envelope modulation (Plomp, 1988). The effects of different time constants on the processed signal are illustrated in this chapter, but the perceptual consequences of different compression schemes are left to other authors.

This chapter begins with a summary of just a few of the many papers that have been published investigating the effects of compression on speech intelligibility and sound quality. It proceeds to a discussion of some signal-processing concerns, and then single-channel compression.

Even though most digital hearing aids use multichannel compression, a single-channel system is useful for illustrating the effects of the rule that determines the amount of amplification as a function of signal level, the effects of a volume control on a compressor, and the procedures used to estimate the signal level. Multichannel compression is then presented, and the temporal and frequency-domain behavior of a multichannel system are described. A multichannel system can be implemented using a filter bank or using an FFT approach, and FFT-based compressors are discussed next. Filter banks and FFT compressors can add distortion to the processed signal, but much of the distortion can be avoided using a side-branch structure. An old idea in signal processing, but new in hearing aids, is to use digital frequency warping to modify the frequency analysis in the digital hearing aid to more closely match that of the human auditory system. The chapter concludes with an explanation of frequency warping and its use as the basis for compression.

Does Compression Help?

One of the justifications for compression is compensation for recruitment. But Plomp (1994) comments that recruitment is not necessarily bad; he claims that it increases the speech envelope modulation depth and reduces the interaction between sounds. To test the effects of recruitment, Nejime and Moore (1997) simulated a hearing loss in normal-hearing subjects. They used dynamic-range expansion to simulate recruitment and spectral smearing to simulate the reduced frequency resolution found in impaired ears. They found that the simulated recruitment, when combined with NAL-R amplification, did not reduce speech intelligibility in stationary noise when compared with normal hearing. Thus, the assumption that syllabic compression is needed to compensate for recruitment does not appear to be valid as long as the speech is amplified above threshold.

Experiments measuring the perceptual benefits for dynamic-range compression have given mixed results. For example, Neuman et al. (1994), in a study of listener preferences, found that compression ratios less than 2:1 were preferred for all conditions. The linear system (compression ratio of 1:1) was preferred for the multitalker babble by those listeners with a residual dynamic range greater than 30 dB, whereas those subjects with a residual dynamic range of less than 30 dB preferred a compression ratio of 1.5:1 or 2:1. However, Souza et al. (2005) found that listeners with severe hearing loss had lower intelligibility and preference scores for a three-channel compression system than for compression limiting. Humes et al. (1999) compared analog linear to two-channel wide dynamic-range compression aids, and found that the compression instrument gave better speech intelligibility for sentence test materials at 50 or 60 dB SPL in quiet, but that the linear instrument gave better intelligibility for the materials at 75 dB SPL in babble at a SNR of 10 or 5 dB. However, Walden et al. (2000) found improved intelligibility and listener preferences for a wide dynamic-range compression hearing aid over one with just compression limiting.

The best number of channels to use in multichannel compression systems is also unclear. Keidser and Grant (2001) found that increasing the number of channels from one to four had no significant effect on speech intelligibility, and most subjects did not have a preference in paired-comparison tests. Moore et al. (1999) found that the number of compression channels had no significant effect on the speech reception threshold (SRT) for a single interfering talker, although multichannel compressors showed a small (less than 1 dB) but significant advantage compared to linear amplification. For modulated noise, the compression conditions also showed small but statistically significant benefits over linear amplification, and the one-channel compressor showed a small (0.7 dB) but not significant advantage over the multichannel systems. Van Buuren et al. (1999) compared compression systems having 1, 4, and 16 channels for compression ratios ranging from 0.25:1 to 4:1. For the hearing-impaired subjects, the SRT was lower (better) for the single-channel system than for the four-channel system, which in turn was better than the 16-channel system, although the differences were small. Pleasantness for speech and music were both highest for the single-channel compressor and lowest for the 16-channel system for compression ratios greater than 1:1. Plomp (1994) found that, for speech-shaped stationary noise at a SNR equal to SRT + 2 dB, the speech intelligibility for hearing-impaired listeners decreased as the number of compression channels was increased from one to 16, and the higher the compression ratio, the greater the loss in intelligibility.

The parameters in a compression system are the number of frequency channels, and the compression ratios, attack times, and release times in each frequency band. It may well be that the optimum compressor adjustment is a function of the type and amount of background noise or interference and the characteristics of the individual hearing loss. Identifying different sound environments for the purpose of adjusting compression or other signal-processing system parameters is the subject of Chapter 12. This chapter focuses on the design and signal-processing behavior of wide dynamic range compression systems.

Algorithm Design Concerns

As with any algorithm design, a dynamic-range compressor involves several engineering tradeoffs. It is important to realize that there is no single best compressor design. Each system involves tradeoffs between processing complexity, frequency resolution, time delay, and quantization noise. The most important processing concerns are the system frequency resolution and the processing time delay. Most digital compression systems use multiple frequency bands. For any given processing approach, increased frequency resolution comes at the price of increased processing delay.

FREQUENCY RESOLUTION

One concern in designing a multichannel compressor is to match the frequency resolution of the digital system to the resolution of the human auditory system. For example, several hearing-aid fitting procedures are based on loudness scaling in the impaired ear (Dillon et al., 1997), and the estimation of loudness presupposes an auditory frequency analysis. Digital frequency analysis, such as the discrete Fourier transform, typically provides constant-bandwidth frequency resolution. The frequency resolution of the human auditory system, however, is more accurately modeled by a filter bank having a nearly constant bandwidth at low frequencies but with bandwidth becoming proportional to frequency as the frequency increases (Moore & Glasberg, 1983; Zwicker & Terhardt 1980).

PROCESSING DELAY

A second concern in designing a compression system for a hearing aid is the overall processing delay. Time delays can cause coloration effects to occur in the user's ear when the hearing-aid user is talking. When talking, the talker's own voice reaches the cochlea with minimal delay via bone conduction and through the hearing-aid vent. This signal interacts with the delayed and amplified signal produced by the hearing aid to produce a comb-filtered spectrum at the cochlea. An example of the filter that results when a signal is combined with a delayed version of itself with a delay of 10 msec is plotted in Figure 8-1. The comb filter for this delay has peaks at multiples of 100 Hz, and deep valleys in between the peaks. If the fundamental frequency for a vowel overlays one of the peaks it will be audible, but if the fundamental lies in one of the valleys the speech will be strongly attenuated. Shifts in the vowel fundamental frequency will therefore result in amplitude modulation of the signal. Delays as short as 3 to 6 msec are detectible (Agnew & Thornton, 2000; Stone & Moore, 2002), and overall delays in the range of 15 to 20 msec can be judged disturbing or objectionable (Stone & Moore, 1999, 2002, 2005). These delay effects are also a factor in designing binaural systems as discussed in Chapter 13.

The system frequency-dependent delay can also introduce audible artifacts when listening to speech even when the user of the hearing aid

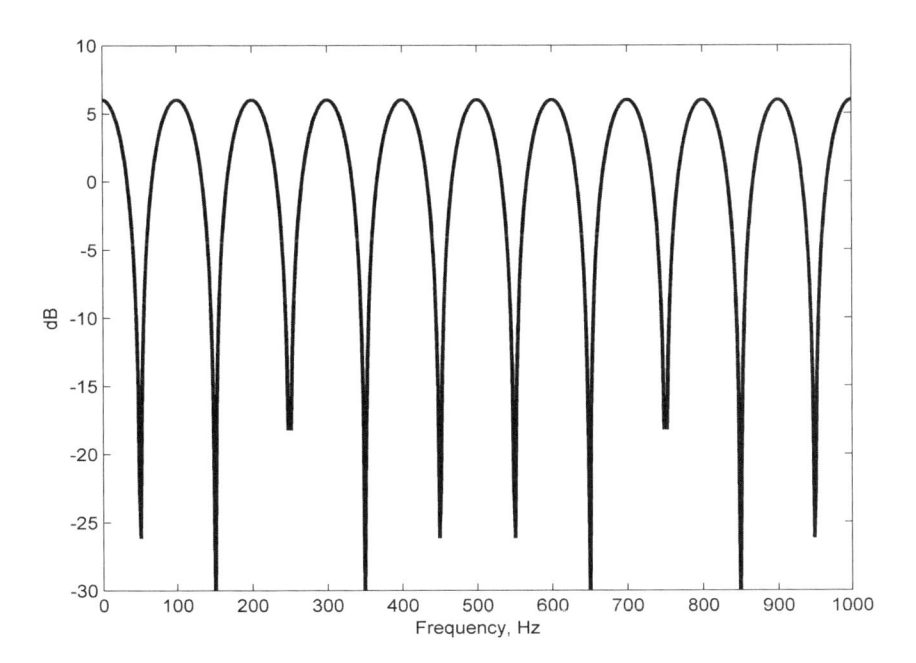

Figure 8-1. Magnitude frequency response for a signal combined with a delayed version of itself for a delay of 10 msec.

is not talking. For example, a click is converted into a descending chirp when passed through a cascade of all-pass filters having a group delay that is greater at low frequencies than at high frequencies. Relatively short delays can be detected for click stimuli when the group delay varies across frequency. Blauert and Laws (1978) passed clicks through all-pass filters giving increased delay in narrow frequency regions, and found that normal-hearing subjects can detect delays as short as 1 msec at 2 kHz, with the detection threshold increasing to 2 msec at 8 kHz or 1 kHz. Kates and Arehart (2005) found that the threshold of detection using a click stimulus was about 2 msec for normal-hearing listeners when the low frequencies were delayed relative to the high frequencies, and about 4 msec for hearing-impaired listeners.

Group-delay detection thresholds for speech are greater than for clicks. Kates and Arehart (2005) found that the detection thresholds in their experiment were approximately doubled when the click stimulus was replaced by speech for both the normal-hearing and hearing-impaired listeners. Based on results using one normal-hearing subject, Greer (1975) reported that for narrow-band all-pass filters the detection thresholds for speech sounds were 4 to 8 msec for a plosive, 8 to 16 msec for a vowel, and 16 to 32 msec for a fricative. For broader all-pass filters, having bandwidths approximately equal to the filter center frequency, the detection thresholds were 2 to 4 msec for a plosive, 2 to 4 msec for a vowel, and 4 to 8 msec for a fricative. The frequency-dependent group delay also can interfere with speech intelligibility, but at delays that greatly exceed the detection thresholds. Stone and Moore (2003) found that hearing-impaired listeners' identification of nonsense syllables decreased by a small but significant amount as the low-frequency delay was increased from no delay to a 24-msec delay compared to the delay at high frequencies.

In summary, overall delays as short as 3 msec and frequency-dependent delays as short as 2 msec can be detected for clicks and short-duration speech events, but the detectable delay is much longer for long-duration speech sounds such as vowels. Furthermore, hearing-impaired listeners appear to have greater thresholds than normal-hearing listeners. Based on these results, a hearing aid having a delay less than about 15 msec will, in all likelihood, not cause an objectionable detriment in sound quality or speech production. However, a shorter delay will always be better assuming that no other processing objectives have been compromised.

Single-Channel Compression

The simplest compression system operates on the entire signal without dividing it into separate frequency regions. Most digital hearing aids use multichannel compression, in which different frequency regions are processed independently. However, the basic building blocks of a compressor—the compression rule, volume control, and envelope detection used to control the compression—are the same in the single-channel and multichannel systems. We therefore use the single-channel compressor to introduce these concepts, after which we progress to the more complicated multichannel compression.

INPUT/OUTPUT RULES

The operation of a compressor is typically a two-step process. The compressor determines the signal level using a peak detector or related processing, and the peak-detector output is then used to determine the compression gain. The transformation that gives the signal output level as a function of the peak-detector level is termed the compression rule. The compression rule is normally plotted giving the output level as a function of the input level. As will be shown below, the peak detector output may differ substantially from the instantaneous input signal level during rapid changes in the signal. Thus, the compression rule as normally plotted is accurate only for steady-state signals.

The steady-state input/output relationship for a wide-dynamic-range compression hearing aid is plotted in Figure 8-2. For input levels below the lower compression kneepoint (typically 40–50 dB SPL), the system provides a constant linear gain. The lower kneepoint is intended to allow the amplification of low-intensity speech sounds while preventing the over-amplification of background noise. For input levels above the upper kneepoint (typically 85–100 dB SPL), the system provides compression limiting, in which the output level remains constant despite the changes in the input level. Compression limiting is intended to prevent uncomfortably loud levels from being presented to the user, and also serves to prevent overloading the amplifier circuitry. For input levels between the kneepoints, the system provides dynamic-range compression. The output level increases by 1/CR dB for each dB increase in the input level, where CR is the compression ratio. Thus, for a 2:1 compression ratio, an increase in the signal level of 2 dB results in an increase in the output level of just 1 dB.

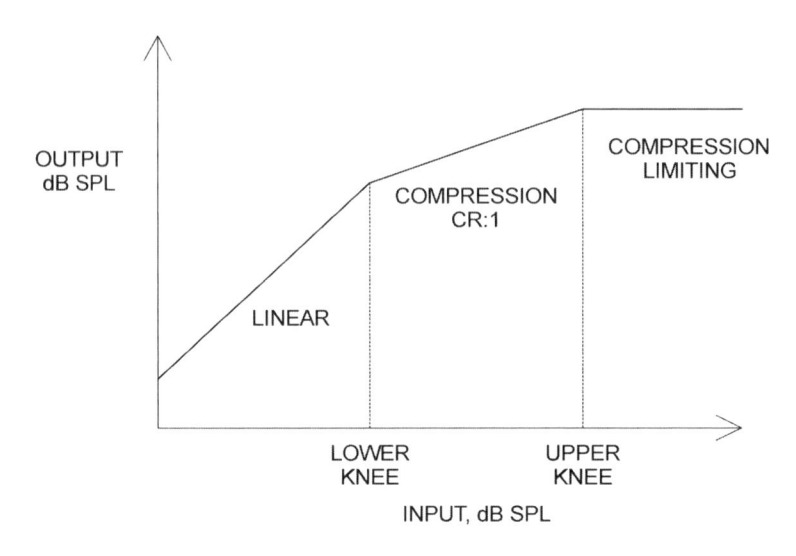

Figure 8-2. Steady-state input/output relationship for a typical hearing-aid compression system.

Other compression rules can also be used in hearing aids. One example is plotted in Figure 8-3. The intent in this system is to suppress background noise. The compression and compression limiting sections of the rule are the same as in Figure 8-2. However, below the lower kneepoint the system reduces the gain as the input level is reduced. The lower the input signal level, the lower the gain provided by the hearing aid. Thus, low level signals, assumed to be background noise, are attenuated relative to the low-level speech. There is a potential problem with expanding low-level signals, however, as the expansion will amplify the peaks more than the valleys in the noise, thus amplifying the noise envelope fluctuations and creating additional annoyance.

A second variation on the compression rule is plotted in Figure 8-4. The intent in this system is to give a more natural perception of loudness at high signal levels. For many hearing-impaired listeners, the perception of loudness at high signal levels is similar to that of normal-hearing listeners (Hellman & Meiselman, 1990). One could therefore argue that the hearing aid, at high input signal levels, should provide linear amplification with 0 dB gain. The compression rule of Figure 8-4 provides compression above the lower kneepoint, but above the upper

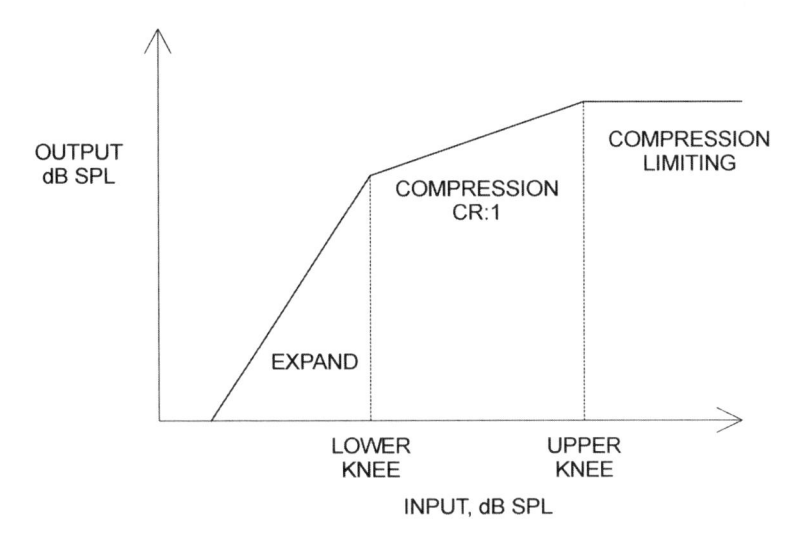

Figure 8-3. Steady-state input/output relationship for a hearing-aid compression system incorporating low-level expansion.

compression kneepoint changes over to linear amplification. Compression limiting then is implemented at signal levels high enough to be uncomfortably loud.

VOLUME CONTROL

Analog hearing aids typically have a volume control, with the volume control placed after the compression stage of the hearing aid (Cole, 1993). The compressor operates in a feedback configuration, as illustrated in Figure 8-5. The block labeled "Detect" determines the signal level, and the block labeled "Comp." compresses the signal level. The hearing-aid designer has several options as to where the volume control is to be placed. Each option, as shown by the A, B, and C in the figure, gives a different family of input/output curves as the volume control is adjusted by the user.

Assume that the compression system is configured as a high-level limiter. Increasing the signal level at control point A increases the output level of the compressed signal and also increases the input level to the compression control circuit. There is therefore an increase in amplitude for signal levels below the limiting threshold, but the limiting threshold is reached sooner. The volume control thus simultane-

230 Digital Hearing Aids

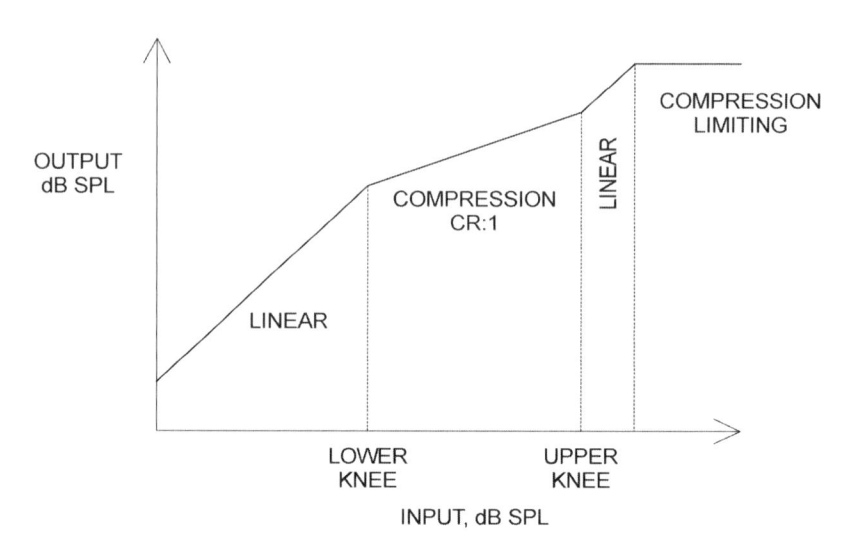

Figure 8-4. Steady-state input/output relationship for a hearing-aid compression system incorporating linear amplification for high-intensity sounds.

ously adjusts the gain and the compression threshold, and a separate trimmer is used to adjust the maximum output level. This operation is termed output automatic gain control (AGC) as the output level is limited.

Increasing the signal level at control point B in Figure 8-5 increases the level of the compressed signal but has no effect on the input level to the compression control circuit. The gain and maximum output levels are simultaneously adjusted by the volume control, but the input-referred compression threshold is unaffected. A separate trimmer adjustment is normally provided for the compression threshold. This operation is termed input AGC. Increasing the signal level at control point C in Figure 8-5 increases the level of the input to the detector but does not affect the level of the compressed signal. Increasing the volume control output at this point increases the signal level at the input to the detector, which in turn causes a decrease in the compression gain and a lower hearing-aid output.

Digital hearing aids typically use feed-forward compression, as shown in Figure 8-6. The signal detection block extracts the incoming signal level, and this level is used to compute the compression gain. A volume control often is not provided in a digital instrument given the assump-

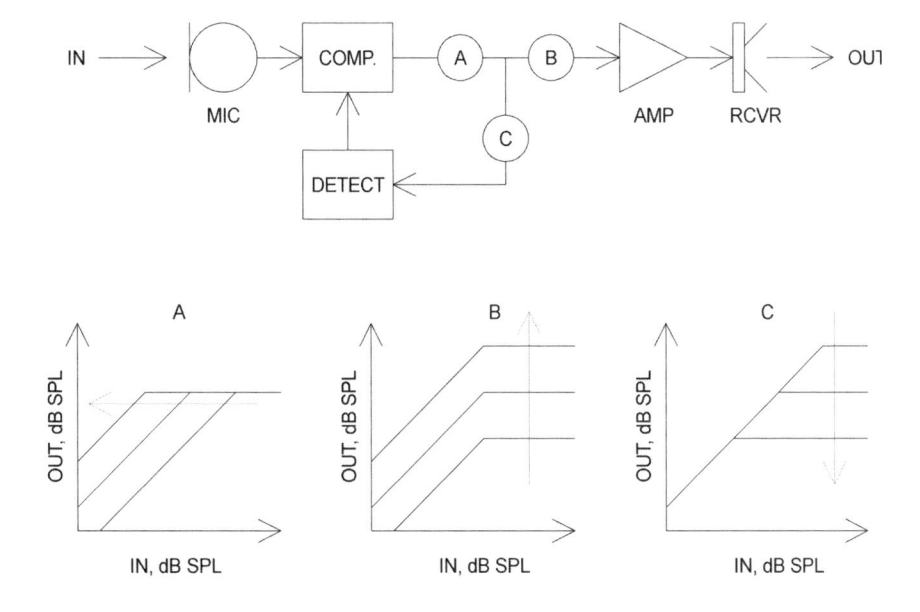

Figure 8-5. Block diagram of a compression hearing aid using feedback compression control. The volume-control gain points are indicated by A, B, and C. The corresponding input/output functions are shown along the bottom of the figure (after Cole, 1993). The arrows show the effects of increasing the gain at the indicated points.

tion that wide-dynamic-range compression will place every sound at a comfortable listening level. If a volume control is provided, however, the placement of the control will affect the compression behavior in a manner similar to that of the feedback compression shown in Figure 8-5. The volume control at position B shifts the level of the compressed signal, whereas a volume control at position A shifts both the input to the compression amplifier and the input to the level detector.

ENVELOPE DETECTION

The envelope detection comprises the dynamic part of the compressor. The output of the envelope detector is the estimate of the signal level, and this estimate forms the input to the compression rule. The dynamic behavior of the compressor therefore depends on the design of the envelope detector.

The envelope detector needs to satisfy several requirements. The

232 Digital Hearing Aids

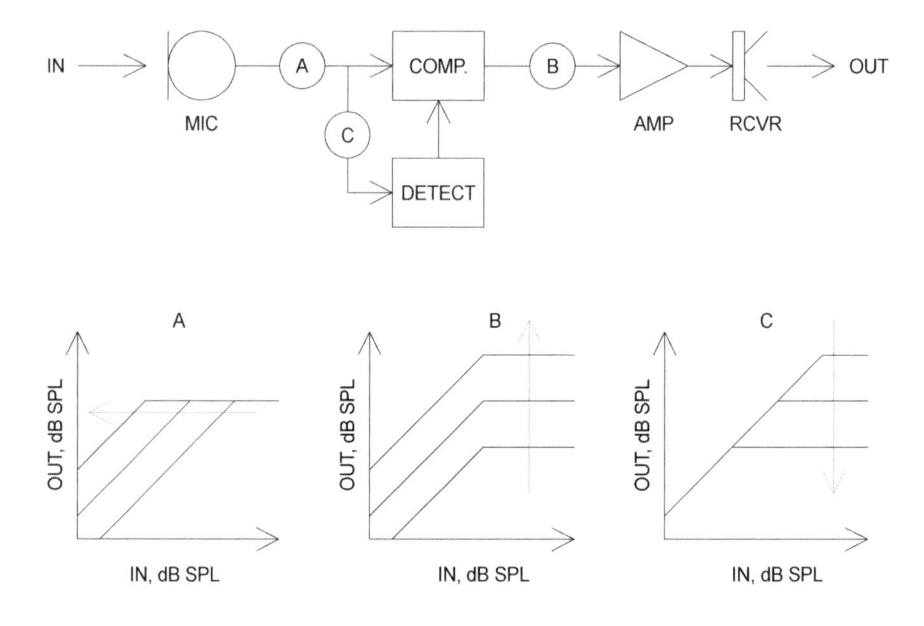

Figure 8-6. Block diagram of a compression hearing aid using feed-forward compression control. The volume-control gain points are indicated by A, B, and C. The corresponding input/output functions are shown along the bottom of the figure. The arrows show the effects of increasing the gain at the indicated points.

detector should have a quick response to rapid increases in the input signal level to prevent saturating the digital arithmetic, overloading the output amplifier, or exceeding the listener's uncomfortable loudness level. At the same time, the detector should smooth out the variations in estimates of noise and steady-state signals to prevent audible amplitude modulation of signals that are perceived as having constant loudness. In general, overamplification of a loud sound is a greater problem than insufficient amplification of a soft sound. Thus, the envelope detector is typically designed to have a fast response to increases in the signal level to prevent overload, and a slow response to decreases in the signal level to reduce audible perturbations in the gain. This behavior gives rise to a peak detector as it tends to track the peaks of the input signal.

The peak detector output is given by:

$$\text{if } |x(n)| \geq d(n-1)$$
$$d(n) = \alpha d(n-1) + (1-\alpha)|x(n)|$$
else   Equation (8.1)
$$d(n) = \beta d(n-1)$$
end

The input signal is $x(n)$, and the peak detector output is $d(n)$. The peak detector uses a fast attack time constant α when tracking increases in the signal level and a slow release time constant β when tracking decreases. As an example, let the ANSI S3.22 (2003) attack time be 5 msec and the release time be 70 msec for a system having a sampling rate of 16 kHz. The value of α is then about 0.65 and the value of β is about 0.97. When the signal level increases above the previous peak detector output, the new peak detector output mixes in a large amount of the input absolute value and rises rapidly toward the new input. When the input is smaller than the previous peak detector output, the new peak detector output decays at a constant rate in dB/sec.

To illustrate the behavior of different envelope detectors, consider the detector response to a short segment of speech. The word "air" spoken by a male talker is plotted in Figure 8-7. The speech segment is predominantly voiced, and the pitch periods are clearly visible. The onset of the word is relatively quick, taking about 40 msec, and the transition to silence at the end takes about 100 msec. The segment is followed by a pause which is filled in by the low-level background noise of the recording.

The results for three different envelope detectors are plotted in Figure 8-8 for the segment of speech shown in Figure 8-7. For the curve labeled "Block RMS," the speech was divided into 8-msec blocks, and the root-mean-squared (RMS) level found for the signal within each block. A rapid response to increases in the signal level is provided by using a short block size. This approach has the advantage of giving the exact signal power within each block, but has the disadvantage that the RMS value cannot be computed until the entire block has been read into digital memory. Thus, the 8-msec block size requires a 8-msec processing delay; this delay, when added to the additional delays in the hearing-aid processing, is too long for most hearing-aid applications. In addition, the block boundaries are not synchronized to the pitch period, so during the vowel there are occasional jumps in the estimated signal

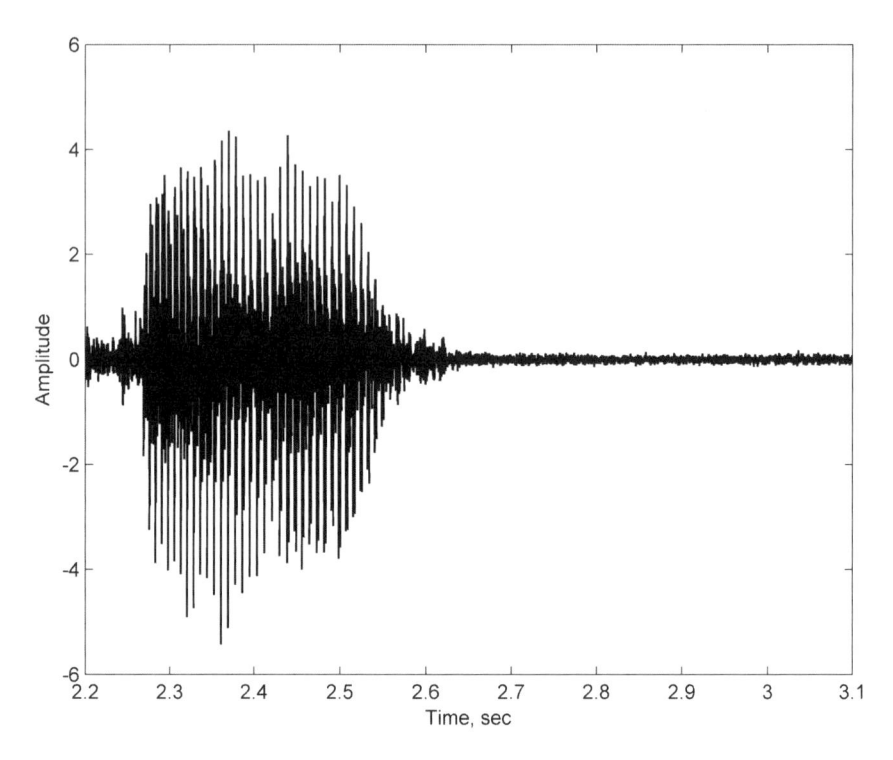

Figure 8-7. Speech segment for the word "air" from the "Rainbow Passage" spoken by a male talker.

level. Similarly, during the noise that follows the word, the block RMS levels vary in response to the fluctuations in the noise as the same minimal smoothing, provided by the block size, is used for decreases in the signal level as is used for increases.

A peak detector with short syllabic time constants was used for the curve labeled "Syllabic." The detector uses a low-pass filter to smooth the magnitude of the signal. The attack time to track increases in signal level was set to 5 msec, and the release time to track decreases in the signal level was set to 50 msec. The envelope of the syllabic peak detector lies about 3 dB above that of the block RMS detector. During the voiced speech, the syllabic peak detector shows some ripple in response to the periodic glottal pulses. At the end of the utterance, the fast release time allows the syllabic peak detector to track the decrease in the signal level as closely as the block RMS detector. In the noise segment, the syl-

Dynamic-Range Compression **235**

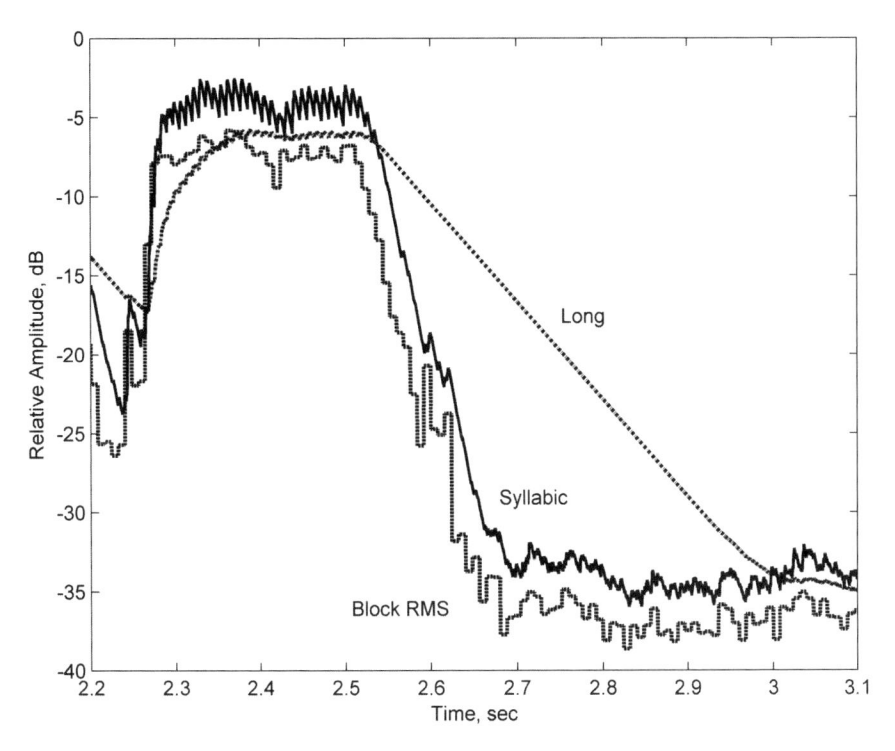

Figure 8-8. Broad-band peak detector output for the speech segment plotted in Figure 8-7. The detector curves are for the root-mean-squared (RMS) level in 8-msec blocks ("Block RMS," *dashed*), syllabic response with an ANSI attack time of 5 msec and a release time of 50 msec ("Syllabic," *solid*), and long time constants with an ANSI attack time of 50 msec and a release time of 250 msec ("Long," *dot-dash*).

labic peak detector shows level variations that are very similar to those shown by the block RMS detector.

The ripples in the peak detector output can be reduced by increasing the attack and release time. A peak detector using an attack time of 50 msec and a release time of 250 msec is indicated in Figure 8-8 by the curve labeled "Long." The longer attack and release times greatly reduce the variance in the estimated signal level during the vowel and noise segments of the utterance. However, the peak detector now responds much more slowly to changes in the input signal level. The long attack time means that the detector takes about 100 msec to respond to the onset of the vowel, during which time the compressor gain may be higher than desired because of the low estimated signal level. Similarly, the estimated signal level remains high at the end of the utterance, which will cause a reduction in gain and output level compared to the syllabic peak detector.

Multichannel Compression

A multichannel compressor, as shown in Figure 8-9, combines a filter bank with compression in each frequency band. In most implementations the compressors operate independently in each channel, although in some systems the compression gains can be grouped across adjacent bands (Kates, 1997; Levitt & Neuman, 1991). The compressed signals in each band are summed to produce the system output. The compressor output involves the response of each frequency band to the signal present in that band, and even simple signals can cause complicated responses.

TEMPORAL RESPONSE

Consider a stepped sinusoid test signal. The ANSI S3.22 (2003) test for compression dynamic behavior uses a sinusoid that jumps 35 dB in level and then returns to the original level. The envelope of a stepped 2-kHz sinusoid is plotted in Figure 8-10. The level increases by 35 dB at 200 msec and then returns to the original level at 500 msec. The frequency of 2 kHz is one of the test frequencies specified in the ANSI (2003) standard, and was chosen because it is within the pass-band of the mid-frequency filter of the three-channel filter bank illustrated in Figure 2-10. The low-frequency band of the filter bank passes signals below 1 kHz, the mid-frequency band from 1 to 2.5 kHz, and the high-frequency band above 2.5 kHz. The system sampling rate is 16 kHz.

The compressor uses independent compression in each of the three frequency bands, and the compression ratio has been set to 2:1 in each of the three channels. The system output to the stepped-sinusoid excitation is plotted in Figure 8-11. The plot has been normalized so that the highest output level is set to 0 dB. The control signal in each channel is the peak-detected filtered input, with an attack time of 5 msec and a release time of 70 msec.

There is obvious overshoot in the output for the jump in the test signal that occurs at 200 msec. The input signal level changes suddenly, but the peak detector output changes more slowly. Thus, the compres-

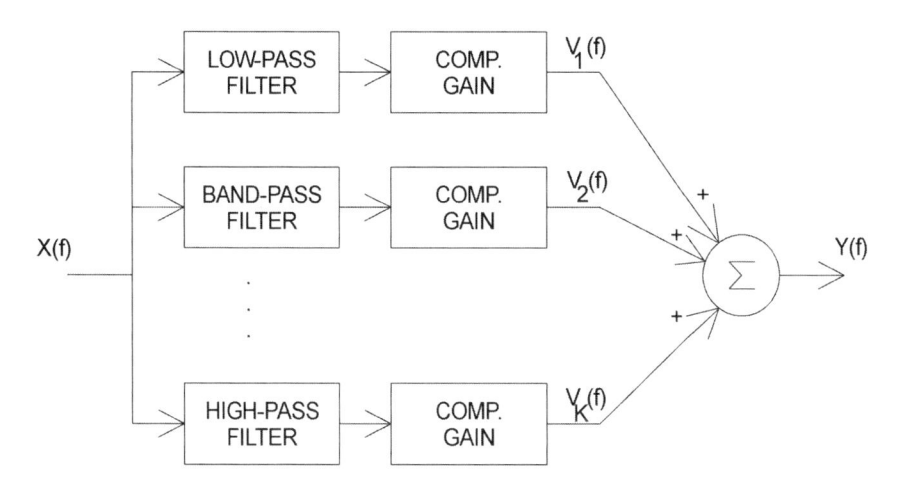

Figure 8-9. Block diagram of a multichannel compression system.

sor gain, as the input jumps, is initially set at the higher gain that corresponds to the lower initial input level. This higher gain applied to the suddenly higher input level causes the overshoot. The peak detector then reacts to the jump in the input signal; the peak detector output increases and the compressor gain goes down until it reaches steady-state for the higher signal level. The speed of the compressor gain adjustment is controlled by the attack time constant.

The sudden decrease in the test signal level that occurs at 500 msec causes the opposite behavior. The compressor gain has stabilized at the lower gain that corresponds to the 35-dB higher signal level. When the signal level is suddenly reduced, the compressor gain is still at the lower gain that corresponds to the high signal level. The lower gain applied to the new lower signal level causes the undershoot in the output. The peak detector then reacts to the reduction in the input signal; the peak detector output decreases and the compressor gain goes up until it reaches steady-state for the lower signal level. The speed of the compressor gain adjustment is controlled by the release time constant.

But notice the small amount of overshoot in the output at 500 msec in Figure 8-11 before the undershoot appears. To understand this effect, look at the individual band outputs plotted in Figure 8-12. The midfrequency band shows overshoot at the jump in the 2-kHz test signal at 200 msec and undershoot when the signal level is suddenly reduced at

238 Digital Hearing Aids

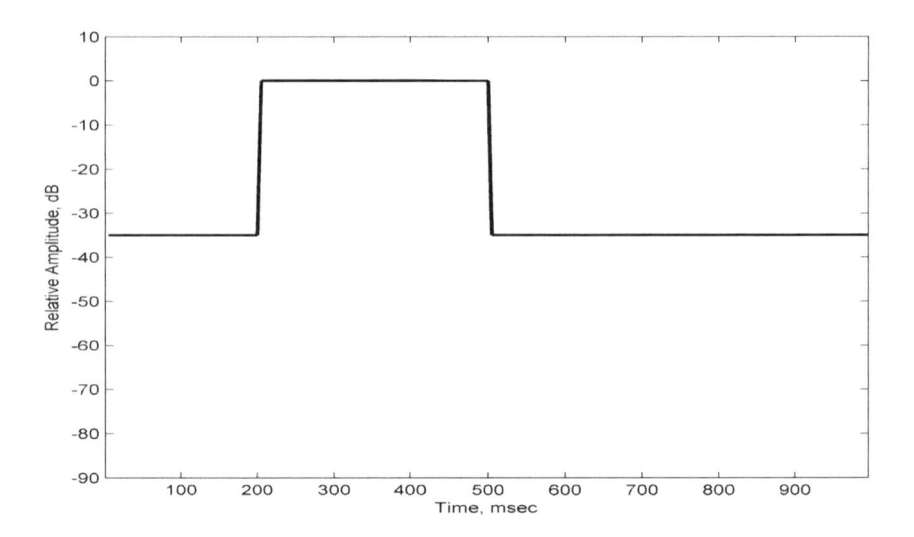

Figure 8-10. Envelope of the stepped 2-kHz sinusoid test signal.

500 msec. The low- and high-frequency bands, however, show spikes in their outputs at both the increase in signal level at 200 msec and sudden reduction at 500 msec. The spikes are the result of the spectral splatter caused by the sudden changes in signal level. Any sudden change, be it an increase or a decrease in signal level, generates a large amount spectral content across a wide frequency range. The greater the change, the greater the amount of spectral splatter.

The low- and high-frequency compression bands initially have high gains corresponding to the low signal levels in these two frequency regions. The jump in signal level at 200 msec then generates spectral content in these two bands which is amplified by the high gain that was established for the low initial input levels. The low- and high-frequency compression bands than adjust to the shift in detected signal level between 200 and 500 msec. At 500 msec the sudden decrease in the test signal level generates out-of-band spectral energy that again is amplified by the compression gains set by the detected signal level prior to the sudden decrease. The low- and high-frequency channel gains then adjust once again to the lower detected levels in each frequency band. Thus, a change in the amplitude of a signal within one frequency band can have consequences at other frequencies, and out-of-band transients can be substantially amplified by the multichannel compression.

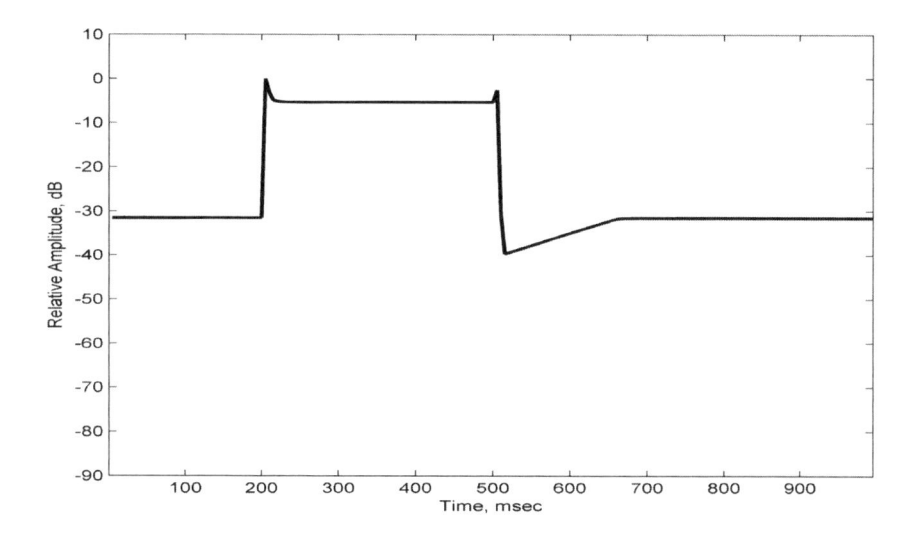

Figure 8-11. Envelope of the output of the three-band FIR filter compressor for the stepped 2-kHz test signal. The compression ratio was set to 2:1 in each frequency band.

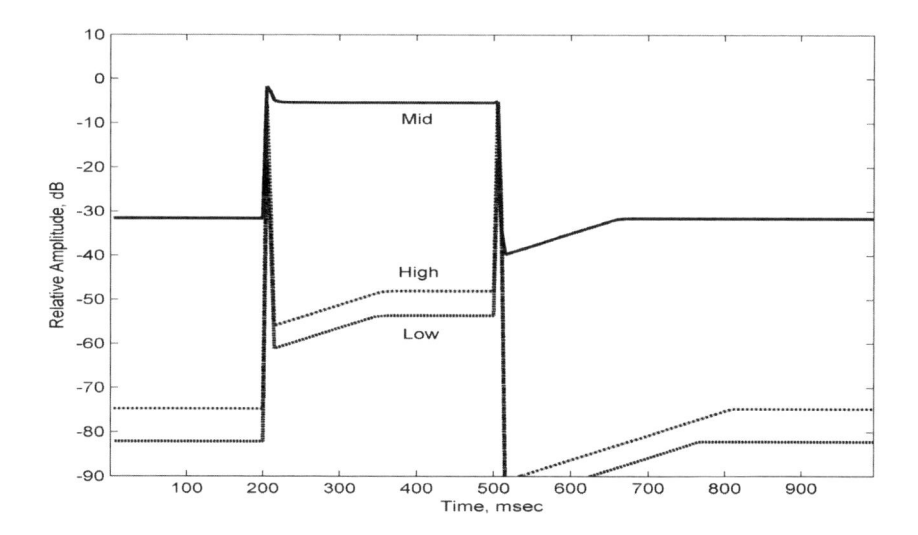

Figure 8-12. Envelope of the output in each of the three compressor bands for the stepped 2-kHz test signal.

SWEPT FREQUENCY RESPONSE

Another aspect of multiband compressor behavior is illustrated by plotting the response to a swept sinusoid. The test signal was a swept sinusoid starting at 200 Hz and continuing up to 8 kHz. The sweep was 5 sec in duration, and the instantaneous frequency as a function of time for the swept sinusoid is plotted in Figure 8-13. The compressor output to the swept sinusoid excitation is plotted in Figure 8-14. All three bands of the compressor were set to a compression ratio of 3:1 with a 5-msec attack time and a 70-msec release time. The response to 1 kHz occurs at 2190 msec and the response to 2500 Hz occurs at 3430 msec into the sweep. There is a response peak of 2 dB at each of these two frequencies, each of which corresponds to the crossover between adjacent frequency bands for the FIR filters plotted in Figure 2-10

The response peaks are the result of the filter gain at the band edges interacting with the compression amplification (Lindemann, 1997). At 1 kHz, for example, the low-frequency band and the mid-frequency band linear-phase filters both have gains of −6 dB relative to their passband responses. The reduced signal level in each frequency band causes an increase in the gain of the compression amplifier in each band compared to the gain that the compressor would have for a signal in the center of its passband. The system output is the sum of the amplified signals in the two bands. With no compression (compression ratio of 1:1), the filter outputs would combine to give the same signal level as would occur for the signal in the center of one of the filter bands. But with the 3:1 compression, the additional compressor gain caused by the reduced signal level in each band results in a peak in the system response when the band outputs are combined.

An additional source of ripple in the compressed output is the ripple in the filter sidelobes. A signal at 4 kHz, for example, will be in the passband of the high-frequency filter but in the stopbands of the mid- and low-frequency filters. The FIR filter-stopbands all have ripple, and the level of the signal in the stopbands is amplified relative to that in the filter passband by the compression. Thus, the multiband compression response to the swept sinusoid amplifies any ripples or irregularities in the filter stopband responses.

Dynamic-Range Compression 241

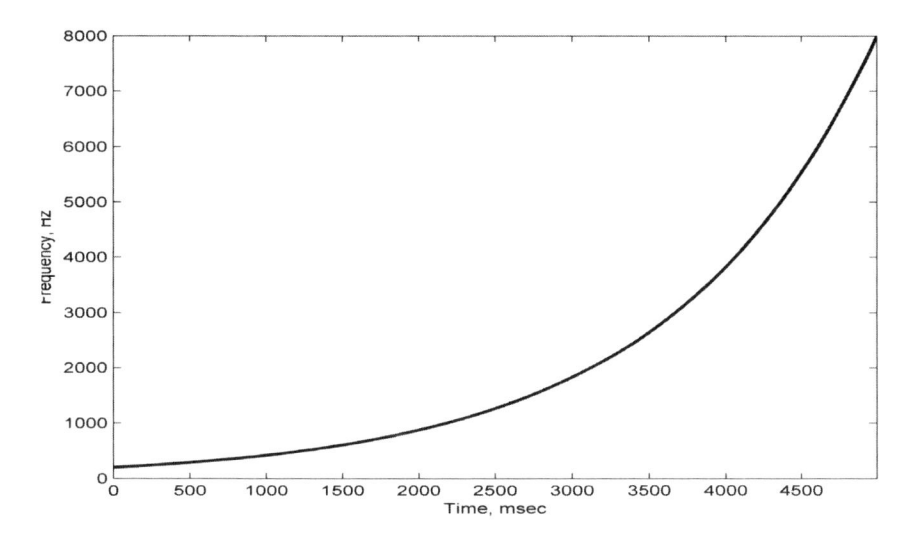

Figure 8-13. Instantaneous frequency as a function of time for the swept sinusoid excitation signal.

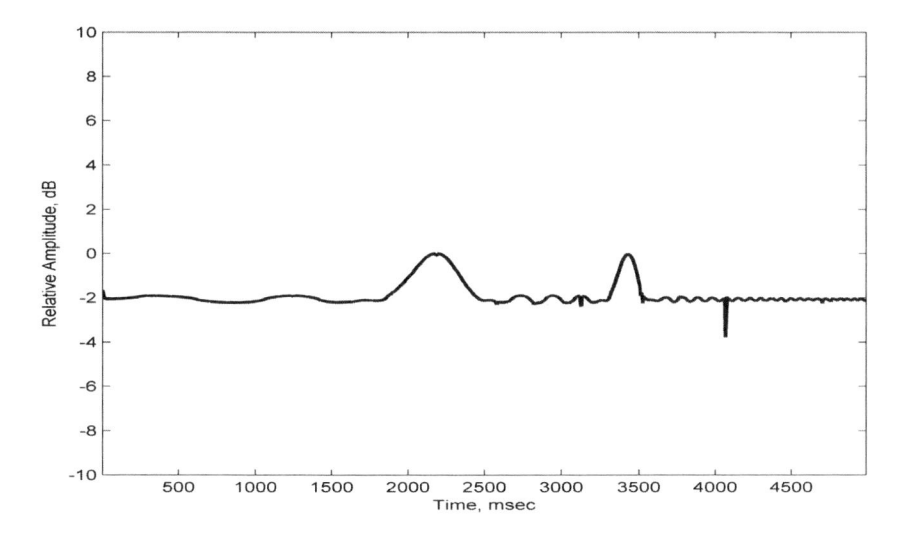

Figure 8-14. Envelope of the output of the three-band FIR filter compressor for an input sinusoid sweep at a constant amplitude. The compression ratio was set to 3:1 in each frequency band. The sweep ran from 200 Hz to 8 kHz; 1 kHz occurs at 2190 msec, and 2.5 kHz occurs at 3430 msec.

Frequency-Domain Compression

The filter bank represents one approach to time-domain processing. The input sequence is convolved with the filters one sample at a time, and the output sequence is formed by summing the filter outputs. An alternative approach is to divide the signal into short segments, transform each segment into the frequency domain using an FFT, compute the compression gains from the computed input spectrum and apply them to the signal, and then inverse transform to return to the time domain.

IDEAL FFT SYSTEM

A block diagram of a frequency-domain compressor is shown in Figure 8-15. The sampling rate has been set to 16 kHz and the FFT size set to 128 samples for purposes of illustration. The FFT implementation uses overlap-add processing as described in Chapter 2. The input fills a data buffer and is windowed and zero-padded. The FFT of the segment is calculated and the power spectrum is then computed from the FFT. For the 128-point FFT used in this example, the power spectrum is computed at a 125-Hz frequency spacing. Power estimates in the desired auditory frequency bands are computed by using individual FFT bins at low frequencies and combining FFT bins to give wider filter bandwidths as the frequency is increased. The power spectrum is computed for each input block of data, so within each auditory filter band a sequence of signal magnitude samples is produced at the block sampling rate. These magnitude samples are peak-detected using the attack and release times adjusted for the block sampling rate.

The compressor gains in each auditory frequency band are computed for the FFT system in the same way as for the individual channels in the time-domain filter-bank approach. The gains are then interpolated across frequency to give a gain value for each FFT bin. Next, the FFT of the input signal is multiplied by the compressor gains to give the compressed signal in the frequency domain. The compressed signal is then inverse transformed to give the time sequence, and the sequences are combined using overlap-add.

The frequency-domain compressor can be considered to be a filtering operation; the spectrum of the input signal is multiplied by the spectrum of the compression filter to give the spectrum of the compressed output signal. However, the compression filter is designed in the frequency domain, so the length of its impulse response is not known. The unknown

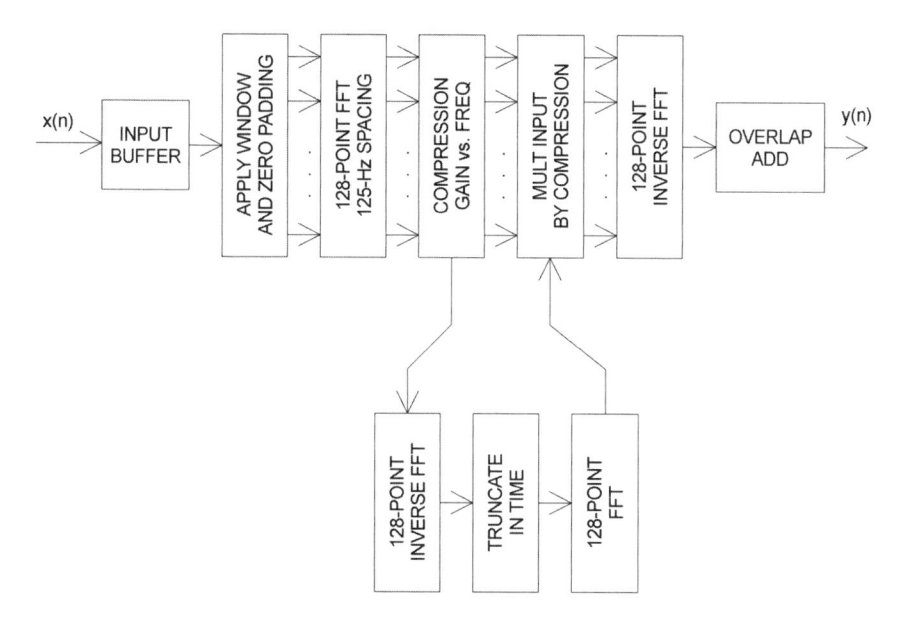

Figure 8-15. Block diagram of an ideal frequency-domain compression system using 128-point FFTs and a sampling rate of 16 kHz.

compression filter length can lead to temporal aliasing, as discussed in Chapter 2. The size of the FFT is set to 128 points in this example. For overlap-add processing, the size of the input sequence L (before zero-padding) and the length of the filter impulse response M must be chosen so that $L+M-1 \leq 128$. For example, if the input segment has length $L = 64$, then the compression filter must have length $M \leq 65$. If M is longer than this amount, the total length of the convolution of the input segment with the filter will exceed the FFT size of 128 samples. The result is that the samples in the convolution that lie beyond 128 samples will be wrapped around to the beginning of the sequence, producing temporal aliasing.

A solution to this problem is to compute the compression filter response in the frequency domain, inverse transform into the time domain, and then truncate the filter impulse response at 65 samples so that temporal aliasing will not occur. The truncated filter is then transformed back into the frequency domain to give the frequency response of a filter that approximates the desired gain-versus-frequency characteristic but for which temporal aliasing has been eliminated.

PRACTICAL FFT SYSTEM

The FFT system with temporal aliasing eliminated requires a total of four FFTs: a forward FFT for the input segment, an inverse FFT for the compression gains, a forward FFT for the truncated compression impulse response, and an inverse FFT for the filtered segment. A practical digital hearing aid, in general, will not have the signal-processing capability to perform four FFTs. The DSP may not be fast enough, or the battery drain may be too great. One solution to this problem is to provide circuitry on the DSP chip that is dedicated to computing the FFT (Gennum, 2005), or to exploit special properties of the FFT and digital filters to design a transform with a reduced operations count (Brennan & Schneider, 1998; Chau et al., 2004).

An additional solution is to compromise on the compression filter design to reduce the number of FFTs needed, as shown in Figure 8-16. Instead of the inverse transform of the compression gains, truncation, and the forward transform, the compression gains are smoothed in the frequency domain. There is a relationship in signal processing that the shorter the impulse response, the smoother the frequency response. Thus, smoothing the compression-gain frequency response is equivalent to an approximate truncation of the impulse response. The smoothing does not produce an exact truncation, so some residual temporal aliasing distortion is possible. A careful selection of the input segment length, FFT size, and frequency-domain smoothing will result in temporal aliasing distortion that cannot be perceived under most listening conditions.

The time delay of the FFT compressor depends on the size of the input buffer and the size of the FFT. The FFT cannot be computed until the input buffer is filled, so there is a processing delay while the input segment is accumulated. In addition, the compression frequency response is specified as a real number greater than zero in each frequency band. A frequency response that is pure real has a corresponding impulse response that is linear-phase. Thus, a set of compression gains for a 128-point FFT has a corresponding compression filter delay equal to 64 samples. If the filter is truncated to fewer than 128 samples, it will still be centered at 64 samples, but will have zeros at its beginning and end. Again, consider a system with a 16-kHz sampling rate and a FFT size of 128 points. If the windowed input segment length is 128 samples with an FFT computed every 64 samples, then the overall signal-processing delay will be 64 samples to fill the input buffer plus

Dynamic-Range Compression 245

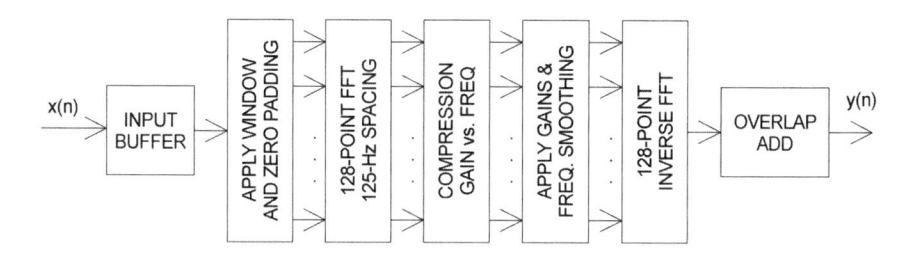

Figure 8-16. Block diagram of a practical frequency-domain compression system using 128-point FFTs and a sampling rate of 16 kHz.

64 samples for the filter impulse response delay, yielding a total delay of 128 samples, or 8 msec.

The delay can be adjusted by changing the size of the input segment and/or that of the FFT. A shorter input segment means that the input buffer will be filled sooner, with a corresponding reduction in the overall delay. However, a shorter input buffer means that the FFTs will have to be computed more often, and the processing capacity of the DSP or the battery drain will need to be increased. The other option is to use a smaller FFT. If the input buffer size is halved and the FFT size halved, then the delay will also be halved without an increase in the computational or power requirements. However, the frequency resolution for a smaller FFT is reduced. For example, if the FFT size is reduced from 128 to 64 points, the frequency resolution will be 250 Hz instead of 125 Hz, and the low-frequency resolution of the compression system will be reduced.

An additional concern in an FFT compressor is quantization noise. The DSP chip in a typical hearing aid uses 16-bit fixed-point arithmetic to reduce the size of the circuit and to reduce power consumption. An FFT involves a large number of multiply-add operations, and for each calculation there is the possibility of round-off error. If the amplitude of the input signal is increased to reduce the relative magnitude of the round-off error, then there is a possibility of overflow because combining two numbers can result in a number twice as large. The FFT computation often involves scaling the input segment during the forward FFT calculation and compensatory scaling during the inverse FFT calculation to prevent overflow while minimizing the quantization noise, but even with these adjustments the quantization noise in a FFT compressor will be higher than for a FIR filter bank.

SIDE-BRANCH STRUCTURE

The side-branch architecture (Williamson, Cummins, & Hecox, 1991) combines the low quantization noise of the FIR filter bank with the efficiency of computing the compression gains in the frequency domain using the FFT. The side-branch system, shown in Figure 8-17, separates the input signal filtering from the frequency analysis and calculation of the compression gains. The side-branch structure is therefore a digital multiband cousin of the simple broadband compressor shown in Figure 8-6. Conversely, the broadband system corresponds to a side-branch compressor with a 1-tap FIR filter that adjusts the overall gain of the input signal. Increasing the number of taps in the FIR filter allows for finer adjustment of the compressor frequency response at the expense of increased processing complexity and system delay. Another way of viewing the side-branch compressor is that it is an FFT system in which the compression filter is transformed into the time domain, with the filtering then performed via time-domain convolution rather than frequency-domain multiplication.

In the implementation shown in Figure 8-17, the input signal fills a $K/2$-sample buffer. The present $K/2$ samples are appended to the previous $K/2$ samples to give a total of K samples which are then windowed to provide the input to the K-point FFT. The signal power spectrum is computed from the FFT bins. As with the FFT compressor, individual bins are used at low frequencies and sums of adjacent bins used at high

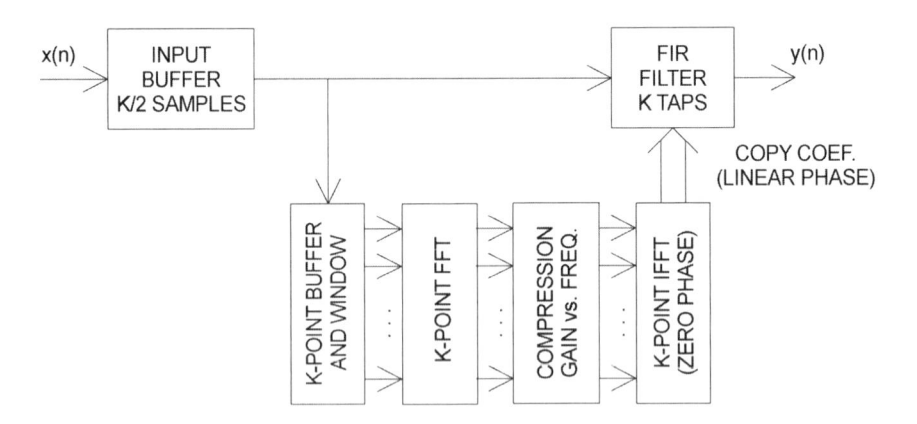

Figure 8-17. Block diagram of the side-branch compressor structure.

frequencies to give the desired auditory frequency bands. The frequency bands are then peak-detected, and the compressor gains as a function of frequency are computed from the peak-detector outputs. The compression gains as a function of frequency are inverse transformed to give the impulse response of the compression filter. Because the gains as a function of frequency are real, the impulse response has even symmetry and yields a linear-phase filter. The impulse response can be windowed if desired to smooth its frequency response. The $K/2$ most-recent input samples are then convolved with the K-point FIR filter to produce the output.

The processing delay for the side-branch compressor is $K/2$ samples to fill the input buffer, plus $K/2$ samples for the linear-phase compression filter. This delay is exactly the same as for the FFT compressor described in the section above. The delay can be reduced by filtering each sample of the input signal as it is acquired, giving a total delay of $K/2+1$ samples. The disadvantage of sample-by-sample filtering is that the compression gains will lag the input signal by up to $K/2$ samples, increasing the chance of overshoot in the compressor output for a jump in the input signal level.

Frequency Warping

One of the problems in building a digital hearing aid is the frequency resolution. Digital frequency analysis inherently embodies a uniform frequency scale, whereas the ear embodies a critical-band frequency scale having increasing bandwidth with increasing frequency. A second concern is the tradeoff between system delay and frequency resolution. Improved frequency resolution in any of the systems described in the previous sections requires longer FIR filters or larger FFTs, resulting in greater system processing delays. Digital frequency warping provides a technique for approximating the frequency resolution of the ear while significantly reducing the overall time delay compared to other processing approaches (Kates, 2003; Kates & Arehart, 2005).

DIGITAL FREQUENCY WARPING

Digital frequency warping is achieved by replacing the unit delays in a digital filter with first-order all-pass filters (Härmä et al., 2000; Oppenheim et al., 1971; Smith & Abel, 1999). The all-pass filter has a flat magnitude frequency response, but has a frequency-dependent group delay. The digital all-pass filter used for the frequency warping is given by

$$A(z) = \frac{z^{-1} - a}{1 - az^{-1}} \quad \text{Equation (8.2)}$$

where a is the warping parameter and z^{-1} is the unit delay operator. In the time domain the all-pass filter becomes:

$$y(n) = -ax(n) + x(n-1) + ay(n-1) \quad \text{Equation (8.3)}$$

where $x(n)$ is the filter input and $y(n)$ is the filter output. The value for the warping parameter that gives a closest fit to the Bark frequency scale is $a = 0.576$ for a 16-kHz sampling rate (Smith & Abel, 1999). The group delay for this choice of parameters is illustrated in Figure 8-18 for a single all-pass filter. The delay at low frequencies exceeds one sample, while the delay at high frequencies is less than one sample.

The warped FIR filter transfer function is the weighted sum of the outputs of each all-pass section:

$$B(z) = \sum_{k=0}^{K} b_k A^k(z) \quad \text{Equation (8.4)}$$

for a filter having K+1 taps (K all-pass sections). A warped FIR filter is compared with the conventional filter in Figure 8-19. Forcing the real filter coefficients $\{b_k\}$ to have even symmetry for a conventional unwarped FIR filter yields a linear-phase filter, in which the filter delay is independent of the coefficients as long as the symmetry is preserved. If the conventional FIR filter has K+1 taps, the delay is K/2 samples. Similarly, forcing even symmetry for the coefficients of a warped FIR filter gives a filter having a fixed frequency-dependent group delay that is also independent of the actual filter coefficient values (Kates, 2003; Kates & Arehart, 2005). If the warped FIR filter has K+1 taps, the group delay is K/2 times that of a single all-pass filter. This filter coefficient symmetry property ensures that no phase modulation occurs as the compressor changes gain in response to the incoming signal. Furthermore, the group delay at the two ears in a binaural fitting will be identical even if different gain-*versus*-frequency responses are

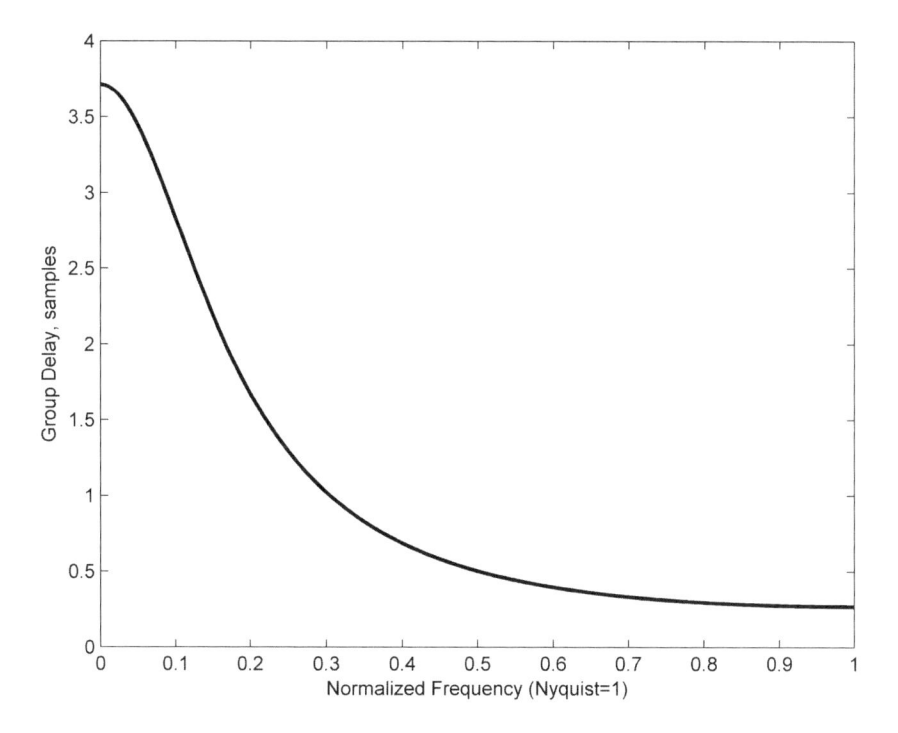

Figure 8-18. Group delay in samples for a single all-pass filter having the warping parameter a = 0.576.

selected, thus guaranteeing that phase localization cues are preserved in a binaural fitting.

WARPED COMPRESSOR SYSTEM

A dynamic-range compression system using warped frequency analysis is presented in Figure 8-20. The basic design is similar to the sidebranch compressor shown in Figure 8-17. The compressor combines a warped FIR filter and a warped FFT. The same tapped delay line is used for both the frequency analysis and the FIR compression filter. The incoming signal $x(n)$ is passed through a cascade of first-order all-pass filters of the form given by Eq. (8.2), with the output of the kth all-pass stage given by $p_k(n)$. The sequence of delayed samples $\{p_k(n)\}$ is then windowed, using a von Hann (raised cosine) or similar window, and an FFT calculated from the windowed sequence. The result of the FFT is a spectrum sampled at a nearly constant spacing on a Bark fre-

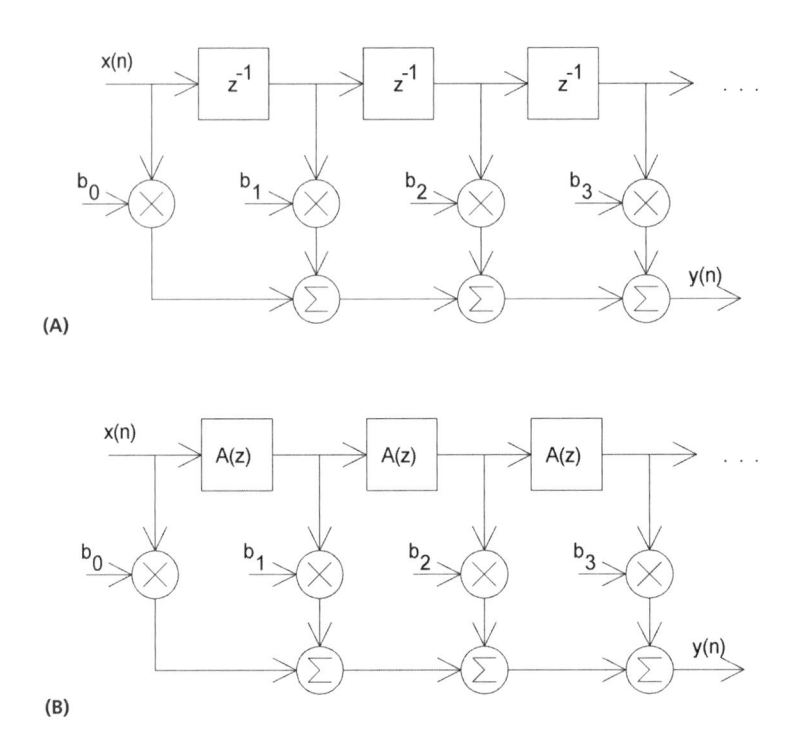

Figure 8-19. Comparison of **A.** conventional FIR filter structure with **B.** its frequency-warped equivalent.

quency scale. The algorithm can be implemented on a sample-by-sample basis or using block data processing. Block processing is typically used, with the FFT computed after a block of samples is read in and processed through the cascade of all-pass filters; the compression gains are therefore updated once per block.

Because the data sequence is windowed, the spectrum is smoothed in the warped frequency domain, giving smoothly overlapping frequency bands. The compression gains are then computed from the warped power spectrum for the auditory analysis bands. The compression gains are pure real numbers, so the inverse FFT to give the warped time-domain filter results in a set of filter coefficients that is real and has even symmetry. The system output is then calculated by convolving the delayed samples with the compression gain filter:

Dynamic-Range Compression 251

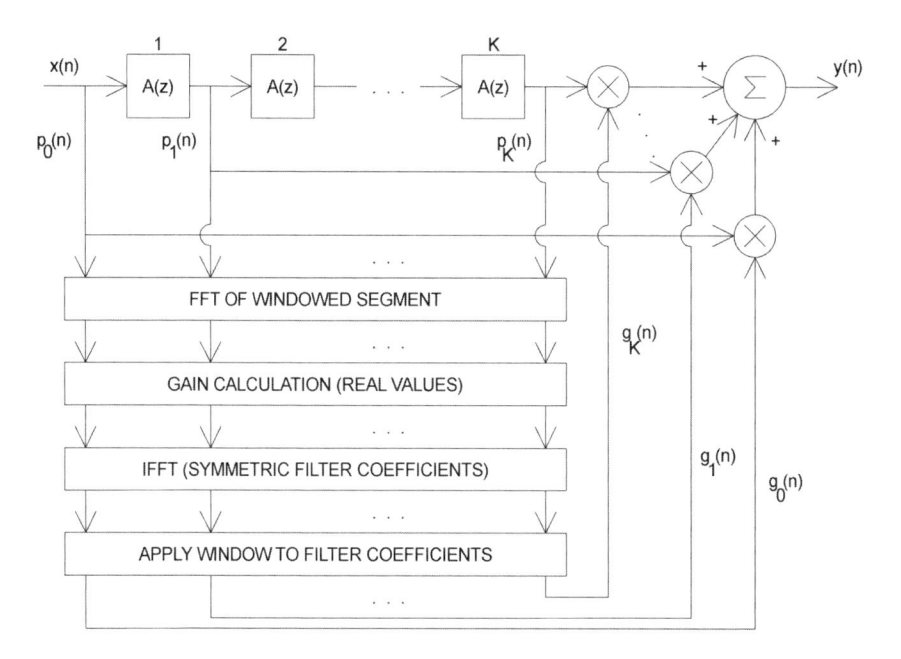

Figure 8-20. Block diagram of a side-branch compression system using frequency warping.

$$y(n) = \sum_{k=0}^{K} g_k(n) p_k(n) \quad \text{Equation (8.4)}$$

where $\{g_k(n)\}$ are the compression filter coefficients.

Consider a warped compressor having a filter with 31 all-pass filter sections. The even coefficient symmetry means that the system will have a group delay equal to that of 15 all-pass filter sections in cascade for any compressor magnitude frequency response. For a system having a flat frequency response and a gain of 0 dB, the filter coefficient $g_{15} = 1$ and all of the other filter coefficients equal zero. If the system input is an ideal impulse (click), the output will be a chirp in which the high frequencies emerge first and the low frequencies emerge later. This system impulse response is shown in Figure 8-21. The relative proportion of signal energy at the different frequencies is unchanged from that of the impulse, which has a flat power spectrum, but the output is dispersed over a duration of approximately 5 msec. A Fourier transform of the

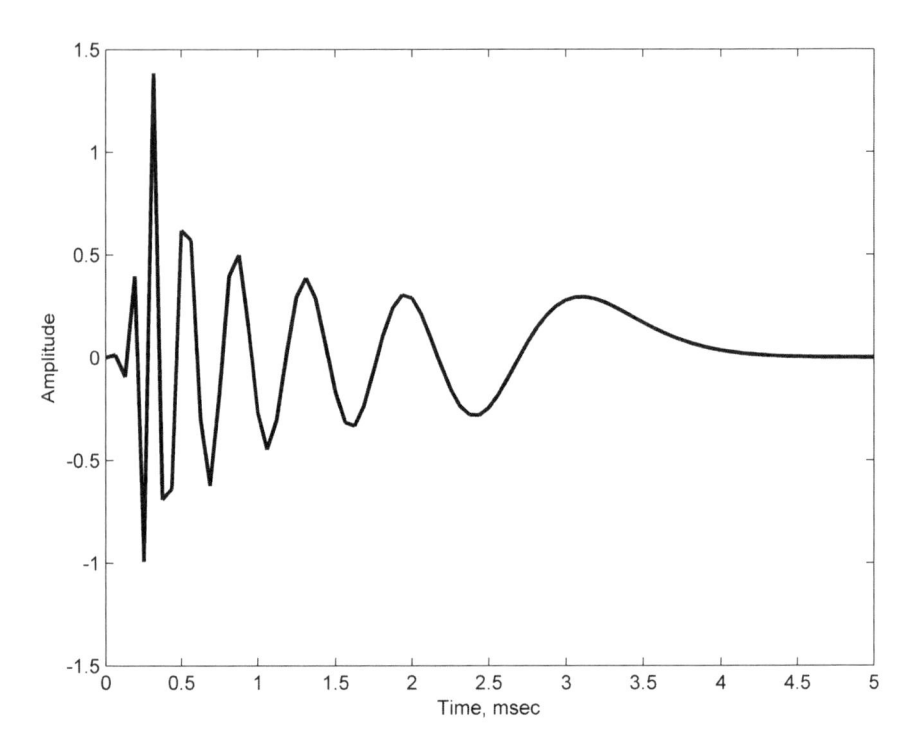

Figure 8-21. Impulse response of the Warp-31 system for a = 0.576 at a sampling rate of 16 kHz. The group delay is equal to that of 15 all-pass filter sections in cascade.

output waveform of Figure 8-22 would show a flat magnitude frequency response.

The frequency analysis performed in Figure 8-20 involves the Fourier transform of the outputs of the cascade of all-pass filters. Compared to a conventional FFT, which has uniform frequency spacing along a linear frequency axis, the warped FFT has better frequency resolution at low frequencies and worse resolution at high frequencies. Why this modification of the frequency resolution occurs is illustrated in Figure 8-22. The delay as a function of frequency is plotted for the input to the warped delay line and for the outputs of the first four all-pass filters. In a conventional FIR filter each of these curves would be a vertical line at 0, 1,...4 samples. However, in the warped system the output sample spacing at low frequencies is much greater than one sample, and at high frequencies is much less than one sample. For an FFT, the longer the

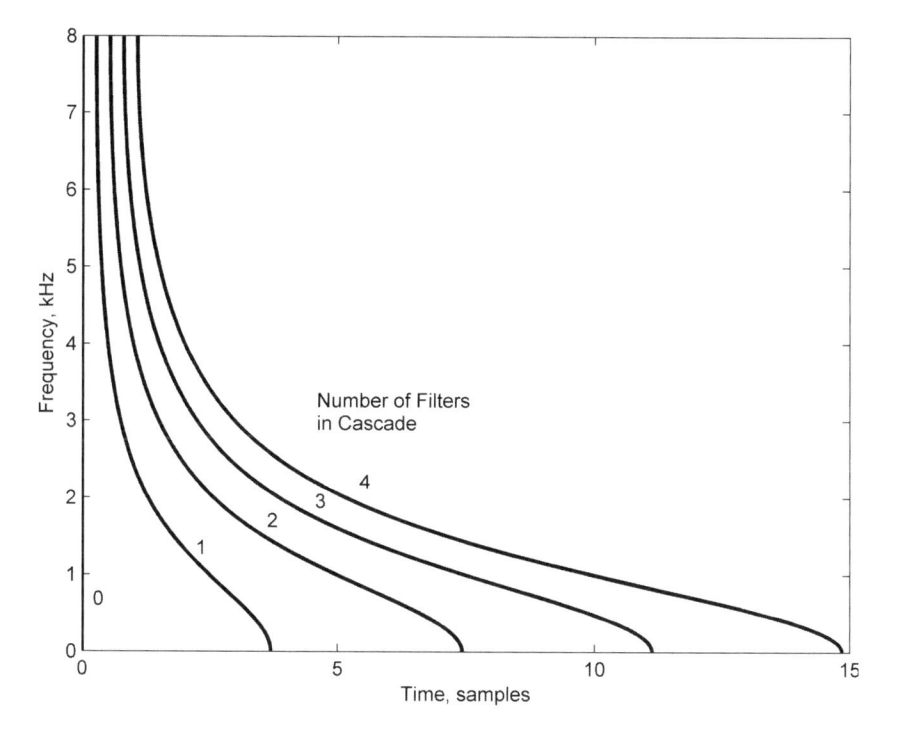

Figure 8-22. Group delay for the all-pass filter outputs for the input and first four filters in a cascade, a = 0.576 for a sampling rate of 16 kHz.

data segment that is analyzed, the better the frequency resolution. At low frequencies, the wider sample spacing means that the set of samples used to compute the FFT spans a much longer time interval than that used for a conventional FFT of the same transform size, and the longer time interval results in better frequency resolution. Conversely, at high frequencies the narrower sample spacing means that the set of samples used to compute the FFT spans a much shorter time interval that that used for a conventional FFT of the same transform size, and the shorter time interval results in poorer frequency resolution.

The resulting frequency resolution for a warped system having 31 all-pass filters is plotted in Figure 8-23. This system, when combined with a 32-point FFT, results in 17 frequency bands from 0 to the system Nyquist frequency (half the sampling rate). To trace out the shape of the equivalent filter responses, the warped system was excited with a

254 Digital Hearing Aids

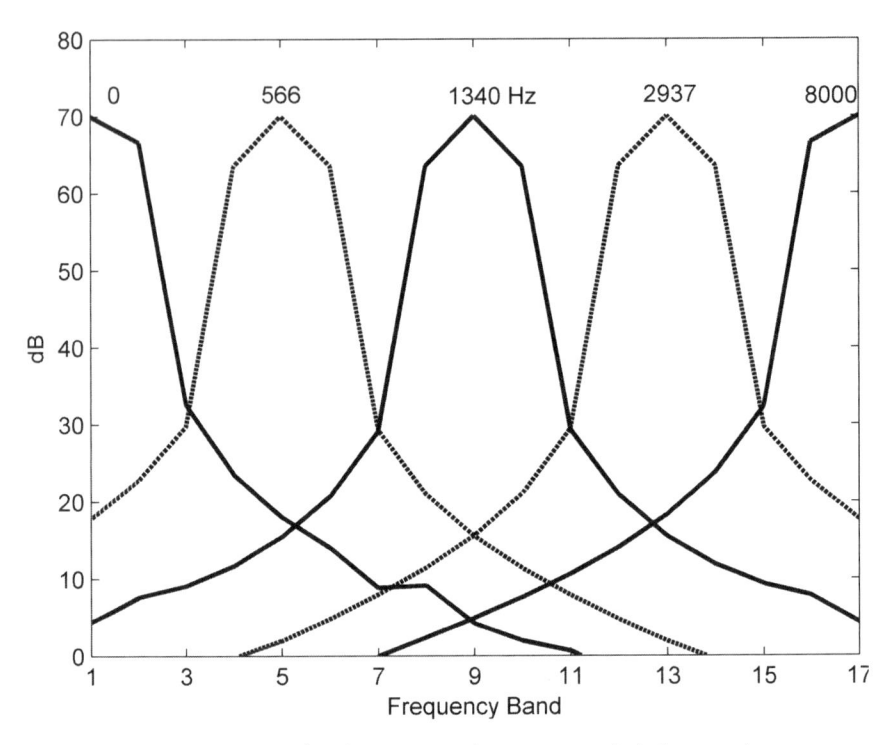

Figure 8-23. Power spectra for the Warp-31 frequency analysis for steady-state sinusoidal excitations at the indicated warped FFT bin center frequencies. The excitation signal is at a level of 70 dB SPL.

series of 17 sinusoids, each one at the center frequency of a warped FFT analysis bin. The signal magnitude in each FFT bin was recorded for all 17 sinusoids, and then plotted in the figure for five of the 17 bands. The shapes of the power spectra for the different excitation frequencies are essentially shifted versions of the same basic response. The response at the adjacent frequency band is about 5 dB below the response at the excitation frequency, and the average slope of the response over the first octave is about 50 dB/octave Replacing the von Hann with a different window shape will modify the spectral response in manner comparable to the effects of the window on a conventional FFT.

In comparison with a conventional FIR system having the same FIR filter length, the warped compression system will require more computational resources because of the all-pass filters in the tapped delay line.

However, in many cases the warped FIR filter will be shorter than the conventional FIR filter needed to achieve the same degree of auditory frequency resolution.

SYSTEM DELAY COMPARISON

Two compression systems were simulated for the performance evaluation. The systems operated at a 16-kHz sampling rate and were simulated in MATLAB. The first compressor is the side-branch system of Figure 8-17. For a short system delay, a 16-sample buffer is used for the block time-domain processing, and the signal is processed by a 31-tap FIR filter. The frequency analysis uses a 32-point FFT operating on the present and previous 16-point data segments. A window is used to provide adequate FFT smoothing at low frequencies, and overlapping FFT bins are summed to give the analysis bands at high frequencies. This system has a total of 9 frequency analysis bands, with a low-frequency resolution of 500 Hz. The frequency resolution can be improved by increasing the FFT size, but the system delay will also be increased. The compression gains are calculated in the frequency domain, and the gains inverse transformed to give the symmetric compression filter used to modify the incoming signal.

The second compressor is the warped FIR side-branch system of Figure 8-20 in which a 16-sample data buffer and a 32-point FFT are used in conjunction with a 31-tap warped FIR filter. This compressor is essentially the frequency-warped version of the side-branch compressor of Figure 8-17. The input data segment is windowed with a 32-point von Hann window, and no frequency-domain smoothing is applied to the spectrum. The compression gains are smoothed by applying a 31-point von Hann window to the compression filter after the gain values are transformed into the time domain. We will call this system the Warp-31 compressor (Kates & Arehart, 2005).

The Warp-31 compressor provides frequency analysis with a separation of approximately 1.3 Bark. There are a total of 17 bands covering the positive frequencies, including 0 and π radians. The low-frequency bands are approximately spaced at multiples of 135 Hz, with the spacing increasing to 1800 Hz at the highest frequency. The side-branch compressor using the 32-point FFT, on the other hand, uses the output of the FFT to approximate frequency bands on a Bark scale. The limited resolution of the short FFT with its uniform 500-Hz bin spacing causes a poor match between the side-branch frequency bands and the Bark band spacing at low frequencies. At high frequencies, however, FFT bins can be combined to give a reasonably good match. To achieve the same low-frequency resolution as the Warp-31 system, the side-branch compressor requires an FFT size of 128 points which gives a bin spacing of 125 Hz. The frequency analysis bands for the side-branch using 32-point and 128-point FFTs are compared to those for the Warp-31 system in Table 8-1.

The overall system processing group delay is due to several factors. Certain aspects of the overall system delay, such as the A/D and D/A converter delays, are fixed by the hardware and are not affected by the signal processing. The total software processing delay is the sum of the time required to fill the input buffer, the group delay inherent in the frequency-domain or time-domain filtering operation provided by the

TABLE 8-1. Analysis Frequencies for a Side-Branch (or FFT) System Using a Conventional 128-Point FFT, a 32-Point FFT, and a Frequency-Warped System Using a 32-Point FFT

Side-Branch 128-Point FFT	Side-Branch 32-Point FFT	Warp-31 32-Point FFT
		0
125		135
188		273
313		
438	500	415
625		566
		728
875	1000	907
1188		1108
		1340
1625	1500	1615
2125	2000	1952
		2378
2813	2750	2937
3688	3750	3698
4813	4750	4761
6313	6000	6215
7063	7000	8000

compressor, and the time needed to execute the code before the output signal is available.

The side-branch compressor uses a linear-phase FIR filter, so the delay is independent of frequency. The Warp-31 compressor uses all-pass filters to replace the unit delays in the FIR filter implementation, so this system has a frequency-dependent delay. The total delay for the Warp-31 compressor is an estimate assuming that the hardware delays and the time needed for the code execution will be similar to that needed for the side-branch compressor, with an additional allowance for the all-pass filters. The delay values for the 32-point FFT version of the side-branch compressor are based on measurements of an actual hearing aid, and assume 2.5 msec for the hardware and code execution and 1.0 msec for the 16-sample input buffer.

The group delay for the compression systems is plotted in Figure

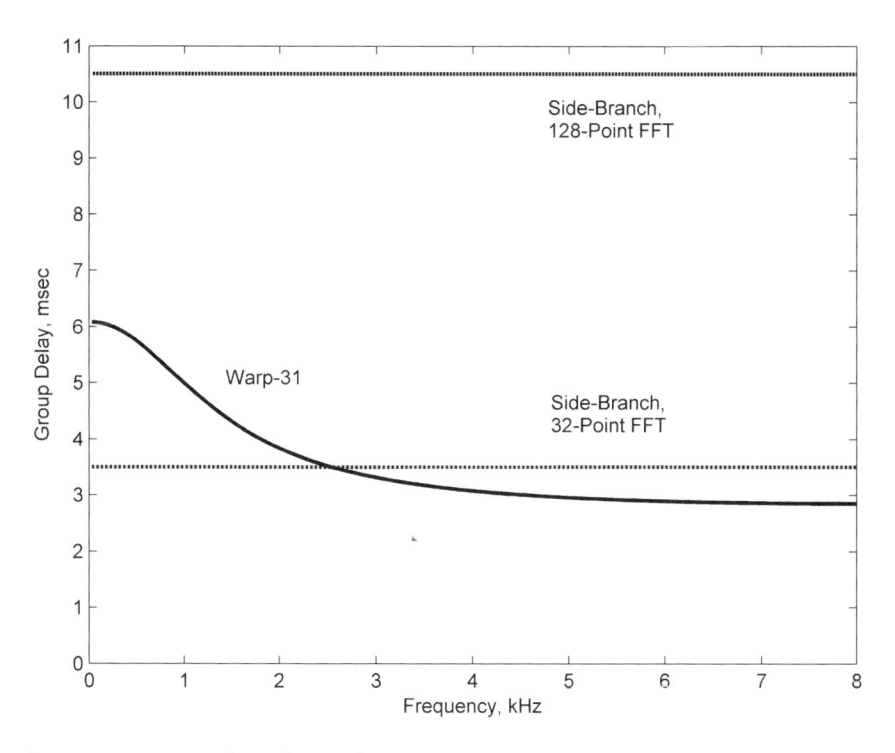

Figure 8-24. Group delay for the frequency-warped compressor and two versions of the side-branch compressor.

8-24. The side-branch system has a constant delay as a function of frequency because of the linear-phase filters used for the processing. The delay is 3.5 msec for an FFT size of 32 points, and increases to 10.5 msec when the FFT size is increased to 128 points. The Warp-31 system has a smooth frequency-dependent delay due to the group-delay characteristics of the all-pass filters used for the warped FIR filtering. The maximum delay for the Warp-31 compressor is 6.1 msec at 0 Hz, with the delay falling to 2.9 msec at high frequencies. Thus, the Warp-31 compressor has delay characteristics similar to those of the side-branch system with a 32-point FFT, while providing frequency resolution that can only be achieved when a 128-point FFT with its much greater delay is used. The warped compressor thus has substantially reduced delay in comparison with a conventional design having comparable frequency resolution.

Concluding Remarks

Multichannel dynamic-range compression is a basic part of digital hearing aids. The design of a digital compressor involves many considerations, including frequency resolution, processing group delay, quantization noise, and algorithm complexity. This chapter has focused on the issues of frequency resolution and group delay. Quantization noise and processing complexity also influence the choice of algorithm and the details of the implementation, but are considered to be beyond the scope of this chapter.

The compression algorithms are directly characterized by the frequency-analysis procedure. Of the various approaches that can be used to design a digital hearing aid, this chapter considered broadband compression, multichannel filter banks, a frequency-domain compressor using the FFT, the side-branch design which separates the filtering operation from the frequency analysis, and the frequency-warped version of the side-branch approach that modifies the analysis frequency spacing to more closely match auditory perception.

The design of the compressor also influences the design of the other aspects of the hearing aid. Because of the limited processing capacity in a digital hearing aid, it is necessary to not duplicate processing steps. Therefore, the frequency analysis used for the multichannel compression also forms the basis for the other processing, such as noise reduction, that may be included. The properties of frequency resolution and group delay described for the compressor approaches will apply to these other algorithms as well. The frequency resolution and group delay thus become fundamental properties of the hearing aid.

References

Agnew, J., & Thornton, J. M. (2000). Just noticeable and objectionable group delays in digital hearing aids. *Journal of the American Academy of Audiology, 11*, 330–336.

ANSI S3.22. (2003). *Specification of hearing-aid characteristics*. New York: American National Standards Institute

Blauert, J., & Laws, P. (1978). Group delay distortions in electroacoustic systems. *Journal of the Acoustical Society of America, 63*, 1478–1483.

Braida, L. D., Durlach, N. I., Lippmann, R. P., Hicks, B. L., Rabinowitz, W. M., & Reed, C. M. (1979). *Hearing aids—A review of past research on linear amplification, amplitude compression, and frequency lowering*. ASHA Monograph No. 10, Rockville, MD: ASHA.

Brennan, R., & Schneider, T. (1998). A flexible filterbank structure for extensive signal manipulations in digital hearing aids. *Proceedings of the 1998 IEEE International Symposium on Circuits and Systems* (pp. 569–572).

Chau, E., Sheikhzadeh, H., & Brennan, R. L. (2004). Complexity reduction and regularization of a fast affine projection algorithm for oversampled subband adaptive filters. *Proceedings of the 2004 International Conference on Acoustics, Speech and Signal Processing*, Montreal, May 17–21.

Cole, W. (1993). Current design options and criteria for hearing aids. *Journal of Speech-Language Pathology and Audiology Monograph*, (Suppl. 1), 7–14.

Dillon, H. (1996). Compression? Yes, but for low or high frequencies, for low or high intensities, and with what response times? *Ear and Hearing, 17*, 287–307.

Dillon, H., Katsch, R., Byrne, D., Ching, T., Keidser, G., & Brewer, S. (1997). The NAL-NL1 prescription procedure for non-linear hearing aids. *National Acoustics Laboratories Research and Development, Annual Report 1997/98* (pp. 4–7). Chatswood NSW, Australia: National Acoustics Laboratories, 1998.

Gennum. (2005). *Voyageur™ open platform DSP system for ultra low power audio processing*. Gennum Corp. Specification Sheet GA3220. Available at http://www.gennum.com/hip/pdffiles/31658DOC.pdf

Greer, W. H. (1975). *Monaural sensitivity to dispersion in impulses and speech*. Ph.D. Thesis, University of Utah, Salt Lake City.

Härmä, A., Karjalainen, M., Savioja, L., Välimäki, V., Laine, U. K., & Huopaniemi, J. (2000). Frequency-warped signal processing for audio applications. *Journal of the Audio Engineering Society, 48*, 1011–1031.

Hellman, R. P., & Meiselman, C. H. (1990). Loudness relations for individuals and groups in normal and impaired hearing. *Journal of the Acoustical Society of America, 88*, 2596–2606.

Humes, L. E., Christensen, L., Thomas, T., Bess, F. H., Hedley-Williams, A., & Bentler, R. (1999). A comparison of the aided performance and benefit provided by a linear and a two-channel wide dynamic range compression hearing aid. *Journal of Speech, Language, and Hearing Research, 42*, 65–79.

Kates, J. M. (1997). Using a cochlear model to develop adaptive hearing-aid processing. In W. Jesteadt, (Ed.), *Modeling sensorineural hearing loss* (pp. 79–92), Mahwah, NJ: Lawrence Erlbaum.

Kates, J. M. (2003). Dynamic-range compression using digital frequency warping. *Proceedings of the 37th Asilomar Conference on Signals, Systems, and Computers*, Pacific Grove, CA., Nov. 9-12, 2003.

Kates, J. M., & Arehart, K. H. (2005). Multi-channel dynamic range compression using digital frequency warping. *EURASIP Journal of Applied Signal Processing, 18*, 3003–3014.

Keidser, G., & Grant, F. (2001). The preferred number of channels (one, two, or four) in NAL-NL1 prescribed wide dynamic range compression (WDRC) devices. *Ear and Hearing, 22*, 516–527.

Levitt, H. & Neuman, A. C. (1991). Evaluation of orthogonal polynomial compression. *Journal of the Acoustical Society of America, 90*, 241–252.

Lindemann, E. (1997). The continuous frequency dynamic range compressor. *Proceedings of the 1997 IEEE Workshop on Applications of Signal Processing to Audio and Acoustics*, New Paltz, NY.

Moore, B. C. J., & Glasberg, B. R. (1983). Suggested formulae for calculating auditory-filter bandwidths and excitation patterns. *Journal of the Acoustical Society of America, 74*, 750–753.

Moore, B. C. J., Peters, R. W., & Stone, M. A. (1999). Benefits of linear amplification and multichannel compression for speech comprehension in backgrounds with spectral and temporal dips. *Journal of the Acoustical Society of America, 105*, 400–411.

Nejime, Y., & Moore, B. C. J. (1997). Simulation of the effect of threshold elevation and loudness recruitment combined with reduced frequency selectivity on the intelligibility of speech in noise. *Journal of the Acoustical Society of America, 102*, 603–615.

Neuman, A.C., Bakke, M. H., Hellman, S., & Levitt, H. (1994). Effect of compression ratio in a slow-acting compression hearing aid: Paired-comparison judgments of quality. *Journal of the Acoustical Society of America, 96,* 1471–1478.

Oppenheim, A. V., Johnson, D. H., & Steiglitz, K. (1971). Computation of spectra with unequal resolution using the fast Fourier transform. *Proceedings of the IEEE, 59,* 299–300.

Plomp, R. (1988). The negative effect of amplitude compression in multichannel hearing aids in the light of the modulation-transfer function. *Journal of the Acoustical Society of America, 83,* 2322–2327.

Plomp, R. (1994). Noise, amplification, and compression: Considerations of three main issues in hearing aid design. *Ear and Hearing, 15,* 2–12.

Smith, J. O., & Abel, J. S. (1999). Bark and ERB bilinear transforms. *IEEE Transactions on Speech and Audio Processing, 7,* 697–708.

Souza, P. E. (2002). Effects of compression on speech acoustics, intelligibility, and sound quality. *Trends in Amplification, 6,* 131–165.

Souza, P. E., Jenstad, L. M., & Folino, R. (2005). Using multichannel wide-dynamic range compression in severely hearing-impaired listeners: Effects on speech recognition and quality. *Ear and Hearing, 26,* 120–131.

Stone, M. A., & Moore, B. C. J. (1999). Tolerable hearing aids delays. I: Estimation of limits imposed by the auditory path alone using simulated hearing losses. *Ear and Hearing, 20,* 182–192.

Stone, M. A., & Moore, B. C. J. (2002). Tolerable hearing aids delays. II: Estimation of limits imposed during speech production. *Ear and Hearing, 23,* 325–338.

Stone, M. A., & Moore, B. C. J. (2003). Tolerable hearing aids delays. III: Effects on speech production and perception of across-frequency variation in delay. *Ear and Hearing, 24,* 175–183.

Stone, M. A., & Moore, B. C. J. (2005). Tolerable hearing aids delays. IV: Effects on subjective disturbance during speech production by hearing-impaired subjects. *Ear and Hearing, 26,* 225–235.

van Buuren, R. A., Festen, J. M., & Houtgast, T. (1999). Compression and expansion of the temporal envelope: Evaluation of speech intelligibility and quality. *Journal of the Acoustical Society of America, 105,* 2903–2913.

Villchur, E. (1973). Signal processing to improve speech intelligibility in perceptive deafness. *Journal of the Acoustical Society of America, 53,* 1646–1657.

Walden, B. E., Surr, R. K., Cord, M. T., Edwards, B., & Olsen, L. (2000). Comparison of benefits provided by different hearing aid technologies. *Journal of the American Academy of Audiology, 11,* 540–560.

Williamson, M. J., Cummins, K. L., & Hecox, K. E. (1991). *Adaptive programmable signal processing and filtering for hearing aids*. U.S. Patent 5,027,410, issued June 25, 1991.

Zwicker, E., & Terhardt, E. (1980). Analytical expressions for critical-band rate and critical bandwidth as a function of frequency. *Journal of the Acoustical Society of America, 68*, 1523–1525.

9

Single-Microphone Noise Suppression

THE PRESENCE OF BACKGROUND NOISE can interfere with the intelligibility of speech and reduce sound quality. The use of directional microphones and microphone arrays, as explained in the previous chapters, is an effective way of reducing the amount of external interference. However, there are situations where one would like to reduce the effects of noise when using a single microphone input to a hearing aid, or would like additional noise reduction beyond that provided by directional microphones. Single-microphone noise suppression algorithms address this problem.

Many different algorithms have been proposed for single-microphone noise suppression. The underlying approach is to determine signal characteristics that differentiate noise from speech, and then design filters based on these characteristics that suppress the noise power while having minimal effects on the speech. This general approach is illustrated in Figure 9-1 for a multichannel noise-suppression system. The signal properties selected for identifying noise generally determine the nature of the suppression algorithm. In this chapter, a variety of single-microphone noise-suppression approaches are described. Some of these approaches were first implemented in analog hearing aids, but the algorithms could easily be programmed in digital instruments and

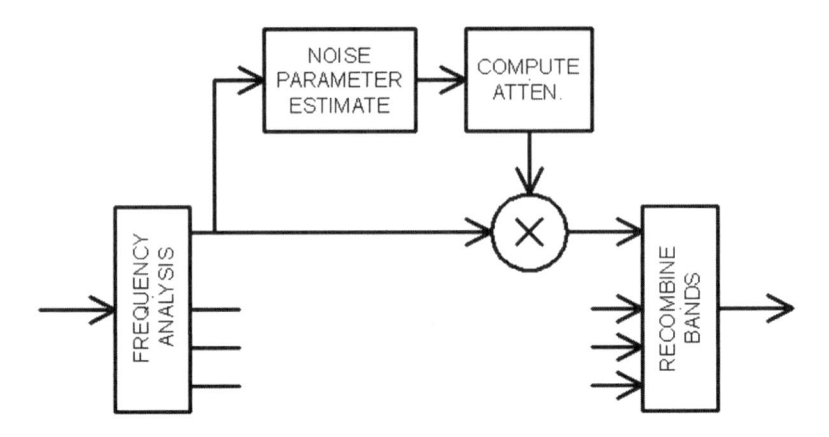

Figure 9-1. Block diagram of a generic multichannel single-microphone noise-suppression system.

the subject test results from the analog implementations are still valid. Two remaining techniques, spectral subtraction and Wiener filters, are important enough to get their own chapter, which follows this one.

This chapter begins with a review of some of the properties of speech and noise signals, followed by a survey of some single-microphone noise-suppression algorithms. The noise is typically less intense than the speech, so low-level expansion is introduced as a technique based on the difference intensity between speech and noise. The temporal properties of the noise signal are often different from those of speech, and differences in the signal envelope behaviors lead to noise-suppression algorithms based on envelope tracking. The spectra of noise signals often differ from those of speech as well, and adaptive low-pass and high-pass filters are designed to exploit these differences. The final approach discussed in this chapter is based on the differences between the envelope modulations of speech and noise, and involves filtering the envelope modulation spectrum.

Properties of Speech and Noise Signals

Noise, in the real world, can be any unwanted sound. When dealing with hearing aids and hearing loss, noise typically means any one of a number of sounds that can interfere with the perception of speech. These noises are generally representative of everyday listening situations, or they have desirable mathematical properties that make them easy to generate in the laboratory.

A noise-suppression algorithm is typically based on a signal property that can be used to distinguish speech from noise. The temporal behavior of a signal is one such property that can be used. The envelope for a segment of speech is plotted in Figure 9-2. The envelope was computed by dividing the signal into 16-msec segments having a 50% overlap. Each segment was weighted with a Hamming window and the power in the windowed segment computed to give the signal envelope for that segment. A new envelope sample was thus computed every 8 msec. The input signal was sampled at 16 kHz, and the envelope samples were computed at a sampling rate of 125 Hz.

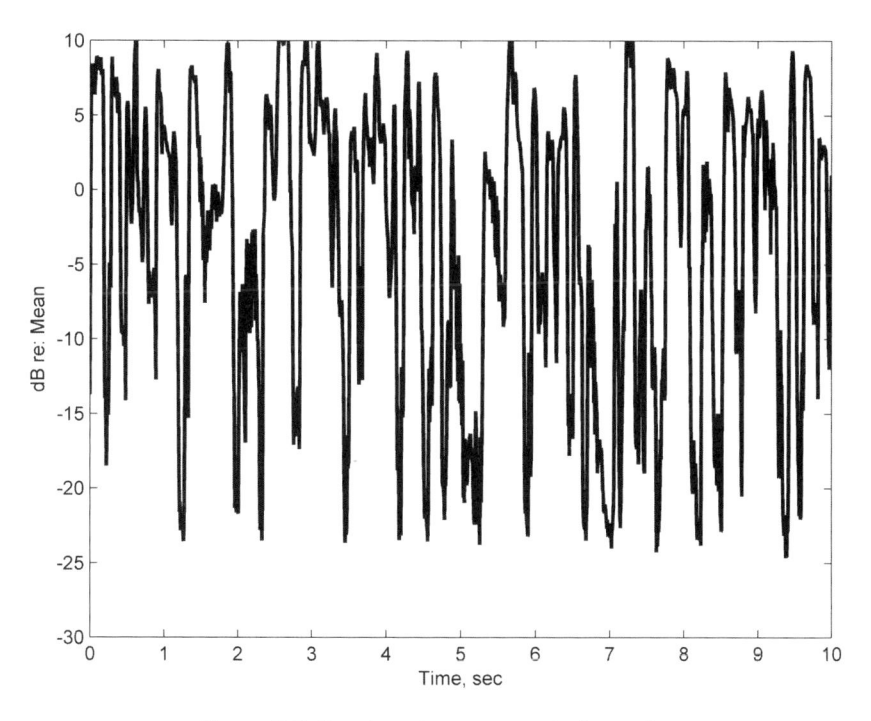

Figure 9-2. Envelope for a segment of speech.

The speech level plotted in Figure 9-2 fluctuates over a wide dynamic range, with peaks ranging up to 10 dB above and valleys 25 dB below the RMS signal level. The wide range of speech level fluctuations is therefore a property that could be exploited by a noise-suppression algorithm. The envelope of a segment of white Gaussian noise is plotted in Figure 9-3 for comparison. The Gaussian noise exhibits very little fluctuation compared to the speech. The Gaussian noise is stationary, which means that its statistics do not change over time; a measurement of the noise power made at one time will still be valid at a later time. The speech signal is nonstationary, as a measurement made during one time interval (e.g., a vowel) would not describe the signal during another interval (e.g., a fricative consonant).

The behavior of many common noises lies in between that of speech and Gaussian noise. The envelope for a segment of multitalker babble is plotted in Figure 9-4, and the envelope for a segment of noise generated by passing automobile traffic is plotted in Figure 9-5. The babble

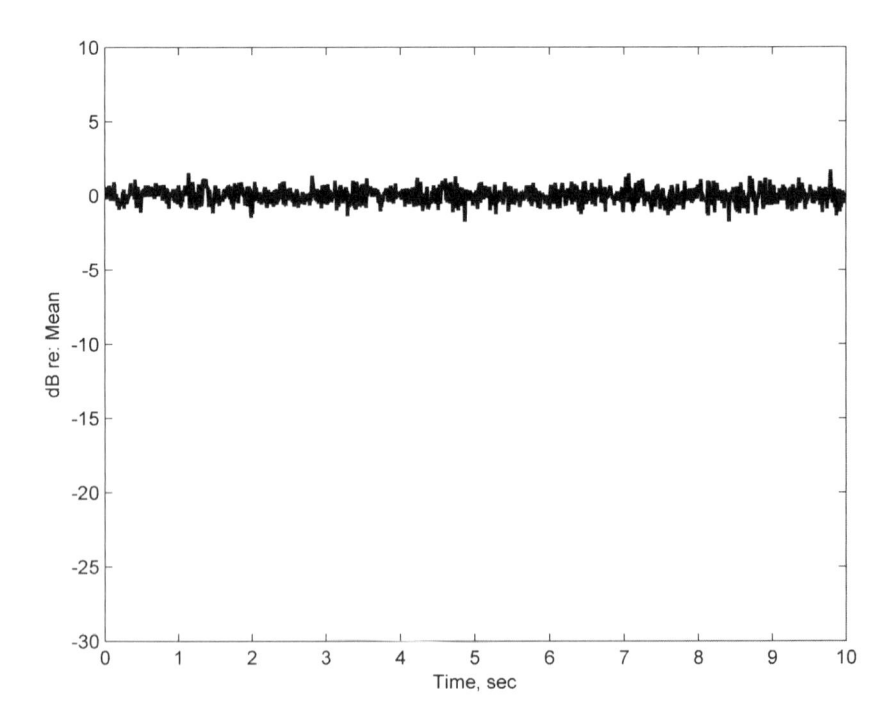

Figure 9-3. Envelope for a segment of white Gaussian noise.

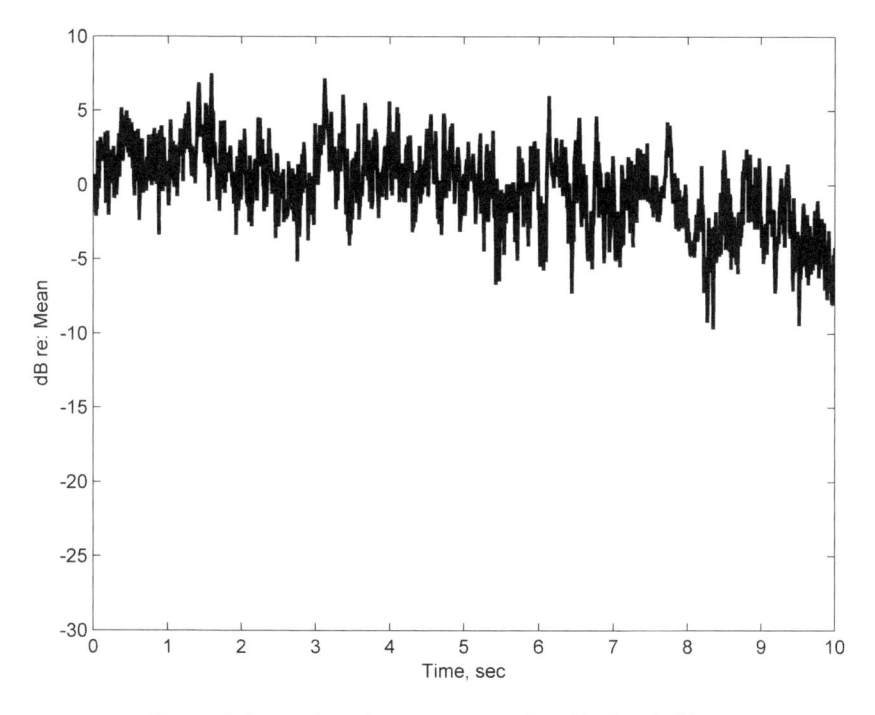

Figure 9-4. Envelope for a segment of multitalker babble.

shows more envelope fluctuations than the Gaussian noise, but the fluctuations are not as pronounced as those for speech. The traffic noise shows large overall changes in level, but the local fluctuations are not as pronounced as those for babble. These noise signals are, in general, nonstationary, but the signal fluctuations tend to be slower than those for speech.

The signal fluctuations can be described by the modulation spectrum, which is the Fourier transform of the envelope samples. The modulation spectrum describes both the rate and intensity of the envelope fluctuations. The modulation spectra for the four signals are plotted in Figure 9-6. The speech shows large envelope fluctuations in the frequency region of 2 to 10 Hz, and the rate of envelope fluctuations then decreases with increasing modulation frequency. The modulation frequency range for speech is considered to be from 2 to 20 Hz (Greenberg & Arai, 2004; Plomp, 1988; Steeneken & Houtgast, 1980). At the other extreme, the stationary Gaussian noise exhibited very little envelope fluctuation, and

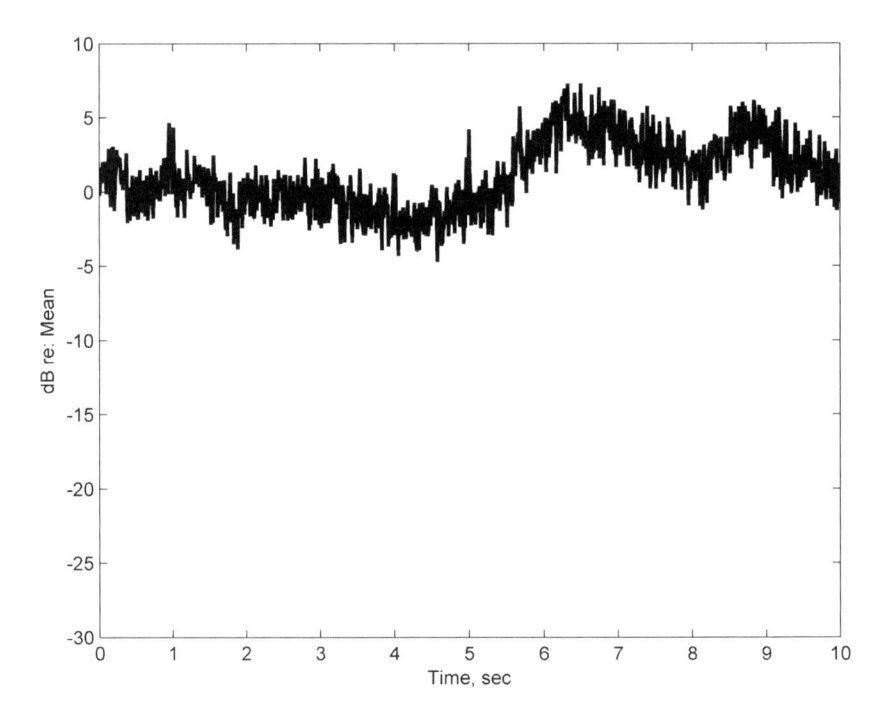

Figure 9-5. Envelope for a segment of noise generated by passing automobile traffic.

its modulation spectrum is correspondingly low with no dominance of any one frequency region. The modulation spectra of babble and traffic noise lie between those of speech and Gaussian noise. Many of the syllabic fluctuations of speech are smoothed over by the overlap of the multiple talkers in the babble, so what remains is a dominant low-frequency modulation component that represents the general rise and fall of the signal level. The traffic noise has fewer fluctuations than the babble, with a low-frequency component near 0 Hz that represents the gradual rise and fall of the signal intensity as a car drives past.

Another signal characteristic that may be useful in distinguishing speech from noise is the average power spectrum. Magnitude spectra for the four signals are presented in Figure 9-7. The Gaussian noise is white, which means that it has a flat spectrum. This spectrum differs considerably from that of speech, which has a concentration of power below 1 kHz in the frequency region corresponding to the first formant. The spectrum for babble is similar to that of the speech segment, but

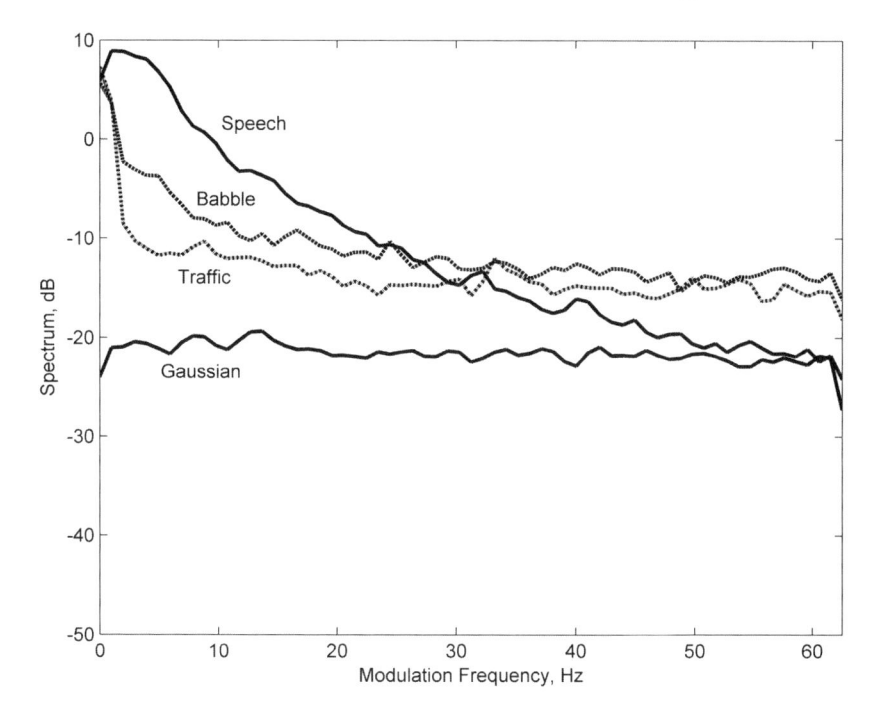

Figure 9-6. Average modulation spectra for the four signals of Figures 9-2 through 9-5. Each plot represents the average of 30 sec of data sampled at 16 kHz.

represents an average over many talkers. Traffic, on the other hand, has a spectrum closer to that of white Gaussian noise.

Another useful technique for analyzing a signal is the spectrogram, which records the time-frequency aspects of the signal. Spectrograms are generally not used in hearing aids, however, because of the storage requirements. Assume that 1 sec of data is needed to characterize a signal as speech or noise. At a 16-kHz sampling rate, short-time spectra would typically be computed using a 256-point FFT, resulting in 129 positive frequency-analysis bins, with a new spectrum computed every 8 msec. To store 1 sec of spectrogram data would thus require 129 bins/spectrum x 125 spectra, resulting in 16,125 words. In a personal computer this amount of memory is trivial, but in a digital hearing aid it would exceed the total data storage available for all of the signal processing implemented in the device. Simpler signal representations are needed for hearing aids.

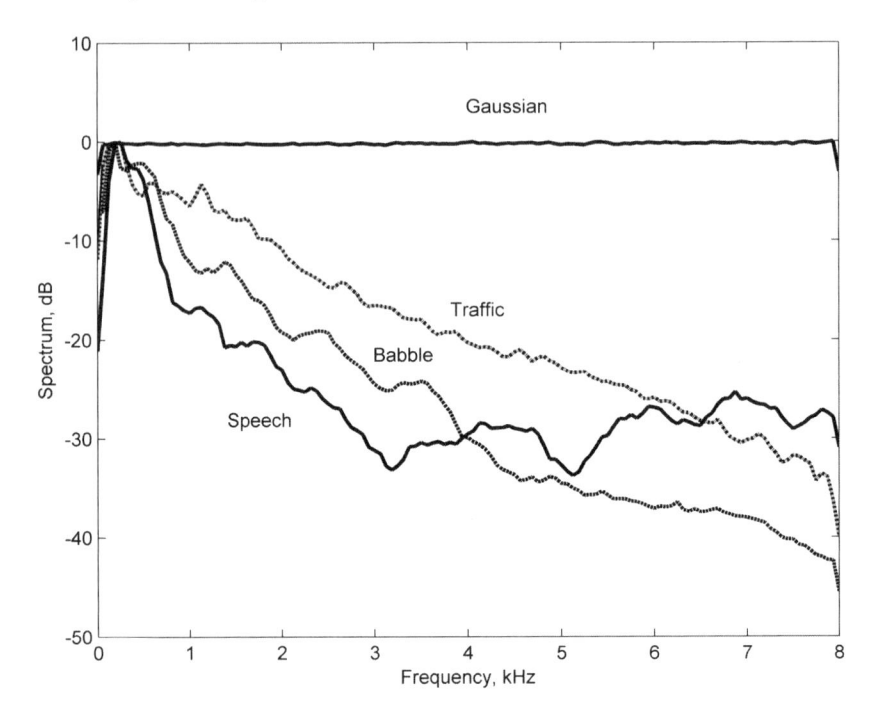

Figure 9-7. Average magnitude spectra for the four signals of Figures 9-2 through 9-5. Each plot represents the average of 30 sec of data sampled at 16 kHz. The plots are normalized by the maximum value for each spectrum.

Low-Level Expansion

The general approach in single-microphone noise suppression is to reduce the gain for that portion of the signal assumed to be noise. One assumption is that speech is more intense than noise, so that high-level signal components are speech and low-level components are noise. This leads to low-level expansion processing, in which low-level signal components are expanded downward. The low-level expansion can be combined with high-level compression, as shown in the input-output relationship diagrammed in Figure 9-8. If the signal level is above the kneepoint, it is compressed by reducing the gain as the signal level is increased. If the signal level is below the kneepoint, it is expanded by reducing the gain as the signal level is reduced. The kneepoint level represents an implicit assumption about the intensity of speech to be

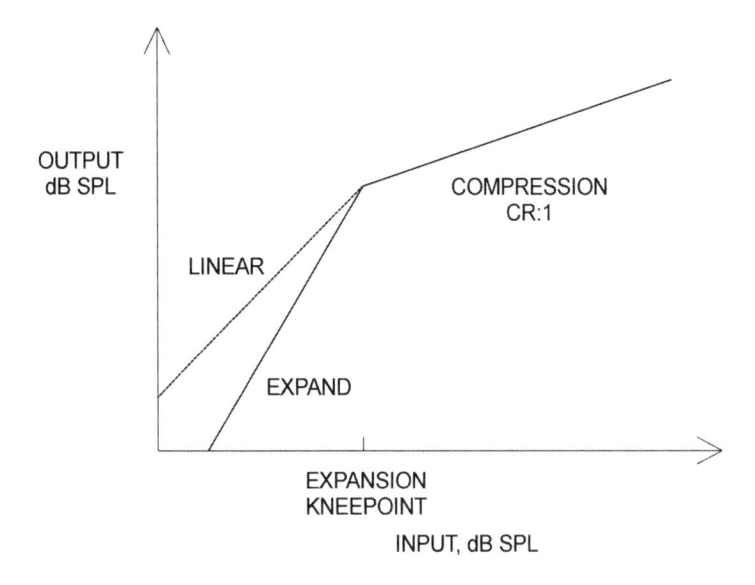

Figure 9-8. Input-output relationship for a system using compression for high-level sounds and expansion for low-level sounds. Linear gain for low-level sounds is indicated by the dashed line.

expected under normal listening conditions. The low-level expansion can be implemented in a broadband (single-channel) system, or in a multiband system in which the expansion is performed independently in each frequency band based on the signal level in that band. The kneepoint depicted in Figure 9-8 is a hard boundary between the expansion and compression portions of the input-output rule, and it is also possible to provide a gradual transition entering into the expansion region (Clarkson & Bahgat, 1991). The expansion portion of the system may also use different time constants than the compression portion.

The problem with low-level expansion is that it may reduce the amplitude of low-level speech sounds along with the noise. In particular, it is worth noting that low-level expansion has been used as a simulation of hearing loss (Duchnowski & Zurek, 1995), so the level of the speech relative to that of the expansion kneepoint is critical. The input-output relationship of Figure 9-8 provides maximum gain for sound intensities at the kneepoint. If the intensity of a speech sound is below the expansion kneepoint, its amplitude will be reduced by the expansion and intelligibility would be expected to suffer.

In an experiment looking at broadband low-level expansion, Plyler et al. (2005a) found that 1:2 expansion reduced speech intelligibility both in quiet, especially for speech input levels near the expansion kneepoint, and also reduced intelligibility for speech in noise. However, on average the hearing-impaired listeners with sloping losses preferred the expanded speech in quiet and in low levels of background noise. They also found (Plyler et al., 2005b) that intelligibility was reduced as the expansion time constants were increased. Fast time constants can attenuate the noise between syllables, reducing the perceived noise level, but can also generate "burbling" artifacts as the gain changes modulate the intensity of the noise. Slow time constants can reduce the severity of the artifacts, but slow down the system response; the onset of a speech sound may be attenuated by the noise suppression gain set for the preceding noise level. Clarkson and Bahgat (1991) studied a multichannel expansion system that used a gradual change in expansion ratio with decreasing signal level, and found a small benefit in intelligibility for speech in noise for normal-hearing listeners.

Envelope Valley Tracking

The signal envelopes plotted in Figures 9-2 through 9-5 showed much greater level fluctuations for speech than for the other signals. This observation has led to noise suppression algorithms based on tracking the signal peak-to-valley ratio. A peak detector follows increases in the signal level with a rapid time constant and decreases in the signal level with a slow time constant. A valley detector works in the opposite direction: signal decreases are followed with a rapid time constant and increases in the signal level with a slow time constant. The difference between the outputs of the peak detector and the valley detector in dB is then the estimated peak-to-valley ratio for the signal. A high peak-to-valley ratio is indicative of speech, and a low peak-to-valley ratio is indicative of noise.

The noise suppression is designed to have unity gain for a high peak-to-valley ratio, and to provide attenuation for a low peak-to-valley ratio. A block diagram of one such system is presented in Figure 9-9. The peaks and valleys are tracked in each band of a multichannel system. The peak-to-valley ratio is computed, and this ratio is the input to a gain-control calculation based on empirical observations on the annoy-

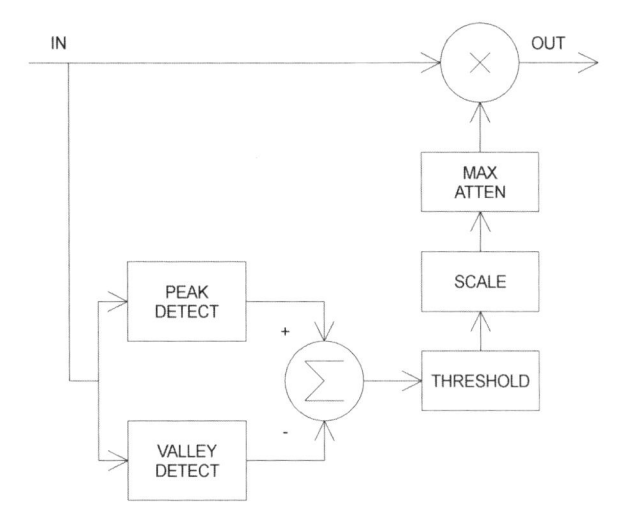

Figure 9-9. Block diagram of one frequency channel of a system that tracks the envelope peaks and valleys in dB and uses the peak-to-valley ratio to control noise attenuation.

ance of the background noise. The gain for the signal in each frequency band is then adjusted based on the attenuation rule, an example of which is shown in Figure 9-10. If the peak-to-valley ratio is sufficiently high, greater than the threshold set to 15 dB in this example, no attenuation is provided. If the peak-to-valley ratio is sufficiently low, below 0 dB in this example, the attenuation is limited to the maximum of 7.5 dB. In between the threshold and 0 dB peak-to-valley ratio, the gain is reduced by 0.5 dB for each 1 dB reduction in the peak-to-valley ratio.

Experiments evaluating this type of processing in general have shown no improvement in intelligibility for speech in noise, but have shown some listener preference for the processed speech. Walden et al. (2000) found that a hearing aid with a directional microphone combined with noise suppression did not improve speech intelligibility in noise over that of the hearing aid with the directional microphone alone. However, subject ratings of speech understanding in noise showed small but insignificant benefits for the processing, and sound comfort showed a significant benefit for the noise suppression. Ricketts and Hornsby (2005) also found no benefit in improving speech intelligibility in noise when noise suppression was used in a hearing aid, but found a significant

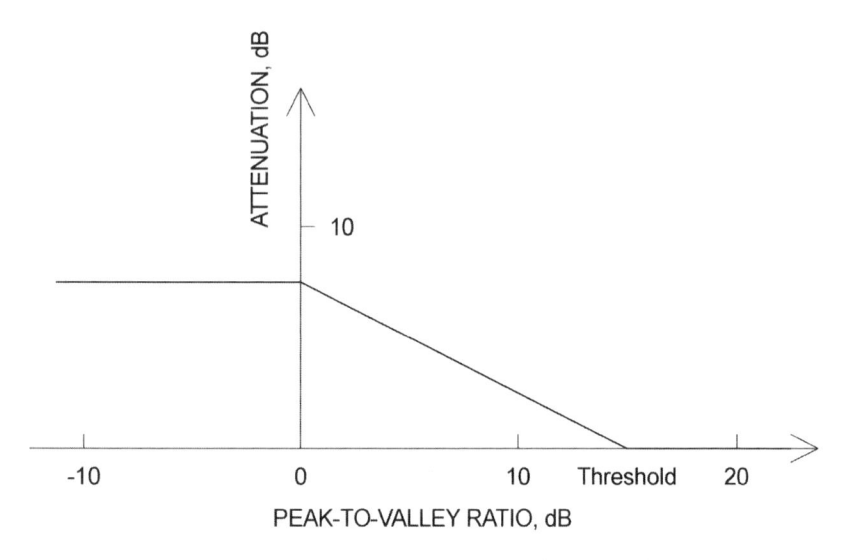

Figure 9-10. Curve giving the signal attenuation as a function of the peak-to-valley ratio in a envelope tracking noise-suppression system presented in Figure 9-9.

listener preference for the processing. Chung et al. (2004), in a study of cochlear implant users, found that the noise suppression offered no improvement in speech intelligibility but significantly improved ease of listening.

Bandwidth Reduction

One of the simplest approaches to suppressing noise is to use a filter to restrict the bandwidth of the system output. If the noise is concentrated in a narrow frequency region, causing a negative SNR, then reducing the gain in that region can attenuate the noise, thus reducing the upward spread of masking and producing a net improvement in speech intelligibility (van Dijkhuizen et al., 1991). Many common noises, such as traffic noise, are concentrated at low frequencies. Other noises are concentrated at high frequencies, an example being the transients caused by jangling a set of keys. Thus, signal-processing strategies have been developed specifically for dealing with noises found at the extremes of the frequency range, the goal being to reduce the effects of the noise while leaving the speech in the mid-frequencies unaltered.

ADAPTIVE HIGH-PASS FILTER

An adaptive high-pass filter is simple enough that it can be implemented in an analog hearing aid. One example was the Siemens 007 ASP (Kates, 1986), an analog in-the-ear (ITE) hearing aid. A block diagram for the noise suppression built into that hearing aid is presented in Figure 9-11. The output from a low-pass filter is monitored to detect the presence of low-frequency noise. The absolute value of the low-frequency output was used, with noise indicated when the output exceeded a threshold that could be adjusted by the dispensor. As the filter output rose above the threshold the low-frequency gain was reduced. The change in the high-pass filter response with increasing noise level is illustrated in Figure 9-12.

Experiments testing the effectiveness of adaptive high-pass filters tend to show a small improvement in speech intelligibility in noise. Bentler et al. (1993) found that the filter reduced the detrimental effects of broadband background noise for hearing-impaired listeners, but did not return the scores to the values observed in quiet. Fabry et al. (1993) found a correlation between the amount of benefit from the high-pass filter and the measured amount of excess upward spread of masking in their subjects, suggesting that the adaptive high-pass filter was improving intelligibility by reducing the masking effects of the low-frequency

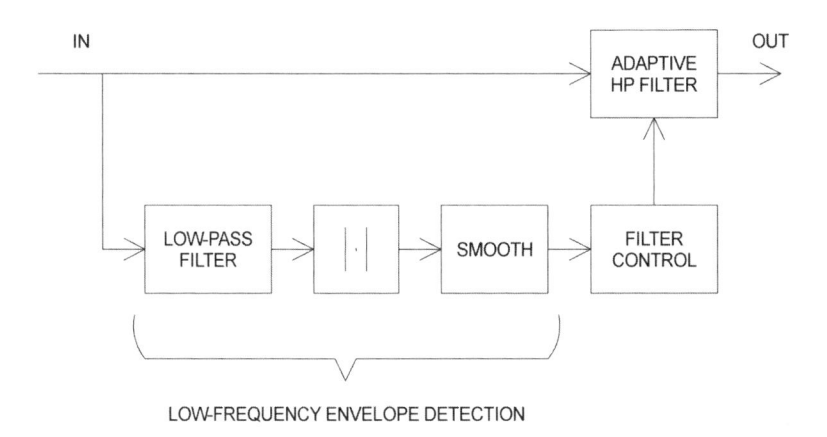

Figure 9-11. Block diagram of an adaptive high-pass filter system intended to suppress low-frequency noise.

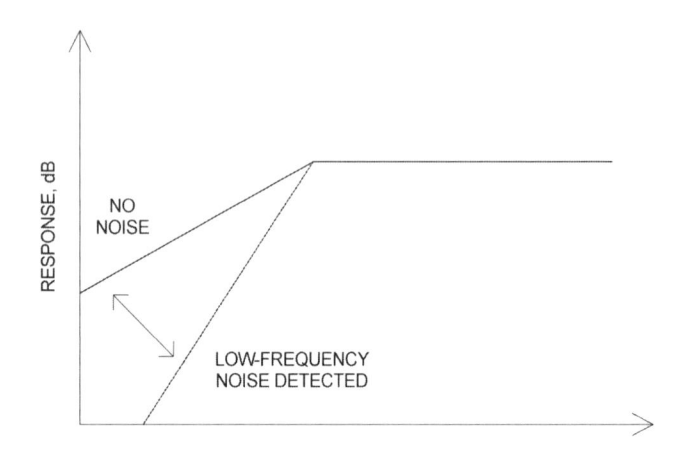

Figure 9-12. Adaptive high-pass filter behavior for the system of Figure 9-11.

noise. Dillon and Lovegrove (1993) found an approximately 1-dB improvement in the SRT when an adaptive high-pass filter was used, with the greatest benefit for low-frequency machine noise.

ADAPTIVE LOW-PASS FILTER

Transient noises can affect the listening comfort for someone using a hearing aid. Transient noise suppression requires an effective procedure for detecting the transients, combined with transient suppression that does not strongly reduce speech intelligibility. As a transient is defined as having a short temporal duration, its spectrum will be concentrated at high frequencies, and a burst of high-frequency energy can be used as a transient indicator.

Gingsjö (1997) proposed and tested the transient reduction system shown in Figure 9-13. The incoming signal is passed through a high-pass filter, rectified, and low-pass filtered to give the envelope of the signal high-frequency component. The high-pass filter response imposes a delay on the envelope estimate, and a compensating delay is provided in the speech signal path. If this delay were not present, the gain reduction triggered by the transient would lag behind the transient in the speech signal. With the delay, the gain is reduced in the signal path in anticipation of the transient and can effectively reduce the transient amplitude.

If the detected high-frequency output exceeds a threshold, the speech is sent through an adaptive low-pass filter to remove the transient, as

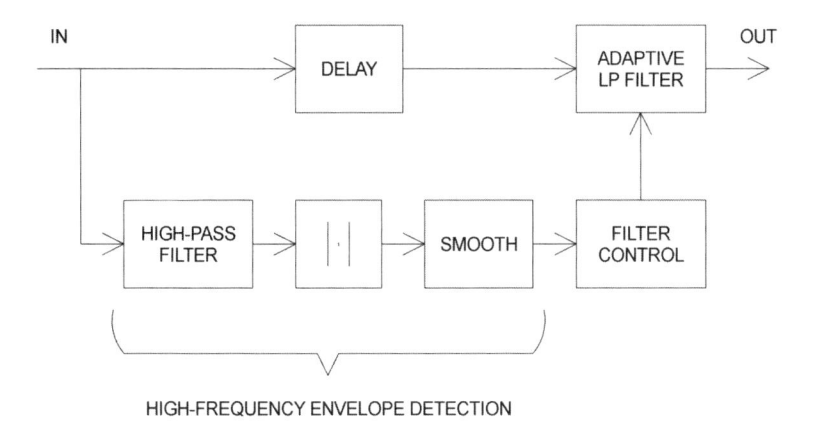

Figure 9-13. Block diagram of an adaptive low-pass filter system intended to suppress high-frequency transient noise.

shown in Figure 9-14. Attenuating the entire broadband signal by 20 dB was also considered in the study. Gingsjö found that a majority of the hearing-impaired subjects preferred the processed speech to unprocessed when transients were present, and that the filtering approach was preferred to the broadband attenuation. When a group of transients was added to speech test material, hearing-impaired subjects showed a small improvement in intelligibility for the processed speech whereas normal-hearing subjects showed a decrement in intelligibility.

"ZETA NOISE BLOCKER"

The "Zeta Noise Blocker" was an early digital noise-suppression circuit implemented in a CMOS integrated circuit (Graupe et al, 1987). The circuit was intended for use with the analog hearing aids available at the time of its introduction. Noise was detected by several means, and the implementation changed with different versions of the integrated circuit (Bentler et al., 1993; Van Tasell et al., 1988). One approach was fitting an autoregressive model to the incoming signal (i.e., modeling the present signal value as a weighted combination of previous sample values) and identifying noise based on the model parameters (Graupe & Causey, 1997). A second approach was monitoring the minima of the signal in different frequency bands and comparing those levels to an absolute threshold or to the average signal level (Graupe & Causey, 1980; Van Tasell et al., 1988). When noise was detected, the circuit

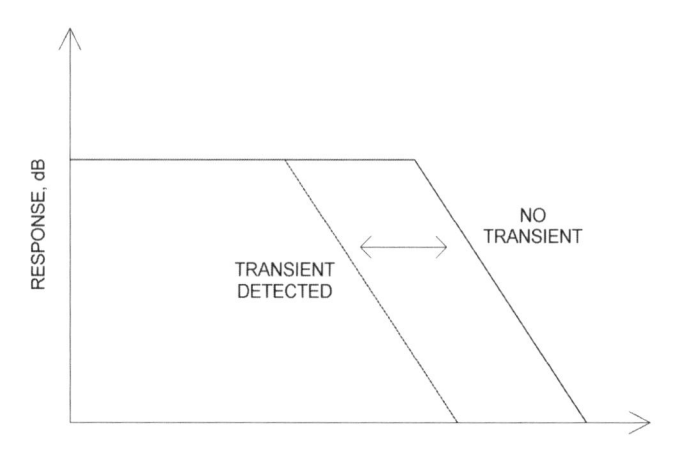

Figure 9-14. Adaptive low-pass filter behavior for the system of Figure 9-13.

responded by restricting the system bandwidth (Bentler et al., 1993; Dillon & Lovegrove, 1993).

Experiments testing the effectiveness of the "Zeta Noise Blocker" gave mixed results. Some showed an improvement for speech intelligibility in various kinds of noise, including narrow-band low-frequency noise, cafeteria noise, multitalker babble, and white noise (Stein & Dempsey-Hart, 1984; Wolinsky, 1986). However, in both of these favorable experiments the subjects were allowed to adjust the hearing-aid volume control. It is possible that the observed improvements in intelligibility were the results of increased speech audibility and/or reduced hearing-aid distortion as the volume control was adjusted. In experiments in which the hearing-aid volume control was kept fixed, no improvement in intelligibility was found for speech presented in stationary speech-shaped noise (Bentler et al., 1993; Van Tasell et al., 1988), although some improvement in intelligibility was found for noise concentrated at low frequencies (Dillon & Lovegrove, 1993).

Envelope Modulation Filters

The speech envelope-modulation spectrum plotted in Figure 9-6 shows much more speech modulation power in the region from 2 to 10 Hz than is present in the noise signals. Above a modulation frequency of

20 Hz the speech envelope modulations continue to fall off in intensity, whereas the noise modulation spectra remain restively flat as the modulation frequency increases. These differences between the speech and noise modulation spectra form the basis of several related approaches to noise suppression. The idea is to filter the modulation spectra to preserve the speech envelope modulations in the 2 to 20 Hz range while reducing the amplitude of the modulations outside this speech range. These modulation-filtering techniques have not been implemented in hearing aids, but they represent an interesting approach to noise suppression.

Langhans and Strube (1982) investigated several different versions of envelope modulation filtering. A block diagram of one system is presented in Figure 9-15. The incoming signal was sampled at a 10-kHz sampling rate and analyzed using a short-time Fourier transform. The block size was 400 samples (40 msec), windowed with a Hamming widow and padded out to 512 samples with zeros. The FFT frame rate was 100 Hz, so envelope modulations up to 50 Hz can be represented in the modulation spectrum.

In the processing, the FFT magnitude is combined across frequency bins to produce a critical-band spectrum. A new spectrum is produced every 10 msec, and the output in each critical band is sent though a modulation filter, shown here as a band-pass filter although a low-pass filter was also used in some experiments. The ratio of the filtered envelope to the unfiltered envelope is the gain in that critical band that is applied to the signal. The unfiltered envelope is delayed to compensate for the group delay of the envelope-modulation filter so that the unfiltered and filtered envelopes are synchronized. The magnitude in each FFT bin is then multiplied by the envelope-modulation gain as a function of frequency and recombined with the original phase to produce the enhanced signal. Again delays are provided for the magnitude and phase to compensate for the group delay of the envelope-modulation filter. The time-domain signal for each speech segment is computed from the inverse FFT of the modified spectrum, and the output waveform is produced by combining the segment outputs using overlap-add.

In one experiment, Langhans and Strube (1982) used the modulation filter to compensate for reverberation. In a reverberant environment, the speech modulation depth is reduced by the reflections overlapping the desired speech signal. Langhans and Strube therefore designed a modulation filter having a modulation gain rising to 9.5 dB at low fre-

280 Digital Hearing Aids

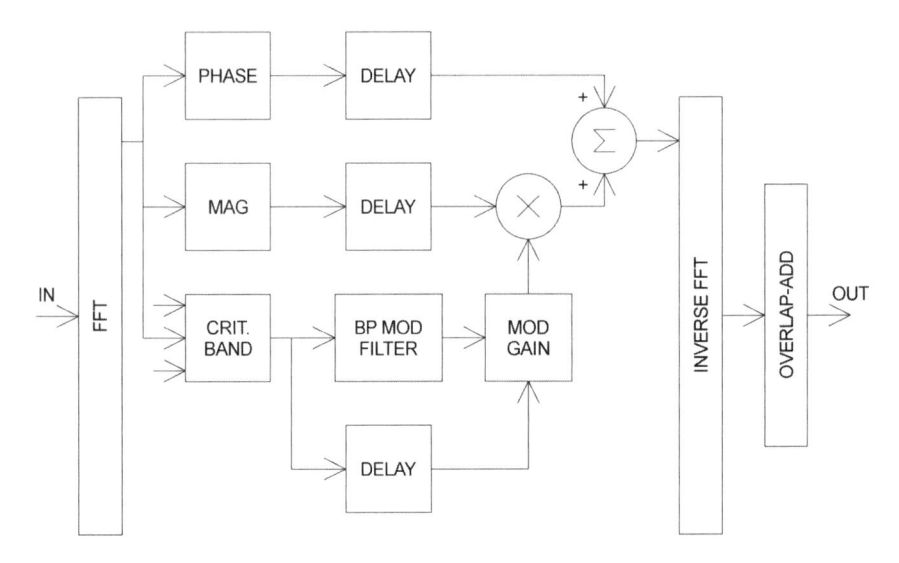

Figure 9-15. Noise suppression using envelope modulation filtering (Langhans & Strube, 1982). The envelope filtering for one frequency band is shown.

quencies and which then decayed to zero for modulation frequencies above 40 Hz. However, a group of normal-hearing subjects showed no improvement in intelligibility.

In a second experiment, they used a band-pass filter to enhance the envelope of speech combined with additive stationary noise. The modulation in each critical band is reduced by the noise, and the objective of the filter was to restore the modulation depth of the noisy speech to match that of the original speech. The gain of the band-pass filter was set to 1 for modulations at 0 Hz, and was set to:

$$M(k) = \frac{S(k) + N(k)}{S(k)} \quad \text{Equation (9.1)}$$

for the critical bands above 0 Hz where k is the critical band index, $M(k)$ is the modulation filter gain, $S(k)$ is the signal power, and $N(k)$ is the noise power. The modulation-filter gain decayed to zero above 40 Hz. This form of modulation filtering improved the measured SNR by 3 dB, but produced no improvement in intelligibility for normal-hearing subjects.

Langhans and Strube (1982) then tried a modulation filter based on a logarithmic transformation of the signal magnitude. This system is illustrated in Figure 9-16. The critical band output is converted to dB and then filtered as before. The difference between the filtered and original log critical band outputs give the filter gain in dB. This difference in dB is then exponentiated to give the linear enhancement gain, and the remainder of the enhancement processing is the same as in Figure 9-15. The band-pass filter had a gain of 0.05 at 0 Hz, gains of 5 dB from 2 to 16 Hz, and dropped to a gain of 1 above 18 Hz. The authors were interested in investigating this form of processing as a compression/expansion scheme for a hearing aid, and presented the test materials to normal-hearing subjects having a hearing loss simulated by additive noise. The processing greatly improved speech intelligibility for the simulated loss compared to the unprocessed stimuli, but no comparison with linear amplification was provided.

A related approach is the RASTA algorithm proposed by Hermansky and Morgan (1994). The bulk of their paper is devoted to investigat-

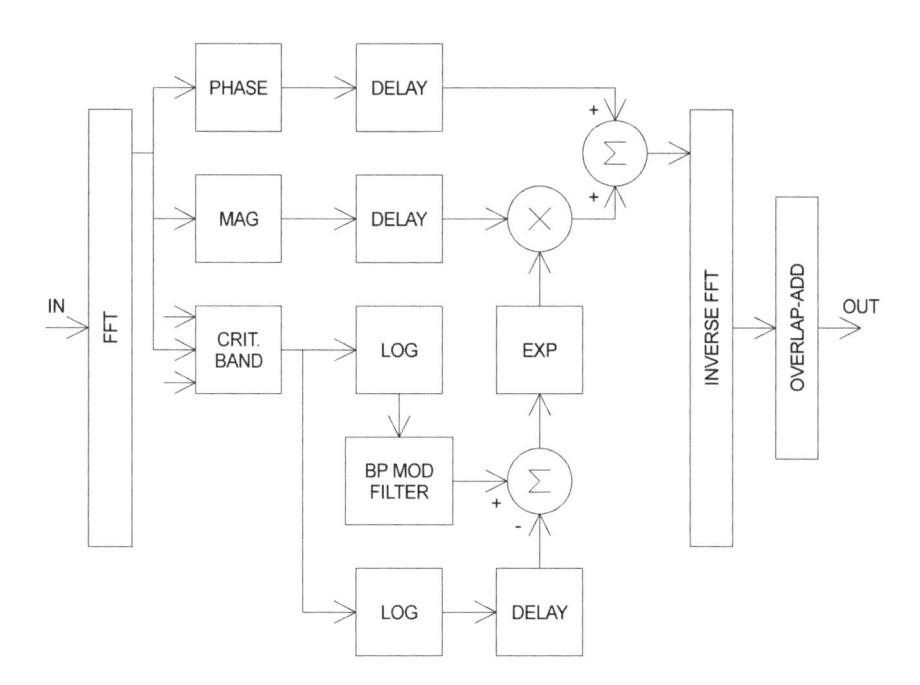

Figure 9-16. Noise suppression using log envelope modulation filtering (Langhans & Strube, 1982). The envelope filtering for one frequency band is shown.

ing a system similar to that shown in Figure 9-16 as a preprocessor for computer speech recognition. They used 31.25-msec segments with a Hamming window, with a new segment selected every 7.8125 msec. Their system used an envelope-modulation filter having a pass band from 1 to 10 Hz, and they found noticeable improvements in the accuracy of isolated digit recognition. For listening to noisy speech, they replaced the logarithmic operation shown in Figure 9-16 with a cube-root operation. The resultant system is shown in Figure 9-17. The cube root of the magnitude in each FFT bin was taken, the resultant signal band-pass filtered, and the filter output was then raised to the third power to produce the modified signal envelope. The band-pass filter passed the frequencies from 1 to 15 Hz. Only informal listening results are mentioned in their paper, and they indicate no apparent improvement in intelligibility, a reduction in the amplitude of steady-state and impulsive background noises, and the presence of processing artifacts that affected sound quality.

Envelope modulation filtering can also be implemented using a filter bank to replace the FFT. In a group of related papers (Arai et al., 2002; Arai et al., 2004; Hodoshima et al. 2004; Kitamura et al., 2000; Kusumoto et al., 2000), researchers at Sophia University in Japan have investigated the effects of envelope modulation filtering on reducing the effects of reverberation on speech intelligibility. The basic system (Kitamura et al., 2000) is illustrated in Figure 9-18. The incoming signal is divided into one-third octave bands by the filter bank, and the envelope in each frequency band is extracted using a Hilbert transform filter. A Hilbert transform filter provides a phase shift of 90 degrees; if the input to the filter is $cos(2\pi fn)$, the output will be $sin(2\pi fn)$. Squaring and adding the input and output signals together and taking the square root of the sum then gives the envelope of the signal. The envelope is band-pass filtered, after which the signal in the frequency band is resynthesized by multiplying the filtered envelope by the carrier frequency, which is a sinusoid at the center frequency of the band. The filtered envelope thus modulates the amplitude of the tone at the carrier frequency. The peaks of the envelope modulation filters range from 10 Hz at high frequencies down to 4 Hz at low frequencies. In another version of the processing, the band-pass filter was replaced by a high-pass filter. The gain for the band was reduced when the output of the filter indicated a nearly steady-state envelope, and was kept at 0 dB when the filter output indicated a fluctuating envelope.

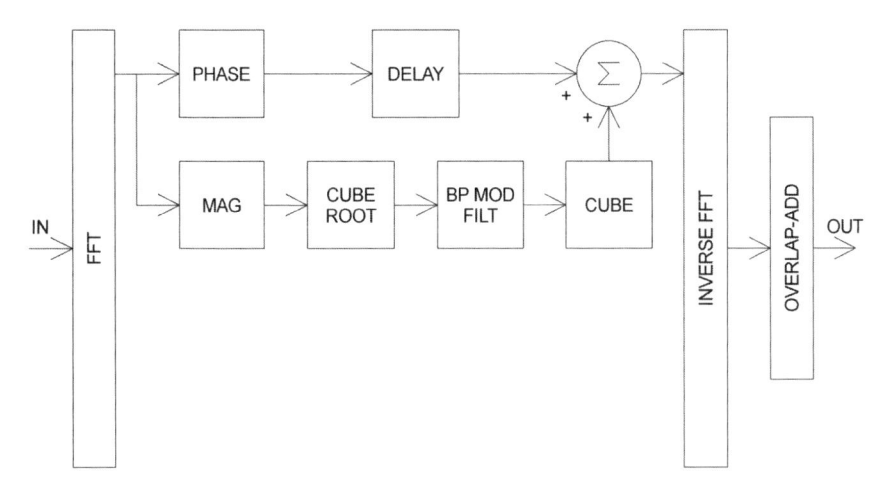

Figure 9-17. Noise suppression using the RASTA method of envelope modulation filtering (Hermansky & Morgan, 1994). The envelope filtering for one frequency band is shown.

Their results in improving speech intelligibility and quality in reverberation are summarized in Arai et al. (2004). In a preference test using the band-pass envelope modulation filter for processing reverberant speech, Kusumoto et al. (2000) found that their group of four hearing-impaired listeners preferred the processed speech. Kitamura et al. (2000) found a small improvement in intelligibility for the one hearing-impaired subject that was tested, and an improvement in quality of 1.25 on a 5-point scale for a group of two normal-hearing subjects. In an experiment using the steady-state suppression, Arai et al. (2002) found a small but not statistically significant improvement in intelligibility for a group of 12 normal-hearing subjects, and Hodoshima et al. (2004) found a significant improvement in intelligibility for identifying Japanese nonsense syllables when testing a group of 24 normal-hearing subjects. A small improvement in intelligibility was observed for a single elderly hearing-impaired subject under similar test conditions (Arai et al., 2004). However, in another experiment involving the same subject no improvement in intelligibility was found.

Ghitza (2001) has pointed out that reconstructing a signal from the smoothed envelope and original phase does not remove the high modulation frequencies from the signal. Even though the envelope is smoothed, the modulation information is still contained in the phase. Thus, the sys-

284 Digital Hearing Aids

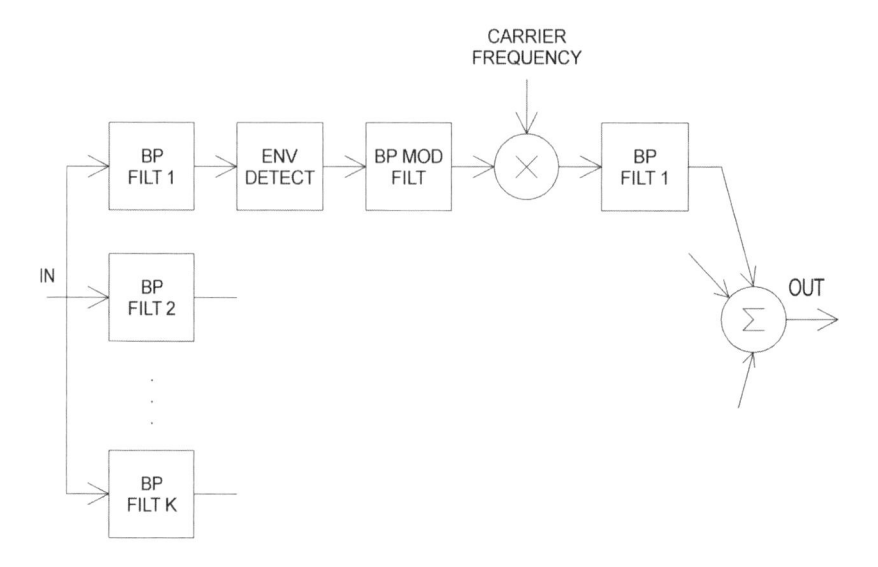

Figure 9-18. Noise suppression using the Hilbert transform procedure of Kitamura et al. (2000). The envelope filtering for one frequency band is shown.

tems of Langhans and Strube (1982) and Hermansky and Morgan (1994) incompletely remove the noise modulations from the speech. Ghitza (2001) also has pointed out that a signal reconstructed from a band-limited envelope and carrier has a much wider bandwidth than expected. Interactions between the outputs in the different frequency bands can then generate audible distortion (Atlas & Janssen, 2005). Thus, the performance of the system illustrated in Figure 9-18 could be limited by band interaction effects, although these effects should be minimized by the presence of the second band-pass filter in each frequency band applied just before the processed signals are added together.

Atlas and colleagues at the University of Washington (Atlas & Janssen, 2005; Li & Atlas, 2005; Schimmel & Atlas, 2005; Sukittanon et al., 2005) are developing an envelope modulation filtering approach designed to avoid the problems identified by Ghitza (2001). Their system can be considered to be a modification of the system presented in Figure 9-18, and a block diagram of this modified system is shown in Figure 9-19. The dominant frequency in each band is identified and the frequency estimate is smoothed. This smoothed frequency is used for the carrier instead of the nominal center frequency of the band, and

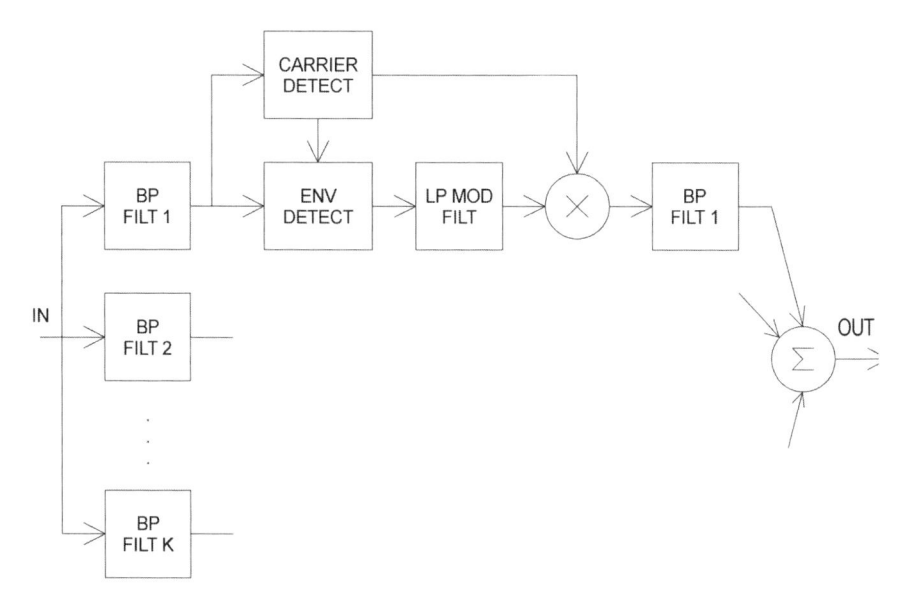

Figure 9-19. Noise suppression using coherent demodulation envelope filtering (Li & Atlas, 2005). The envelope filtering for one frequency band is shown.

the carrier frequency can vary over time. The envelope in each band is extracted by coherent demodulation, in which the signal within the band is multiplied by the time-varying carrier. The multiplication takes a signal component at the carrier frequency and shifts it down to 0 Hz, and the frequencies to either side of the carrier become low-frequency components that represent the signal envelope. The envelope is filtered and the signal within the band is reconstructed by multiplying the smoothed envelope by the carrier to shift it back up in frequency. The system output is then summed across the frequency bands.

In preliminary experiments, Souza et al. (2005) investigated the potential benefits of the processing for cochlear implant and hearing aid users. The unprocessed speech, speech enhanced using the system of Figure 9-19 with time-varying carrier frequencies in each band, and the same system with fixed carrier frequencies in each band were compared. The time-varying carrier frequencies were extracted off-line and matched to utterances of each talker. The fixed carrier frequencies result in a system similar to that of Figure 9-18, in which the Hilbert transform was used to extract the envelope in each band. The filtering applied to the signal envelopes was not specified. The results for a simulated cochlear implant system gave an improvement in SRT of about 20 dB for the time-varying carrier frequencies in comparison with the unprocessed speech, but no improvement for the fixed carrier frequencies. For a group of five hearing-impaired subjects, the fixed carrier frequencies resulted in poorer performance on the SRT compared to the unprocessed speech, whereas the time-varying carrier frequencies gave improvements in the SRT for four out of the five subjects with a mean improvement of about 4 dB.

Concluding Remarks

The noise-suppression algorithms discussed in this chapter are based on reducing the gain for signal components deemed to be noise. The suppression can occur in the time domain by reducing the amplitude of low-level sounds, reducing the signal bandwidth, or in the envelope modulation domain by restricting the envelope modulation rate to the 2 to 20-Hz range typical of speech. The best any of these approaches could do in improving speech intelligibility was equivalent to about a 1-dB reduction in SNR. Larger benefits for the processed speech were found in listener preferences. So the real benefit for noise suppression may not be in improving intelligibility, but in reduced listening effort; listeners may still make the same mistakes, but they don't have to work as hard in making them.

The disappointing results for noise suppression lead one to wonder why these algorithms don't work better than they do. One reason may be that each algorithm concentrates on one specific aspect of speech or noise, but does not take into account the interaction of the processing with other aspects of the speech signal. For example, downward expansion will reduce the amplitude of low-intensity noise, but will also reduce the intensity of low-intensity speech sounds. A second concern is distortion and artifacts introduced by the processing. Unintended side effects may undo the benefit that could otherwise be obtained from the processing approach.

The algorithms discussed in this chapter cannot remove the noise from the speech. They only attenuate those time intervals or spectral regions that appear to be noisy and are assumed to make a minimal contribution to speech intelligibility. But there is a fundamental rule in signal processing, which is that filtering a signal can never add information but only remove it. It is hard to improve intelligibility by removing information from the signal. The benefits of noise suppression will only be found by compensating for the imperfect signal processing in the impaired ear, and this is surprisingly difficult to do.

References

Arai, T., Kinoshita, K., Hodoshima, N., Kusumoto, A., & Kitamura, T. (2002). Effects of suppressing steady-state portions of speech on intelligibility in reverberant environments. *Acoustic Science and Technology*, 23, 229–232.

Arai, T., Yasu, K., & Hodoshima, N. (2004). Effective speech processing for various impaired listeners. *Proceedings of the 2004 International Conference on Acoustics*, II (pp. 1389–1392), Kyoto.

Atlas, L., & Janssen, C. (2005). Coherent modulation spectral filtering for single-channel music source separation. *Proceedings of the IEEE International Conference on Acoustics, Speech, and Signal Processing*, IV (pp. 461–464), Philadelphia.

Bentler, R. A., Niebuhr, D. P., Getta, J. P., & Anderson, C. V. (1993). Longitudinal study of hearing aid effectiveness. I: Objective measures. *Journal of Speech and Hearing Research*, 36, 808-819.

Chung, K., Zeng, F-G., & Waltzman, S. (2004). Using hearing aid directional microphones and noise reduction algorithms to enhance cochlear implant performance. *Acoustic Research Letters Online*, 5, 56–61.

Clarkson, P. M., & Bahgat, S. F. (1991). Envelope expansion methods for speech enhancement. *Journal of the Acoustical Society of America*, 89, 1378–1382.

Dillon, H., & Lovegrove, R. (1993). Single-microphone noise reduction systems for hearing aids: A review and evaluation. In G. A. Studebaker & I. Hochberg, Eds. *Acoustical factors affecting hearing aid performance*. Boston: Allyn and Bacon.

Duchnowski, P., & Zurek, P. (1995). Villchur revisited: Another look at automatic gain control simulation of hearing loss. *Journal of the Acoustical Society of America*, 98, 3170–3181.

Fabry, D. A., Leek, M. R., Walden, B. E., & Cord, M. (1993). Do adaptive frequency response (AFR) hearing aids reduce upward spread of masking? *Journal of Rehabilitation Research and Development*, 30, 318–325.

Ghitza, O. (2001). On the upper cutoff frequency of the auditory critical-band envelope detectos in the context of speech perception. *Journal of the Acoustical Society of America, 110*, 1628-1640.

Gingsjö, A. L. (1997). *On transient noise and its reduction in hearing aids.* Ph.D. Thesis, Chalmers University of Technology, Göteborg, Sweden. (Tech. Report 319, Dept. of Applied Electronics, School of Electronics Computer Engineering)

Graupe, D., & Causey, G. D. (1977). *Method of and means for adaptively filtering near-stationary noise from speech.* U.S. Patent 4,025,721, issued May 24, 1977.

Graupe, D., & Causey, G. D. (1980). *Method and means for adaptively filtering near-stationary noise from an information bearing signal.* U.S. Patent 4,185,168, issued Jan. 22, 1980.

Graupe, D., Grosspietsch, J. K., & Basseas, S. P. (1987). A single-microphone-based self-adaptive filter of noise from speech and its performance evaluation. *Journal of Rehabilitation Research and Development, 24*, 119–126.

Greenberg, S., & Arai, T. (2004). What are the essential cues for understanding spoken language?" *IEICE Transaction on Information and Systems,* E87-D, 1059–1070.

Hermansky, H., & Morgan, N. (1994). RASTA processing of speech. *IEEE Transactions on Speech and Audio Processing, 2*, 578–589.

Hodoshima, N., Inoue, T., Arai, T., Kusumoto, A., & Kinoshita, K. (2004). Suppressing steady-state portions of speech for improving intelligibility in various reverberent environments. *Acoustic Science and Technology, 25*, 58–60.

Kates, J. M. (1986). Signal processing for hearing aids. *Hearing Instruments, 37*, 19–21.

Kitamura, T., Kinoshita, K., Arai, T., Kusumoto, A., & Murahara, Y. (2000). Designing modulation filters for improving speech intelligibility in reverberant environments. *Proceedings of the 6th International Conference on Spoken Language Processing, 3* (pp. 586–589), Beijing, Oct. 16–20, 2000.

Kusumoto, A., Arai, T., Kitamura, T., Takahashi, T., & Murahara, Y. (2000). Modulation enhancement of speech as a preprocessing for reverberant chambers with the hearing-impaired. *Proceedings of the International Conference on Acoustics, Speech, and Signal Processing, II* (pp. 253–256), Istanbul, June 5–9, 2000.

Langhans, T., & Strube, H. W. (1982). Speech enhancement by nonlinear multiband envelope filtering. *Proceedings of the IEEE International Conference on Acoustics, Speech, and Signal Processing,* (pp. 156–159), Paris, May 1982.

Li, Q., & Atlas, L. (2005). Properties of modulation spectral filtering. *Proceedings of the IEEE International Conference on Acoustics, Speech, and Signal Processing, IV* (pp. 521–524), Philadelphia.

Plomp, R. (1988). The negative effect of amplitude compression on multichannel hearing aids in the light of the modulation-transfer function. *Journal of the Acoustical Society of America, 83*, 2322–2327.

Plyler, P. N., Hill, A. B., & Trine, T. D. (2005a). The effects of expansion on the objective and subjective performance of hearing instrument users. *Journal of the American Academy of Audiology, 16*, 101–113.

Plyler, P. N., Hill, A. B., & Trine, T. D. (2005b). The effects of expansion time constants on the objective performance of hearing instrument users. *Journal of the American Academy of Audiology, 16*, 614–621.

Ricketts, T. A., & Hornsby, B. W. Y. (2005). Sound quality measures for speech in noise through a commercial hearing aid implementing "Digital Noise Reduction." *Journal of the American Academy of Audiology, 16*, 270–277.

Schimmel, S., & Atlas, L. (2005). Coherent envelope detection for modulation filtering of speech. *Proceedings of the IEEE International Conference on Acoustics, Speech, and Signal Processing, I* (pp. 221–224), Philadelphia.

Souza, P., Atlas, L., Schimmel, S., Rubenstein, J., Drennan, W., & Won, J. H. (2005). Coherent modulation enhancement: Improving performance in noise for hearing aids and cochlear implants. *Journal of the Acoustical Society of America, 117*, 2535.

Steeneken, H. J. M., & Houtgast, T. (1980). A physical method for measuring speech-transmission quality. *Journal of the Acoustical Society of America, 67*, 318–326.

Stein, L. K., & Dempsey-Hart, D. (1984). Listener-assessed intelligibility of a hearing aid self-adaptive filter. *Ear and Hearing, 5*, 199–204.

Sukittanon, S., Atlas, L. E., Pitton, J. W., & Filali, K. (2005). Improved modulation spectrum through multi-scale modulation frequency decomposition. *Proceedings of the IEEE International Conference on Acoustics, Speech, and Signal Processing, IV* (pp. 517–520), Philadelphia.

van Dijkhuizen, J. N., Festen, J. M., & Plomp, R. (1991). The effect of frequency-selective attenuation on the speech-reception threshold of sentences in conditions of low-frequency noise. *Journal of the Acoustical Society of America, 90*, 885–894.

Van Tasell, D. J., Larsen, S. Y., & Fabry, D. A. (1988). Effects of an adaptive filter hearing aid on speech recognition in noise by hearing-impaired subjects. *Ear and Hearing, 9*, 15–21.

Walden, B. E., Surr, R. K., Cord, M. T., Edwards, B., & Olson, L. (2000). Comparison of benefits provided by different hearing aid technologies. *Journal of the American Academy of Audiology, 11*, 540–560.

Wolinsky, S. (1986, October). Clinical assessment of a self-adaptive noise filtering system. *Hearing Journal*, pp. 29–32.

10
Spectral Subtraction

CHAPTER 9 PRESENTED several different approaches to noise suppression based on how the noise spectrum or envelope modulation differed from that of speech. This chapter concentrates on spectral subtraction. The basic idea is to estimate the noise spectrum, and then subtract it from the noisy speech spectrum to get an improved estimate of the original speech spectrum. The estimated speech spectrum is then used to reconstruct an enhanced signal waveform.

The speech is assumed to be degraded by additive noise, as shown in Figure 10-1. In an ideal world, we would estimate the noise signal and subtract it from the noisy speech to reconstruct the clean speech signal. But separating the noise from the noisy speech in this way requires access to the original noise signal, and the noise signal is generally not available. All that is available is the noisy speech. The best that can be done is to estimate the statistics of the noise from observations of the noisy speech, and to then try to produce an enhanced signal that has statistics closer to the original clean speech signal. This process is shown in the block diagram of Figure 10-2 (reprinted from Chapter 9), where the estimated noise parameters are used to adjust the gain in each of the analysis frequency bands. One can think of spectral subtraction as starting with a distribution of noisy speech magnitude samples measured over some time interval, and then adaptively adjusting the gain in each frequency band so that the distribution of the processed magnitude samples more closely represents that of the clean speech.

292 Digital Hearing Aids

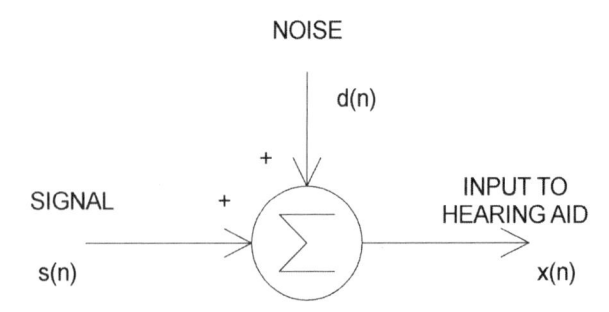

Figure 10-1. Block diagram illustrating additive noise being combined with the speech signal.

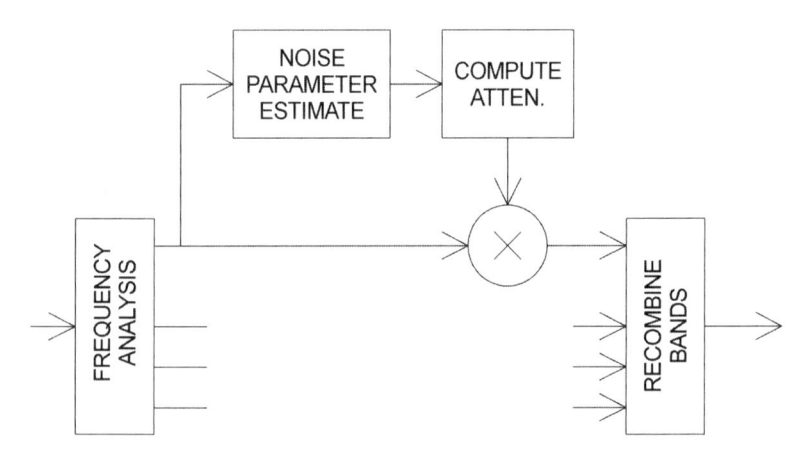

Figure 10-2. Block diagram of a generic multichannel single-microphone noise-suppression system.

The chapter begins with a section on noise estimation, as the accuracy of the spectral subtraction depends on the accuracy of the estimated noise properties. One of the earliest approaches to noise suppression was the Wiener filter, which is described next. The Wiener filter assumes that the speech and noise are stationary (signal statistics such as the signal power do not change over time), which is not the case in the real world. The adaptive Wiener filter is intended to deal with slowly fluctuating speech and noise, and is closely related to spectral subtraction. Spectral subtraction is discussed next, and several different forms of the basic signal-processing strategy are presented. The chapter concludes with a summary of perceptual experiments evaluating the effectiveness of spectral subtraction in improving the intelligibility and quality of noisy speech.

Noise Estimation

Spectral subtraction requires an accurate estimate of the noise power in each frequency band. Two general approaches to noise estimation can be found in the literature. Early work concentrated on identifying signal segments containing voiced speech, termed a voice activity detector (VAD). The noise power estimate is held constant during the voiced speech segments and updated during the nonspeech segments. The reader is referred to Marzinzik and Kollmeier (2002) for a review of this approach. Recent research has concentrated on continuously updating the noise power estimate without using a VAD. These newer approaches are attractive for hearing aids as they do not require the extra computations needed for a VAD. Three noise-estimation approaches that do not use a VAD are discussed in this section.

All of the noise-estimation schemes, those that use a VAD and those that do not, are based on the assumption that the noise is stationary, that is, the noise statistics do not change over time. The noise power estimate is updated when conditions are favorable for doing so, and the estimate is held with minimal change during those signal intervals that are more likely to be speech. The stationarity assumption is thus an assumption that the noise power estimate will be valid even during those time intervals where it is not being updated. If the noise level is fluctuating rapidly, this stationarity assumption will be violated and the error in the estimated noise power will reduce the effectiveness of the spectral subtraction algorithm.

VALLEY DETECTION

The simplest approach to noise power estimation is to use valley detection in each frequency band. In valley detection the estimated signal level is decreased rapidly when the signal level decreases but increased slowly when the signal level increases. The valley detector is thus the opposite of the peak detector given by *Eq. (8.1)*. The valley detector output is given by:

if $|x(n)| \leq v(n-1)$
$v(n) = \alpha v(n-1) + (1-\alpha)|x(n)|$
else   Equation (10.1)
$v(n) = (1+\frac{1}{\beta})v(n-1)$
end

where the input signal is $x(n)$ and the valley detector output is $v(n)$. The valley detector uses a fast attack time constant α when tracking decreases in the signal level and a slow release time constant β when tracking increases. In a multichannel system, a valley detector would be implemented in each frequency band.

An example of valley detection is presented in Figure 10-3 for a segment of speech. The noise is multitalker babble at a SNR of 20 dB. The noise alone is present for the first 250 msec of the signal, after which the speech is present. The figure gives the output of a frequency band centered at 728 Hz and having a bandwidth of about 340 Hz. The light gray curve is the signal envelope given by computing the signal power in 1-msec segments. The output of a peak detector having an attack time of 5 msec and a release time of 70 msec is given by the dashed black line, and the output of a valley detector having an attack time of 50 msec and a release time of 500 msec is given by the solid black line. The valley detector output rises slowly during the initial noise-only portion of the signal. It then drops slightly during the first pause in the speech, rises again during the following voiced segment, and proceeds to fall and rise in synchrony with the speech during the remainder of the utterance. Longer attack and release times for the valley detector would smooth out these fluctuations; for example, Arslan et al. (1995) recommend adjusting the valley detector to increase at a rate of 3 dB per second for increasing signal levels and to decrease at a rate of 12 dB per second for decreasing signal levels. But even with the longer time constants, the same behavior of rising during voiced speech and falling during speech pauses would be present.

MINIMA STATISTICS

A more elegant approach to estimating the noise power is to test each sample of the signal envelope in each frequency band. The signal sample is used to update the estimated noise power if the signal sample has a

Spectral Subtraction **295**

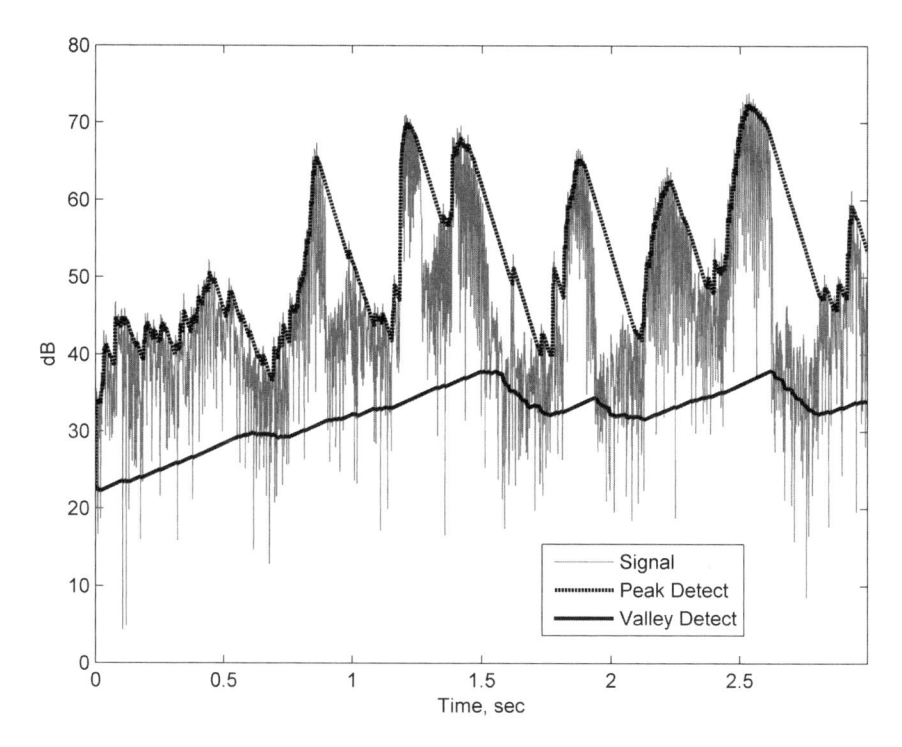

Figure 10-3. Peak detection (attack time 5 msec, release time 70 msec) and valley detection (attack time 50 msec, release time 500 msec) for a segment of speech in additive low-pass filtered noise at an SNR of 20 dB. Results for the 728-Hz band are shown.

higher probability of being noise than speech. A reasonable assumption is that the speech samples in dB are drawn from a Gaussian probability density function, and that the noise samples in dB are drawn from a Gaussian probability density function having a lower mean. Figure 10-4 gives a histogram of samples in dB taken every millisecond from the end of the noisy speech signal plotted in Figure 10-3 for the 728-Hz frequency band. An approximate fit of a pair of Gaussian probability density functions to this histogram is shown in Figure 10-5. The noise probability density function has a mean of 40 dB SPL and a standard deviation of 8 dB, and the speech probability density function has a mean of 60 dB SPL and a standard deviation of 7 dB. The ratio of the amplitudes of the two probability density functions represents the relative occurrence of the noise and speech samples in noisy speech.

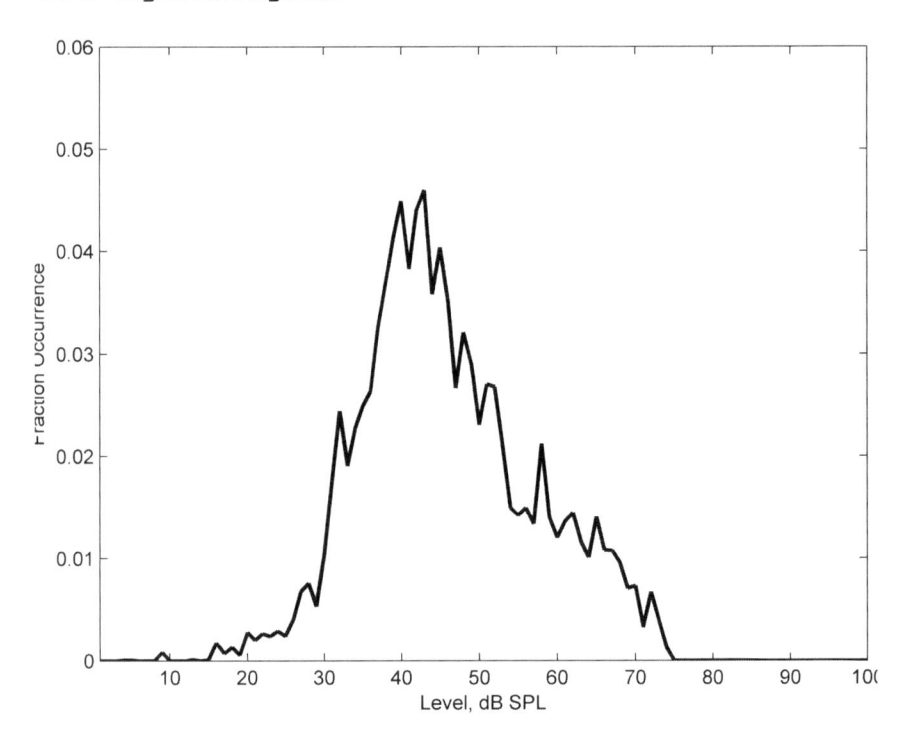

Figure 10-4. Log-level histogram of the noisy speech signal in the 728-Hz band at the end of the segment shown in Figure 10-3.

The noise power estimate is updated using an adaptive averaging operation (Cohen & Berdugo, 2002; Doblinger, 1995; Martin, 2001). Let $|N(k,m)|$ be the noise magnitude estimate for frequency band k and processing block m, and let $|X(k,m)|$ be the incoming noisy signal magnitude. The noise update is given by:

$$|N(k,m)| = \mu(k,m)|N(k,m-1)| + [1-\mu(k,m)]|X(k,m)|$$

Equation (10.2)

The averaging time constant $\mu(k,m)$ depends on the amplitude of the signal envelope sample $|X(k,m)|$. A fast averaging time is used for low-intensity samples that have a high probability of being noise, and a slow averaging time is used for high-intensity samples that have a high prob-

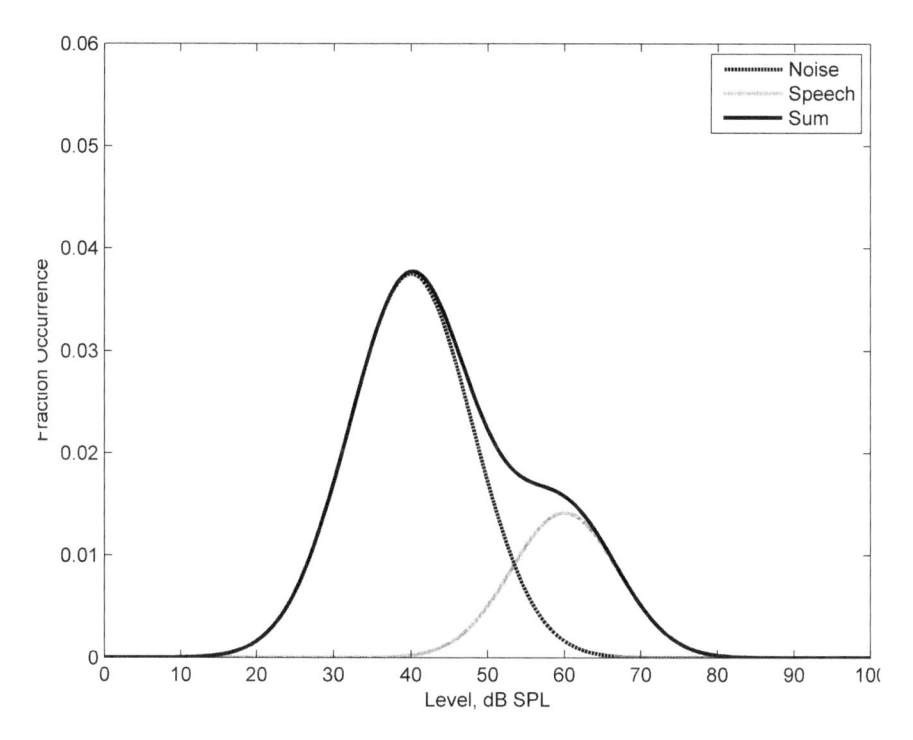

Figure 10-5. Gaussian probability density functions approximating the distribution of signal levels for speech and noise in the histogram plotted in Figure 10-4. The noise distribution has a mean of 40 dB SPL and a standard deviation of 8 dB. The speech distribution has a mean of 60 dB SPL and a standard deviation of 7 dB.

ability of being speech. Intermediate time constant values are used for intermediate signal envelope amplitudes.

A simplified version of this approach is the algorithm described by Hirsch and Ehrlicher (1995). Let $|N(k,m)|$ again be the noise magnitude estimate for frequency band k and processing block m, and let $|X(k,m)|$ be the incoming noisy signal magnitude. Their algorithm is given by:

$$\text{if } |X(k,m)| > b|N(k,m-1)|$$
$$|N(k,m)| = |N(k,m-1)|$$
$$\text{else} \qquad \qquad \text{Equation (10.3)}$$
$$|N(k,m)| = a|N(k,m-1)| + (1-a)|X(k,m)|$$
$$\text{end}$$

This algorithm replaces the adaptive averaging time constant used in Eq. (10.2) with just two values: a short time constant for samples assumed to be noise or an infinitely long time constant for samples assumed to be speech. The selection of which time constant depends on the signal level compared to an adaptive threshold. The algorithm averages the incoming signal into the noise estimate if the signal power is close to or less than that of the existing noise estimate, and holds the new noise estimate to the previous value if the signal power exceeds the noise estimate by the preset threshold b.

The noise level estimate produced by the Hirsh and Ehrlicher (1995) algorithm is plotted in Figure 10-6 for the same noisy speech segment plotted in Figure 10-3. The low-pass filter time constant in Eq. (10.3) was chosen to be 200 msec, and the threshold value b was set to 2. The estimated noise level quickly adapts to the actual noise level during the initial noise-only portion of the noisy speech signal. The noise estimate is then held constant during the more intense speech portions of the signal, but continues to adapt during the less intense portions of the signal where the babble dominates. The result is a nearly constant noise level estimate despite the fluctuations in the speech amplitude.

HISTOGRAM

It is clear from Figures 10-4 and 10-5 that the histogram of signal levels plotted in dB contains useful information about the noise amplitude. The histogram bin containing the greatest number of samples is a good estimate of the noise level if there are more noise samples than speech samples. As the speech and noise levels change over time, the histogram must also track these level changes. The histogram should therefore be "leaky," with the importance of old signal samples slowly decaying and new samples given the greatest weight. Let $H(k,m)$ be the current histogram of the signal levels in dB in frequency band k processing block m. The histogram contains L bins, each encompassing a different signal level in dB, so an individual bin would be denoted by $h(k,m,l)$. Each bin contains the relative count of the number of occurrences of that level in the signal. The noisy signal level $|X(k,m)|$ in dB is then assigned to the closest histogram bin; call this bin index i. The algorithm for updating the histogram is then:

Spectral Subtraction 299

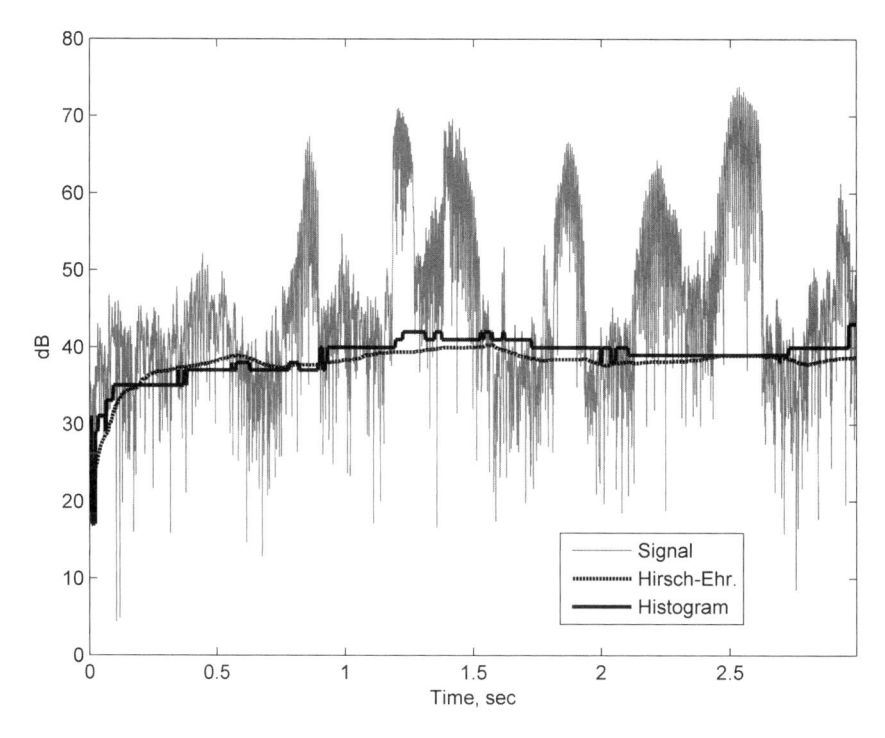

Figure 10-6. Noise detection using the Hirsch-Ehrlicher (1995) algorithm and a log-level histogram approach for a segment of speech in additive low-pass filtered noise at a SNR of 20 dB. The 728-Hz band is shown.

$$h(k,m,l) = \eta h(k,m-1,l) \text{ for } 1 \leq l \leq L$$
$$h(k,m,i) = h(k,m,i) + (1-\eta)$$
Equation (10.4)

where $\eta < 1$. The contents of all of the histogram bins are decayed with a long time constant, thus reducing the influence of old samples, and then the histogram bin corresponding to the current signal envelope sample is incremented. The plot of Figure 10-4 is actually the histogram updated using Eq. (10.4) with a time constant of 1 sec and plotted at the end of the 3 seconds of noisy speech

To use the histogram for noise estimation, one must identify the peak of the noise distribution given that only the distribution of the noisy speech is available. Several different approaches have been proposed (McAulay & Malpass, 1980; Stahl et al., 2000; Van Compernolle, 1987).

A simple method is to compute the mean of the time-varying histogram computed using Eq. (10.4) for each processing block, and then find the peak at or below the mean. If only noise is present, the distribution of the signal levels in dB can be approximated by a single Gaussian distribution, and the peak will be near the mean of the histogram. Selecting the peak of the histogram will therefore find the peak of the underlying distribution and will give the mean noise level $|N(k,m)|$. If speech is present, the distribution will be similar to the sum of two Gaussians, as shown in Figure 10-5, and the mean of the histogram will lie above the peak of the noise distribution. Searching below the mean for the peak will again return the mean noise level.

The noise level estimate produced by this histogram approach is plotted in Figure 10-6 along with the estimate produce by the Hirsch-Ehrlicher (1995) algorithm. The histogram bins are 1-dB wide and no smoothing has been applied to the noise estimate, so the histogram noise level is quantized in 1-dB steps. There appears to be very little difference between the histogram estimate and that produced by the Hirsch-Ehrlicher algorithm for this signal. The estimate rises quickly to the actual noise level during the initial noise-only portion of the noisy speech signal, and then holds a relatively constant noise estimate despite the fluctuations of the speech.

Wiener Filter

The Wiener filter (Wiener, 1949) is one of the oldest techniques for suppressing noise in a noisy signal. The Wiener filter requires separate estimates of the speech and noise powers. The filter design also assumes that the speech and noise are stationary. In practical terms, this assumption means that the Wiener filter can be designed for the average speech and noise, but cannot take into account the speech or noise fluctuations.

The basic idea for the Wiener filter is illustrated in the block diagram of Figure 10-7. The speech signal $s(n)$ is corrupted by additive noise $d(n)$ to form the input signal $x(n) = s(n) + d(n)$. This noisy signal is then filtered by the Wiener filter $G(f)$ to give the output $y(n)$. The criterion for the design of the Wiener filter is to minimize the mean-squared error between the clean input and the filtered output:

Spectral Subtraction

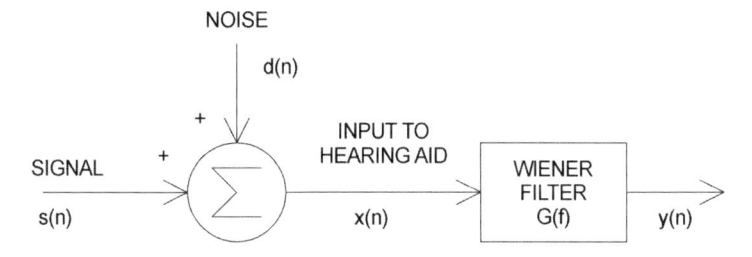

Figure 10-7. Block diagram showing a Wiener filter used to process the input of a hearing aid.

$$\varepsilon = \sum_n [s(n) - y(n)]^2 \quad \text{Equation (10.5)}$$

The Wiener filter thus filters the noisy speech x(n) to form the closest possible match to the clean speech s(n). The solution to the filter design problem in the continuous frequency domain is:

$$G(f) = \frac{|S(f)|^2}{|S(f)|^2 + |D(f)|^2} \quad \text{Equation (10.6)}$$

where S(f) is the long-term average speech spectrum and D(f) is the long-term average noise spectrum. In practice the speech and noise spectra are not available, so the Wiener filter is usually approximated from the noisy signal spectrum X(f) and the estimated noise spectrum N(f):

$$G(f) \approx \frac{|X(f)|^2 - |N(f)|^2}{|X(f)|^2} \quad \text{Equation (10.7)}$$

The Wiener filter maximizes the signal-to-noise ratio (SNR) of the noisy speech averaged over the entire signal. However, the minimum mean-squared error criterion used in the Wiener filter design does not directly involve any aspects of auditory perception. The assumption in applying the Wiener filter to speech is that the mathematical optimization will also lead to improvements in speech perception. The Wiener filter can be effective if the noise is stationary and concentrated in narrow frequency regions or in regions that do not contain much speech energy (Lim, 1986). In most problems of interest, however, the speech and noise both fluctuate in amplitude and the noise spectrum substantially overlaps the speech spectrum. Signal processing for these conditions requires a Wiener filter that varies over time to reflect the effect of the noise on different speech sounds (Levitt et al., 1993). The time-varying Wiener filter is discussed in the next section as it can be considered to be a form of spectral subtraction.

Spectral Subtraction

Spectral subtraction refers to a family of related noise-suppression algorithms. In these algorithms the estimated noise spectrum (or a function of the noise spectrum) is subtracted from the noisy speech spectrum to produce an estimate of the clean speech spectrum. Early forms of spectrum subtraction, including adaptive Wiener filters, magnitude spectrum subtraction, and power spectrum subtraction are described in the next section. These forms of spectral subtraction had problems, in particular, residual noise components termed "musical noise" comprising sinusoids at random frequencies that appear and then disappear in the processed speech (Boll, 1979; Cappé, 1994) as the amount of signal attenuation fluctuates. Improvements in spectral subtraction, described next, have concentrated on improving the noise estimation and on reducing the musical noise in the processed speech.

CLASSICAL APPROACHES

Spectral subtraction works on the short-time spectrum of the noisy speech, as shown in Figure 10-2. The incoming signal is divided into blocks. Each block is windowed and the short-time FFT is computed from the windowed data sequence. The magnitude spectrum of the noise is estimated, as described above, and the noise-suppression gain as a function of frequency is computed from the magnitude spectrum of the noisy signal and the estimated noise magnitude spectrum. The gain function $G(f)$ is applied to the noisy spectrum to give the estimated clean speech spectrum, and the modified spectrum is inverse transformed to give the time waveform of the enhanced signal. In general the signal blocks have an overlap of 50% and the processed waveform is synthesized using the overlap-add procedure. The enhanced signal has a modified envelope, but retains the noisy phase.

The Wiener filter given by Eq. (10.7) is based on the long-term average estimated noise and noisy speech spectra. An adaptive Wiener filter can be created by replacing the long-term average noisy speech spectrum $X(f)$ with the short-term spectrum $X(k,m)$ and the long-term noise estimate $N(f)$ with an estimate $N(k,m)$ that is allowed to track changes in the noise level. The resultant gain $G_W(k,m)$ for frequency band k and block m can be written as:

$$G_W(k,m) = \frac{|X(k,m)|^2 - |N(k,m)|^2}{|X(k,m)|^2} = 1 - \frac{|N(k,m)|^2}{|X(k,m)|^2} \qquad \text{Equation (10.8)}$$

Another approach is power spectral subtraction (Lim & Oppenheim, 1979). Assume that the noise and speech are uncorrelated. The noisy speech power spectrum can then be represented as the sum of the speech power spectrum and the noise power spectrum, $|X(k,m)|^2 = |S(k,m)|^2 + |D(k,m)|^2$. Using the estimated noise spectrum to replace the actual noise spectrum leads to

$$|\hat{S}(k,m)|^2 \approx |X(k,m)|^2 - |N(k,m)|^2 \qquad \text{Equation (10.9)}$$

The gain needed to get the noisy speech power spectrum to match the clean speech power spectrum is then

$$G_P^2(k,m) = \frac{|\hat{S}(k,m)|^2}{|X(k,m)|^2} = 1 - \frac{|N(k,m)|^2}{|X(k,m)|^2} \qquad \text{Equation (10.10)}$$

The gain for power spectral subtraction is thus the square root of the Wiener filter gain:

$$G_P(k,m) = \sqrt{1 - \frac{|N(k,m)|^2}{|X(k,m)|^2}} \qquad \text{Equation (10.11)}$$

Another approach is magnitude spectral subtraction (Boll, 1979). The gain for magnitude spectral subtraction is given by:

$$G_M(k,m) = 1 - \frac{|N(k,m)|}{|X(k,m)|} \quad \text{Equation (10.12)}$$

In all of the spectral subtraction gain equations Eq. (10.8), Eq. (10.11), and Eq. (10.12), it is possible for the estimated noise level to be greater than the short-term spectrum for the signal block. When this occurs, the spectral subtraction would compute a negative gain, which is not physically meaningful. All of the algorithms therefore replace a negative gain with zero.

The gain for these three spectral subtraction approaches is plotted in Figure 10-8 as a function of the SNR. For low noise levels (high SNR), the algorithms all give gains near 0 dB. If the noise level is low, there is no need to attenuate the signal. As the noise level increases the signal attenuation also increases, but the algorithms differ in the degree to which the noisy signal is attenuated as a function of SNR. The magnitude spectral subtraction provides the greatest attenuation, whereas the power spectral subtraction provides the least.

GENERAL EQUATION

The spectral subtraction given by Eqs. 10.8, 10.11, and 10.12 can be combined into a single general formulation (Berouti et al., 1979; Virag, 1999):

$$G(k,m) = \begin{cases} \left[1 - \alpha \frac{|N(k,m)|^\gamma}{|X(k,m)|^\gamma}\right]^{1/\delta} & \text{if } \frac{|N(k,m)|^\gamma}{|X(k,m)|^\gamma} < \frac{1}{\alpha + \beta} \\ \left[\beta \frac{|N(k,m)|^\gamma}{|X(k,m)|^\gamma}\right]^{1/\delta} & \text{otherwise} \end{cases}$$

Equation (10.13)

All of the classical spectral subtraction algorithms described above use $\alpha = 1$ and $\beta = 0$ when expressed in this formulation. The Wiener filter is

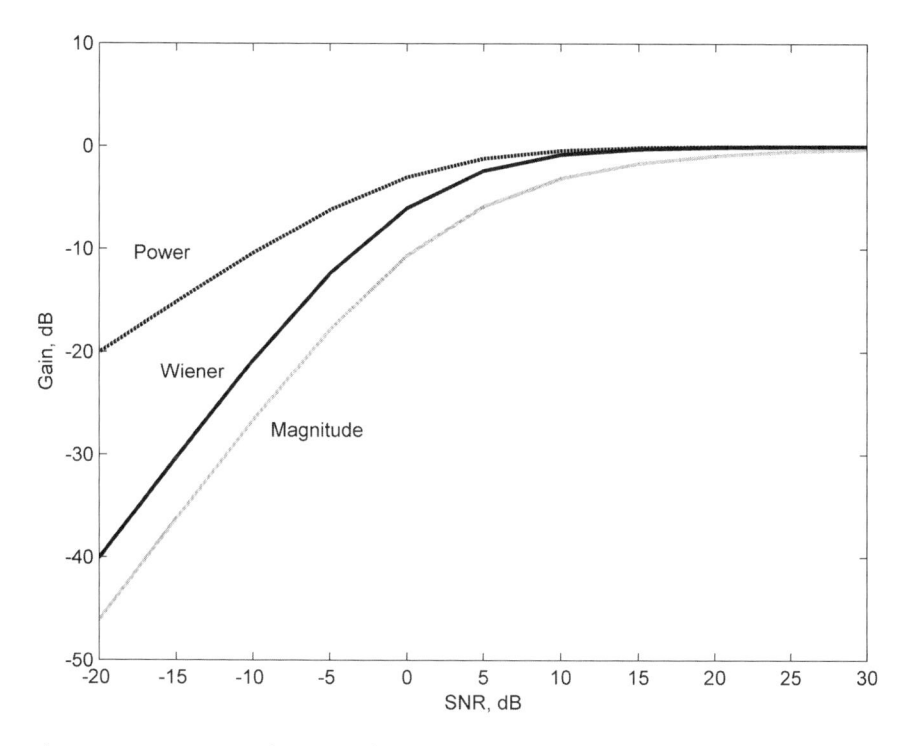

Figure 10-8. Gain as a function of the signal-to-noise ratio (SNR) for different versions of spectral subtraction.

given by $\{\gamma = 2, \delta = 1\}$, power spectral subtraction by $\{\gamma = 2, \delta = 2\}$, and magnitude spectral subtraction by $\{\gamma = 1, \delta = 1\}$.

The general formulation adds two additional factors. One is an oversubtraction factor $\alpha \geq 1$ and the other is the attenuation floor $0 \leq \beta < 1$. The oversubtraction factor α increases the signal attenuation at poor SNRs beyond the amount shown in Figure 10-8, which reduces the amplitude of the background noise when no speech is present. The attenuation floor β limits the maximum attenuation that the algorithm produces. Increasing β increases the background noise level but reduces the gain fluctuations that can contribute to musical noise at low signal levels. Setting β within the range of −10 to −20 dB re: 1 can provide audible noise suppression while reducing the amount of musical noise. A further variation is to make the factor α time-dependent. Virag (1999) has proposed making α a function of the estimated SNR; α is large at poor SNRs when speech is absent, thus increasing the background noise suppression, and α is reduced at good SNRs when speech is present to reduce the amount of distortion introduced by the spectral subtraction. In her implementation α ranged from 6 at poor SNRs to 1 at very good SNRs.

An alternative technique to reduce musical noise is to average the spectral subtraction gains across signal blocks. Gustafsson et al. (2001) propose using an adaptive averaging time constant for the suppression gains. If the spectrum in the current signal block is similar to that of the previous block, a long averaging time constant is used on the assumption that the signal is noise; noise spectra will be very similar from one block to the next. If the spectrum in the current block differs significantly from that in the previous block, a short averaging time constant is used to allow the suppression gain to change rapidly in response to the presence of speech.

NONLINEAR EXPANSION

An approach related to spectral subtraction is to compute a suppression gain based on the signal and estimated noise powers. One such function that has been successfully used (Clarkson & Bahgat, 1991; Eger et al., 1984; Tsoukalas et al., 1997) is given by:

$$G(k,m) = \frac{1}{1+v\left[\frac{|N(k,m)|}{|X(k,m)|}\right]^{\gamma}} \quad \text{Equation (10.14)}$$

The family of gain curves given by Eq. (10.14) is plotted in Figure 10-9. The curves are drawn for different combinations of γ and v. The value of controls the maximum attenuation provided by the expansion when only noise is present; increasing v increases the maximum attenuation. The value of γ controls the rate at which the gain changes with SNR; increasing γ reduces the SNR range in dB needed to go from minimal attenuation to nearly full attenuation. For curve (i) $\gamma = 1$ and $v = 10$, (ii) $\gamma = 2$ and $= \sqrt{10}$, (iii) $\gamma = 1$ and $v = 10$, (iv) $\gamma = 2$ and $v = 10$, (v) $\gamma = 2$ and $v = 100$.

This family of gain functions has the advantage that the gain remains constant at poor SNRs, whereas the gain curves plotted in Figure 10-8 continue to decrease forever as the SNR decreases. If a signal segment is just noise, the SNR will be negative and the gain from Eq. (10.14)

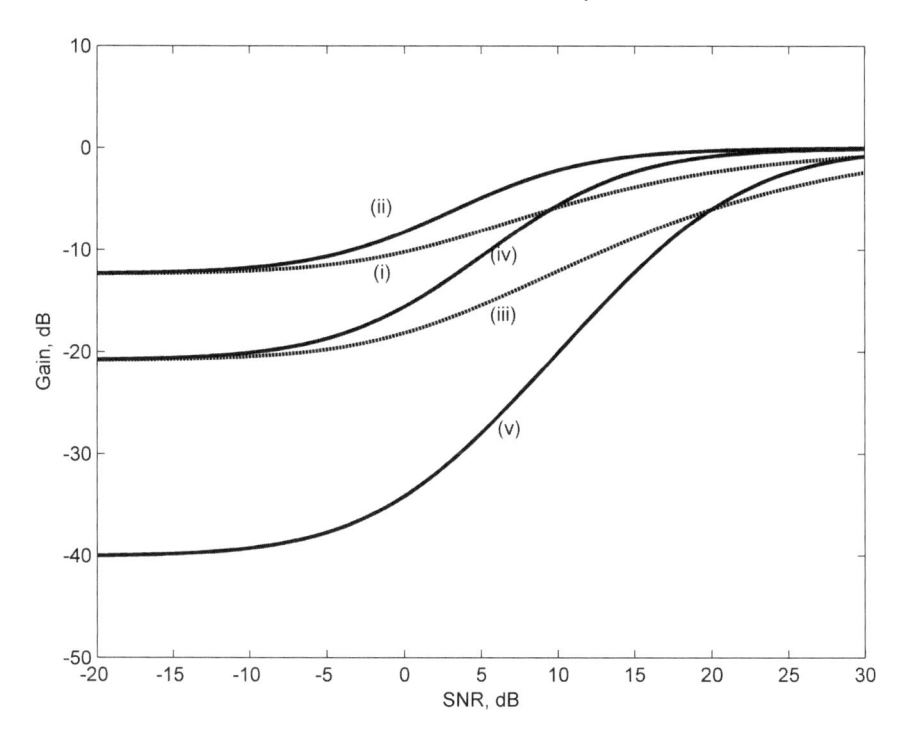

Figure 10-9. Gain versus the instantaneous SNR for the nonlinear expansion approach. The curves are for different settings of the gain rule given by Eq. (10.14) and are described in the text.

will barely fluctuate. This constant gain for signals dominated by noise will minimize the musical noise and gain-modulation artifacts in the processed signal.

EPHRAIM-MALAH ALGORITHM

The noise suppression gain given by Eq. (10.13) depends on the instantaneous SNR given by the ratio of noisy signal $|X(k,m)|$ in block m to the estimated average noise power $|N(k,m)|$. If the SNR is good $|X(k,m)| \gg |N(k,m)|$, and fluctuations in the signal level will only cause small changes in the gain when expressed in dB re: 1. However, as the SNR approaches 0 dB, we get $|X(k,m)|/|N(k,m)| \approx 1$. If $\alpha = 1$, as in the classical spectral subtraction algorithms, the gain will be approximately 0. Small changes in $|X(k,m)|$ will then cause large changes in the gain expressed in dB. These large relative gain fluctuations are one

308 Digital Hearing Aids

of the causes of the musical noise artifacts in spectral subtraction (Cappé, 1994; Marzinzik, 2000).

An alternative approach to spectral subtraction is to assume that the noise samples come from a Gaussian probability distribution and that the speech samples come from a second independent Gaussian distribution. The gain is set close to 0 dB if a given sample appears to come from the speech distribution, and the gain is reduced if the sample appears to come from the noise distribution (Ephraim & Malah, 1984; McAulay & Malpass, 1980; Wolfe & Godsill, 2001). The resultant suppression gain rule depends on the SNR, and lies between the power spectral subtraction and Wiener filter gain rules plotted in Figure 10-8.

Where these statistical approaches differ from classical spectral subtraction is in how the SNR is calculated. The estimated SNR is a combination of two terms, the a priori SNR and the a posteriori SNR. Assume that the clean speech spectrum $S(k,m)$ and the noise spectrum $D(k,m)$ are known. The a priori SNR is then given by:

$$\varepsilon_{priori}(k,m) = \frac{E[|S(k,m)|^2]}{E[|D(k,m)|^2]} \quad \text{Equation (10.15)}$$

where E[ ] is the expectation operation, typically implemented as the long-term average. The a posteriori SNR estimate uses the noisy signal measurements, and it is given by:

$$\varepsilon_{post}(k,m) = \frac{|X(k,m)|^2 - |N(k,m)|^2}{|N(k,m)|^2} = \frac{|X(k,m)|^2}{|N(k,m)|^2} - 1$$

Equation (10.16)

The SNR estimate used in the Ephraim and Malah (1984) algorithm is a linear combination of the a priori and the a posteriori SNR estimates (Cohen, 2004; Hendriks et al., 2005). In practice, the a priori SNR is not known, so it is approximated by using the speech signal estimate and the noise power estimate from the previous block:

$$\varepsilon(k,m) = \alpha \frac{|\hat{S}(k,m-1)|^2}{|N(k,m-1)|^2} + (1-\alpha)\max\left[\frac{|X(k,m)|^2}{|N(k,m)|^2} - 1, 0\right]$$

Equation (10.17)

The averaging factor α, $0 < \alpha < 1$ controls the tradeoff between noise reduction and signal distortion. A value of α close to 1 smoothes the SNR estimate, thus reducing the processing artifacts but reducing the ability of the estimate to track changes in the signal level. A small value of α gives a rapid response to changes in the signal level but will cause more processing artifacts.

At a good SNR, the SNR calculation is close to that used in classical spectral subtraction and depends primarily on the instantaneous signal level and the estimated average noise level. At poor SNRs, however, the SNR calculation averages the instantaneous SNR value over many signal blocks, thus smoothing the SNR estimate and the resultant suppression gain. The smoothed gain has reduced fluctuations compared to classical spectral subtraction. The effect of the averaging on the estimated SNR is plotted in Figure 10-10. During the noise-only portion of the signal the averaged SNR is much smoother than the instantaneous SNR. Once the speech starts, however, the Ephraim and Malah (1984) algorithm reduces the amount of averaging and the estimated SNR is very close to the instantaneous SNR used in classical spectral subtraction.

In practice, the Ephraim and Malah (1984) algorithm has been found to give reduced musical noise artifacts when compared to classical spectral subtraction (Cappé, 1994; Marzinzik, 2000). But it is also possible to use the Ephraim and Malah approach to estimate the SNR without implementing the rest of their algorithm or their gain-reduction rule. Combining the SNR estimation procedure of *Eq. (10.17)* with the Wiener filter given by *Eq. (10.8)* also results in a reduction in musical noise (Hendriks et al., 2005), strongly suggesting that the benefit of the Ephraim and Malah approach is in the smoothed SNR estimate and not in the theory used to derive the noise suppression.

AUDITORY MASKING

Up to this point, the spectral subtraction algorithms have been based on mathematical properties of the speech and noise, and have ignored the fact that a human will be listening to the processed signal. The goal of

310 Digital Hearing Aids

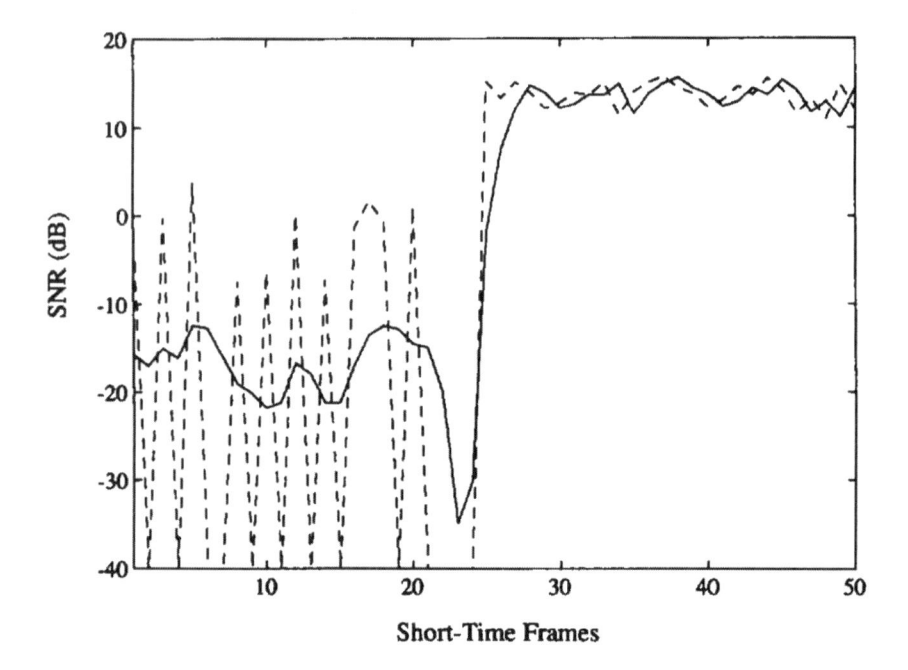

Figure 10-10. Estimated SNRs in successive signal blocks (denoted as short-time frames) for the Ephraim and Malah (1984) noise suppression algorithm. The dashed line gives the SNR computed from the instantaneous signal envelope samples, and the solid line gives the averaged SNR computed using the algorithm. For the first 25 blocks the signal contains only noise. For the next 25 blocks speech is present at a SNR of 15 dB (from Cappé, 1994).

the processing is to render the noise inaudible. One aspect of spectral subtraction, and also the Ephraim and Malah (1984) algorithm, is that a large amount of suppression is provided by the gain rule at poor SNRs. But gain reductions that push the noise level below the audible threshold are actually counterproductive. The changes in the suppression gain from one signal block to the next modulate the envelope of the signal, and this modulation can generate audible processing artifacts. The more the gain varies from one block to the next the greater the envelope modulation, so limiting the maximum amount of signal attenuation to that which just renders the noise inaudible will limit the modulation depth imposed by the processing and reduce the probability of generating audible artifacts such as musical noise.

Limiting the maximum signal attenuation requires implementing a model of noise audibility. The spectral subtraction attenuation is computed for the frequency band, and the reduced noise level is compared to the threshold of audibility in that band. If the attenuation is greater than that needed to place the noise at the audible threshold, the attenuation is reduced so that the noise level matches the threshold (Azirani et al., 1995; Tsoukalas et al., 1997; Virag, 1999).

To compute the model of audibility, the signal spectrum is first grouped into auditory analysis bands, such as critical bands (Zwicker & Terhardt, 1980) or equivalent rectangular bandwidths (ERBs) (Moore & Glasberg, 1983). Auditory masking for the noisy speech signal is then computed using the masking model of Johnston (1988), which takes into account the spread of excitation across auditory filter bands and whether the excitation is tonal or noiselike in nature. For hearing-impaired listeners, the maximum of the auditory masking function or the impaired auditory threshold is then taken as the noise threshold (Natarajan et al., 2005).

A FUNDAMENTAL COMPROMISE

Spectral subtraction involves multiplying the noisy speech signal $X(k,m)$ by a gain factor $G(k,m)$. The processed output is given by:

$$Y(k,m) = G(k,m)[S(k,m) + D(k,m)] \quad \text{Equation (10.18)}$$

The reduced noise level is given by $G(k,m)D(k,m)$, and the speech distortion is given by the change in the speech amplitude $[1-G(k,m)]S(k,m)$. If $G(k,m)$ is close to 1, there will be minimal modification to the speech signal along with only a small reduction in the noise level. If $G(k,m) \approx 0$, the speech signal will be substantially modified, but there will be a large reduction in the noise level. Thus, no matter what procedure is used to estimate the noise level or compute the suppression gain, there still remains a tradeoff between the amount of noise suppression and the amount of signal distortion. For any spectral subtraction algorithm, increasing the amount of noise suppression will increase the amount of speech distortion. Thus, designing a signal processing algorithm and adjusting the parameters will always involve a compromise between noise suppression and distortion, and the effects of the algorithm on intelligibility and sound quality will depend on the choices made.

Algorithm Effectiveness

Jamieson et al. (1995) looked at the effects of an adaptive Wiener filter on different kinds of noise and different SNRs. The noises included white Gaussian noise, white noise low-pass filtered at 1 kHz, and multitalker babble. Both normal-hearing and hearing-impaired listeners took part in the experiments. An SRT test using a closed set of spondees showed significantly improved intelligibility for the Wiener filter for both the normal-hearing and hearing-impaired subjects listening in low-pass filtered noise, and no benefit for the white noise or babble. No statistically significant intelligibility benefit was observed for the Wiener filter for any noise condition or group of listeners for isolated vowel-consonant-vowel (VCV) test materials. Preference testing used continuous discourse (female talker), and both the normal-hearing and hearing-impaired listeners preferred the processed material at positive SNRs, had no preference at a SNR of 0 dB, and preferred the unprocessed material at negative SNR values.

A study of spectral subtraction was reported by Levitt et al. (1993). The test stimuli were nonsense syllables in a background of multitalker babble at an SNR of 15 dB. The speech was pre-emphasized with a 6-dB/octave slope. In one version of the processing magnitude spectral subtraction was applied to the entire signal spectrum. In the second version of the processing the spectral subtraction was applied to the speech spectrum below 2800 Hz and the spectrum at higher frequencies was left unprocessed. The split-band processing gave slightly higher speech recognition scores than the full-band processing, but neither version of spectral subtraction was more intelligible than the unprocessed stimuli. Both versions of spectral subtraction were preferred to the unprocessed materials about 70 percent of the time.

Marzinzik (2000) investigated the spectral subtraction scheme proposed by Ephraim and Malah (1984). The test stimuli were sentences in three kinds of noise: industry noise recorded on a factory floor, cafeteria babble, and stationary speech-shaped noise. Intelligibility for the normal-hearing subjects in cafeteria babble showed no significant difference between the processed and unprocessed stimuli. Intelligibility for the hearing-impaired subjects showed a slight nonsignificant reduction for the processed stimuli in comparison with the unprocessed stimuli for cafeteria babble and speech-shaped noise. Preference judgments for the normal-hearing subjects in cafeteria babble showed a slight preference for the unprocessed over the processed stimuli at both −5 and +5 dB SNRs, although the differences in overall impression were smaller at the higher SNR. The hearing-impaired subjects in industry noise showed no preference at an SNR of 0 dB, and a significant preference for the processed stimuli at an SNR of 10 dB. The hearing-impaired subjects showed no significant preference in the cafeteria babble at either an SNR of 0 or 10 dB. For the speech-shaped noise, the hearing-impaired subjects showed a slight preference for the unprocessed stimuli at an SNR of 0 dB and a slight preference for the processed stimuli at an SNR of 10 dB.

Arehart et al. (2003) evaluated both intelligibility and speech quality for the Tsoukalas et al. (1997) spectral-subtraction approach using both normal-hearing and hearing-impaired listeners. Intelligibility was measured using monosyllables in communication channel (white stationary) noise and highway (low-frequency emphasis, nonstationary) noise. The processed stimuli had a small but significant improvement in intelligibility for the communication noise but not for the highway noise for both groups of subjects. Overall quality judgments using sentence materials for the normal-hearing subjects showed a small improvement for the processed stimuli in the communication noise but not for the highway noise. The hearing-impaired subjects gave higher overall quality ratings to the processed stimuli in all conditions, but the preferences for the processed materials were greater at an SNR of 5 dB than for 0 dB, and were greater for the communication noise than for the highway noise. Further experiments with the same spectral-subtraction algorithm (Natarajan et al., 2005) show a small but not significant benefit in intelligibility for the processed stimuli for both groups of listeners. Both the normal-hearing and hearing-impaired subjects gave the processed speech higher overall quality ratings; however, the benefit of the processing was smaller for crowd noise than for communication channel noise.

A recent study by Hu and Loizou (2006) compared sound quality judgments for 13 speech-enhancement algorithms using normal-hearing listeners. They looked at sentences in four types of noise at 5-dB and 10-dB SNRs. Overall quality judgments appeared to be highest for the Ephraim and Malah (1984) approach and for related algorithms. Judgments were also high for a multiband spectral subtraction approach that smoothed the spectrum across FFT frequency bins before computing the noise suppression gain and then applied power spectral subtraction using an oversubtraction factor that depended on the estimated SNR (Kamath & Loizou, 2002).

Concluding Remarks

This chapter has covered many different approaches to spectral subtraction and related noise-suppression algorithms. Some of the algorithms, such as Wiener filtering (1949) and the Ephraim and Malah (1984) algorithm, are based on theoretical derivations intended to mathematically optimize the separation of the speech and noise. Other algorithms have been designed on more of an ad hoc basis, with the signal processing adjusted to sound as good as possible to the person designing it. The theoretical approach ignores the ear, whereas the ad hoc approach implicitly includes the ear as the algorithm parameters are adjusted based on the results of informal ("Sounds good to me") listening tests. What is interesting is that both approaches to algorithm design have produced comparable results; small improvements in quality and possible improvements in intelligibility for stationary background noise. Ignoring the ear appears to greatly reduce the potential benefit of the theoretically optimum processing, whereas mathematically unsophisticated approaches can be effective if the intuitive design process is effective in including the ear. One can hope that in the future combining mathematical rigor with auditory models will lead to improved spectral subtraction algorithms, but there will always remain the tradeoff between the amount of noise suppression and the amount of signal distortion introduced by the processing.

There still are problems that may limit the effectiveness of spectral subtraction. One problem is nonstationary noise. The basic approach to estimating the noise is to form the estimate during pauses in speech, and then to hold the estimate constant during speech sounds. The assumption is that the noise power will not vary during the speech interval. If the noise fluctuates, the estimate will be in error and the spectral subtraction gain will also be in error. Some types of noise, such as communications channel noise, are nearly stationary and spectral subtraction offers measurable benefits. Other types of noise, such as babble or traffic noise, fluctuate and spectral subtraction may be of only limited benefit.

A second concern is that spectral subtraction affects the magnitude of the signal but not its phase. The envelope is modified to more closely resemble that of the clean speech, but the speech is then reconstructed using the noisy phase. No matter how closely the envelope of the reconstructed signal matches the clean speech, there will still be residual effects of the noise in the phase that have not been removed by the processing.

A further concern is that the spectral enhancement gain changes across processing block boundaries as the estimated SNR changes. Smoothing the gain reduces the fluctuations and thus reduces the audible modulation and processing artifacts such as musical noise introduced by the processing. So there is a processing tradeoff—long smoothing time constants reduce the musical noise, but interfere with the ability of the algorithm to response to rapid changes in the speech level. Short time constants increase the musical noise but also allow the processing to react to the fast onset of a speech sound. Minimizing artifacts while still being able to react to sudden speech onsets is a difficult balancing act that requires as much art as science at the present time.

References

Arehart, K. H., Hansen, J. H. L, Gallant, S., & Kalstein, L. (2003). Evaluation of an auditory masked threshold noise suppression algorithm in normal-hearing and hearing-impaired listeners. *Speech Communication, 40*, 575–592.

Arslan, L., McCree, A., & Viswanathan, V. (1995). New methods for adaptive noise suppression. *Proceedings of the IEEE International Conference on Acoustics, Speech, and Signal Processing, I* (pp. 812–I:815), Detroit, May 9–12, 1995.

Azirani, A. A., Le Bouquin, R., & Faucon, J.-G. (1995) Optimizing speech enhancement by exploiting masking properties of the human ear. *Proceedings of the IEEE International Conference on Acoustics, Speech, and Signal Processing, I* (pp. 800–I:803), Detroit, May 9–12, 1995.

Berouti, M., Schwartz, R., & Makhoul, J. (1979). Enhancement of speech corrupted by acoustic noise. *Proceedings of the IEEE International Conference on Acoustics, Speech, and Signal Processing* (pp. 208–211), April 2–4, 1979, Washington, D.C.

Boll, S. F. (1979). Suppression of acoustic noise in speech using spectral subtraction. *IEEE Transactions on Acoustics, Speech, and Signal Processing, ASSP-27*, 113–120.

Cappé, O. (1994). Elimination of the musical noise phenomenon with the Ephraim and Malah noise suppressor. *IEEE Transactions on Speech and Audio Processing, 2*, 345–349.

Clarkson, P. M., & Bahgat, S. F. (1991). Envelope expansion methods for speech enhancement. *Journal of the Acoustical Society of America, 89*, 1378–1382.

Cohen, I. (2004). On the decision-directed estimation approach of Ephraim and Malah. *Proceedinngs of the IEEE International Conference on Acoustics, Speech, and Signal Processing, I* (pp. 293–I:296), Montreal, May 17–21, 2004.

Cohen, I., & Berdugo, B. (2002). Noise estimation by minima controlled recursive averaging for robust speech enhancement. *IEEE Signal Processing Letters, 9*, 12–15.

Doblinger, G. (1995). Computationally efficient speech enhancement by spectral minima tracking in subbands. *Proceedings of the 4th European Conference on Speech Communication and Technology*, Vol. 2 (pp. 1513–1516), Madrid, Sept 18–21, 1995.

Eger, T. E., Su, J. C., & Varner, W. (1984). A nonlinear processing technique for speech enhancement. *Proceedings of the IEEE International Conference on Acoustics, Speech, and Signal Processing* (pp. 18A.1.1–18A.1.4), San Diego, March 19–21, 1984.

Ephraim, Y., & Malah, D. (1984). Speech enhancement using a minimum mean-square error short-time spectral amplitude estimator. *IEEE Transactions on Acoustics, Speech and Signal Processing, ASSP-32*, 1109–1121.

Gustafsson, H., Nordholm, S. E., & Claesson, I. (2001). Spectral subtraction using reduced delay convolution and adaptive averaging. *IEEE Transactions on Speech and Audio Processing, 9*, 799–807.

Hendriks, R. C., Heusdens, R., & Jensen, J. (2005). Improved decision directed approach for speech enhancement using an adaptive time segmentation. *Proceedings of Interspeech* 2005, 2101–2104.

Hirsch, H. G., & Ehrlicher, C. (1995). Noise estimation techniques for robust speech recognition. *Proceedings of the IEEE International Conference on Acoustics, Speech, and Signal Processing, I* (pp. 153–I:156), Detroit, May 9–12, 1995.

Hu, Y., & Loizou, P. (2006). Subjective comparison of speech enhancement algorithms. *Proceedings of the IEEE International Conference on Acoustics, Speech, and Signal Processing*, Toulouse, May 15–19, 2006.

Jamieson, D. G., Brennan, R. L., & Cornelisse, L. E. (1995). Evaluation of a speech enhancement strategy with normal-hearing and hearing-impaired listeners. *Ear and Hearing, 16*, 274–286.

Johnston, J. D. (1988). Transform coding of audio signals using perceptual noise criteria. *IEEE Journal of Selected Areas in Communication*, 6, 314–323.

Kamath, S. D., & Loizou, P. C. (2002). A multi-band subtraction method for enhancing speech corrupted by colored noise. *Proceedings of the IEEE International Conference on Acoustics, Speech, and Signal Processing*, IV (p. 4164), Orlando, FL, May 13–17, 2002. (Available at: http://www.utdallas.edu/~loizou/speech/mbss2002.pdf).

Levitt, H., Bakke, M., Kates, J., Neuman, A., & Weiss, M. (1993). Signal processing for hearing impairment. *Scandinavian Audiology* (Suppl. 38), 7–19.

Lim, J. S. (1986). Speech enhancement. *Proceedings of the IEEE International Conferece on Acoustics, Speech, and Signal Processing* (pp. 3135–3142), Tokyo, April 7–11, 1986.

Lim, J. S., & Oppenheim, A. V. (1979). Enhancement and bandwidth compression of noisy speech. *Proceedings of the IEEE*, 67, 1586–1604.

McAulay, R. J., & Malpass, M. L. (1980). Speech enhancement using a soft-decision noise suppression filter. *IEEE Transactions on Acoustics, Speech, and Signal Processing*, ASSP-28, 137-145.

Martin, R. (2001). Noise power spectral density estimation based on optimal smoothing and minimum statistics. *IEEE Transactions on Speech and Audio Processing*, 9, 504-512.

Marzinzik, M. (2000). *Noise reduction schemes for digital hearing aids and their use for the hearing impaired.* Doctoral Dissertation, Universität Oldenburg.

Marzinzik, M., & Kollmeier, B. (2002). Speech pause detection for noise spectrum estimation by tracking power envelope dynamics. *IEEE Transactions on Speech and Audio Processing*, 10, 109–118.

Moore, B. C. J., & Glasberg, B. R. (1983). Suggested formulae for calculating auditory-filter bandwidths and excitation patterns. *Journal of the Acoustical Society of America*, 74, 750–753.

Natarajan, A., Hansen, J. H. L., Arehart, K. H., & Rossi-Katz, J. (2005). An auditory masked threshold based noise suppression algorithm GMMSE-AMT [ERB] for listeners. *EURASIP Journal on Applied Signal Processing*, 2005, 2938–2953.

Stahl, V., Fischer, A., & Bippus, R. (2000). Quantile based noise estimation for spectral subtraction and wiener filtering. *Proceedings of the IEEE International Conference on Acoustics, Speech, and Signal Processing*, III (pp. 1875–III·1878), Istanbul, June 5–9, 2000.

Tsoukalas, D. E., Mourjopoulos, J. N., & Kokkinakis, G. (1997). Speech enhancement based on audible noise suppression. *IEEE Transactions on Speech and Audio Processing*, 5, 497-514.

Van Compernolle, D. (1987). Increased noise immunity in large vocabulary speech recognition with the aid of spectral subtraction. *Proceedings of the IEEE International Conference on Acoustics, Speech, and Signal Processing* (pp. 1143–1146), Dallas, TX, April 1987.

Virag, N. (1999). Single channel speech enhancement based on masking properties of the human auditory system. *IEEE Transactions on Speech and Audio Processing, 7,* 126–137.

Wiener, N. (1949). *Extrapolation, interpolation, and smoothing of stationary time series,* Cambridge, MA: MIT Press (formerly Technology Press).

Wolfe, P. J., & Godsill, S. J. (2001). Simple alternatives to the Ephraim and Malah suppression rule for speech enhancement. *Proceedings of the 11th IEEE Workshop on Statistical Signal Processing* (pp. 496–499), Singapore, August 2001.

Zwicker, E., & Terhardt, E. (1980). Analytical expressions for critical band rate and critical bandwidth as a function of frequency. *Journal of the Acoustical Society of America, 68,* 1523–1525.

Spectral Contrast Enhancement

SPECTRAL CONTRAST ENHANCEMENT operates on the signal power spectrum to modify the short-time spectral shape. The processing provides a time-varying filter derived from the signal short-time power spectrum and implemented in the frequency domain. The objective is to compensate for the changes in the shape of the auditory filters often found in the impaired ear. In spectral subtraction, the low-level signal components are suppressed in each frequency band but the intensity of the high-level components is left essentially unaltered. The processing for spectral contrast enhancement may also suppress low-level spectral components in order to increase the spectral contrast between the high- and low-level spectral regions, but more often the processing goal is to sharpen the spectral peaks. Several different approaches to spectral contrast enhancement have been proposed, each based on a different assumption as to what may be the most important aspect of the change in the auditory filter shapes in the impaired ear.

The chapter begins with a review of the effects of cochlear damage on the auditory filters. The changes in the filter shapes lead to several different interpretations as to the dominant effects of the cochlear damage, and these interpretations lead to different processing strategies. Several strategies for spectral contrast enhancement are then presented, including spectral valley suppression using sparse sinusoidal modeling of the signal, raising the spectrum to a power greater than 1 to increase the spectral contrast, spectral filtering operations to sharpen the peaks, processing to compensate for increased upward spread of masking, and filtering to increase the power in the vowel second formant relative to that in the first formant. The chapter concludes with a comparison of some of the different processing strategies. A binaural strategy of dividing the signal into auditory frequency bands and presenting alternating frequency bands to the two ears is described in Chapter 13.

Auditory Filters in the Damaged Cochlea

The goal in spectral contrast enhancement is to modify the short-time spectrum of the signal so as to compensate for the changes in the auditory filters in the impaired ear. The auditory filters are broader in the impaired ear, have a reduced tip-to-tail ratio, and the neural firing patterns at high frequencies can be dominated by low-frequency components of a signal. Perceptual measures indicate that the impaired ear may have excessive upward spread of masking and may benefit from greater spectral contrast in the short-time speech spectrum. These physiologic and perceptual consequences of hearing loss are reviewed in this section.

PHYSIOLOGIC MEASUREMENTS

Tuning Curves

The shape of the auditory filters in the cochlear is typically measured using threshold tuning curves. The measurement procedure involves inserting a probe into an auditory nerve fiber and determining the excitation frequency for which that fiber is maximally sensitive. Sinusoids at a range of frequencies are then used as the excitation, and the signal amplitude at which the fiber response is just above the quiescent neural firing rate is recorded as a function of probe frequency. The resultant curve gives an auditory filter transfer function that is plotted upside down; a low excitation level is needed to get a neural response at the frequency to which the filter is most sensitive, and increasing signal levels are required to elicit a response as the probe frequency is moved away from the center frequency of the filter.

Cochlear damage changes the tuning curves. Versnel et al. (1997)

damaged the cochleas in guinea pigs through noise exposure, and then measured the tuning curves for single auditory nerve fibers. They found that the noise exposure caused several different types of degradation in the tuning curves. Schematic representations of the degraded tuning curves are presented in Figure 11-1. The normal tuning curve is represented by the solid line in each panel, and the degraded tuning curve by the dashed line. Type I is a loss of sensitivity without any change in the overall shape of the tuning curve, and corresponds to the results of partial inner-hair cell destruction (Liberman & Dodds, 1984). Type II reduces the sensitivity at the tip of the tuning curve and increases the auditory filter bandwidth without affecting the low-frequency tail of the tuning curve. Type III reduces the sensitivity at the tip and increases the auditory filter bandwidth combined with an increase in the sensitivity (hypersensitivity) in the tail, and corresponds to partial destruction of the outer hair cells (Liberman & Dodds, 1984). Type IV is a complete loss of neural response, and most likely corresponds to total destruction of both the inner and outer hair cells. Type V is a loss of the response in the tip region combined with hypersensitivity in the tail, and corresponds to complete destruction of the outer hair cells (Liberman & Dodds, 1984).

Versnel et al. (1997) found that the most prevalent type of degradation was type III (38%), and relatively few fibers were found with type IV (10%) or type V (7%). Type I responses were only found below 1 kHz. Type V responses were found only in cases of severe hearing loss (40–60 dB), whereas the other four types of responses were found for both moderate (20–40 dB) and severe losses. These data lead to the conclusion that noise-induced hearing loss affects both outer and inner hair cells in random proportion, and that a severe loss can lead to total destruction of the outer hair cells with the concomitant loss of the mechanical filtering in the cochlea.

Neural Firing Patterns

The changes in the tuning curves can affect the neural responses to speech stimuli. Miller et al. (1997) damaged the cochleas in cats through noise exposure, and then measured the neural firing patterns in response to a synthetic vowel /ɛ/, which had a first formant at 500 Hz, second formant at 1.7 kHz, and third formant at 2.5 kHz. In the normal cochlea, the neural firing patterns for fibers having center frequencies in the vicinity of each formant frequency were synchronized to the period

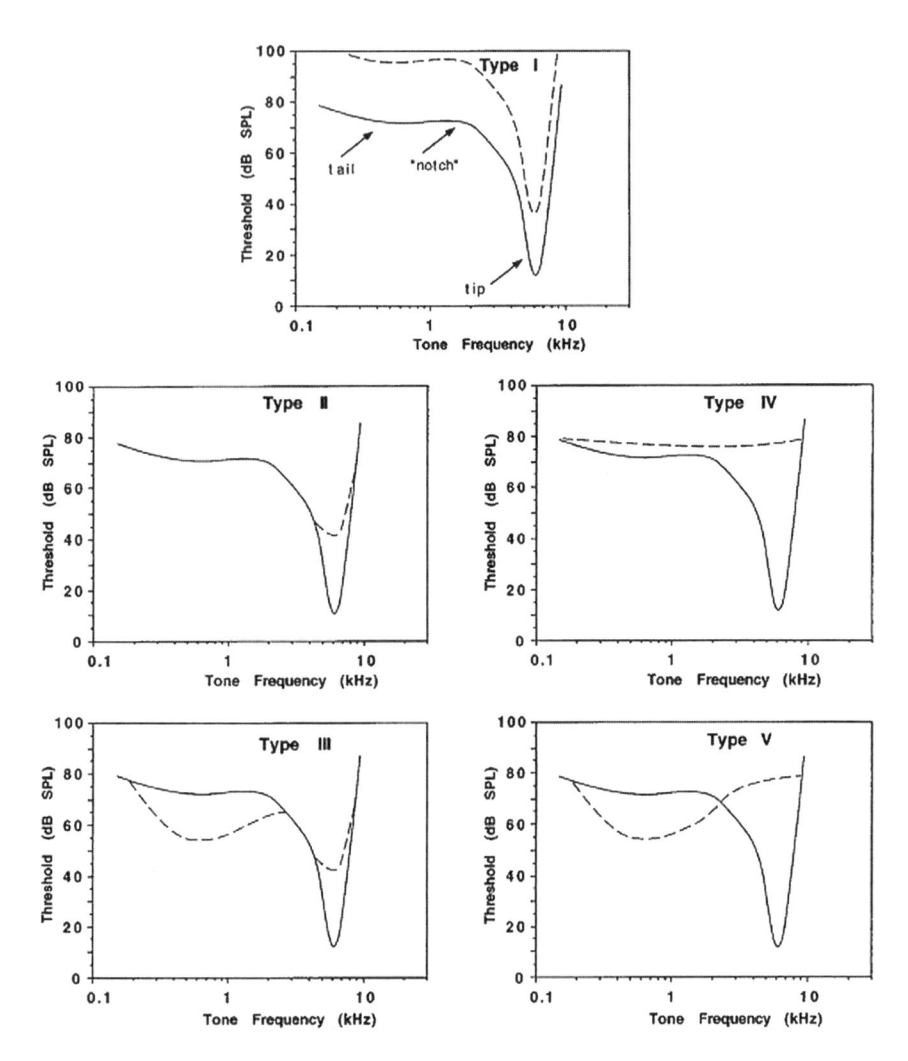

Figure 11-1. Schematic representations of tuning curves found in damaged guinea pig cochleas (from Versnel et al., 1997). The solid line represents the normal tuning curves, and each of the five types indicated by the dashed lines in each panel represents a distinct population of tuning curves resulting from noise-induced hearing damage.

of the formant. The neural response appears to be captured by the strongest frequency component passed by the auditory filter. In the healthy ear this capture results in populations of neurons, located in the cochlea region associated with the frequency of each formant, that all have firing patterns synchronized to the formant period.

In the damaged cochlea, however, the neural firing patterns change as a result of the degraded auditory filters diagrammed in Figure 11-1. The peak level of the first formant of the test stimulus used by Miller et al. (1997) was approximately 8 dB greater than the peak level of the second formant. If the neural firing pattern is to be synchronized to the second formant frequency, the associated auditory filter must have sufficient gain in the vicinity of the second formant compared to the gain for the first formant. In this example, at least 8 dB more gain for the frequency of the second formant would be required. The normal auditory filter having a center frequency in the vicinity of the second formant easily satisfies this requirement; the output of this auditory filter will have a preponderance of power from the second formant and the neural firing pattern will therefore represent the second formant periodicity.

In the damaged cochlea, for example a type III response from Figure 11-1, the gain at the tip is not much higher than for the tail. For a filter having a center frequency in the vicinity of the second formant in our example, the gain at the second-formant frequency of 1.7 kHz may be less than 8 dB greater than the gain at the first-formant frequency of 500 Hz. As a result, even though the auditory filter is nominally tuned to the second formant frequency, the filter output signal will contain more power from the first formant than from the second formant. The first formant captures the neural firing pattern even though the auditory filter is tuned to the frequency of the second formant, and any temporal information used by the auditory system to identify the second formant frequency has been lost.

This neural capture effect is illustrated in Figure 11-2 for a normal ear. The plot is the output of a cochlear model (Kates, 1991a, 1993a, 2002) that incorporates a simplified representation of the cochlear mechanics combined with an inner hair-cell model. The excitation was a synthesized syllable /da/, with formant frequencies starting at 500 Hz, 1.6 kHz, and 2.8 kHz. The contour plot clearly shows the neural firing synchronized to each of the three formant frequencies, with the region of synchronization extending above and below the formant frequency for all three formants. The modeled cochlea was then damaged by eliminating all the outer hair

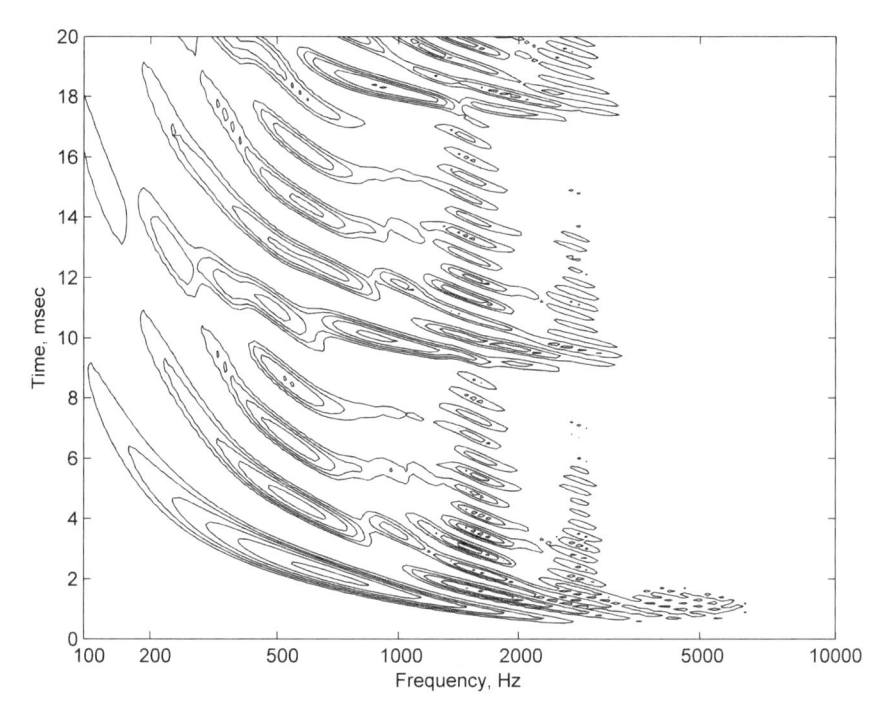

Figure 11-2. Neural firing patterns from the output from a cochlear model of a normal ear for the synthesized syllable /da/.

cells; in the model this causes a substantial reduction in the sensitivity of the tips of the synthesized tuning curves, but does not generate hypersensitivity in the tails. The output of the damaged cochlear model is plotted in Figure 11-3 for the same synthesized /da/ stimulus as used for the normal ear. The firing patterns of all of the neurons have been captured by the first formant, and there is essentially no temporal representation of the second or third formant frequencies.

PERCEPTUAL MEASUREMENTS

The strongest physiologic effect of cochlear damage is the reduction of gain at the tips of the tuning curves, which causes a loss of sensitivity combined with broader auditory filters. In human listeners, the loss of sensitivity is most commonly used to describe the hearing loss. However, broader auditory filters are also found in most listeners with cochlear hearing loss. Glasberg and Moore (1986), for example, measured the

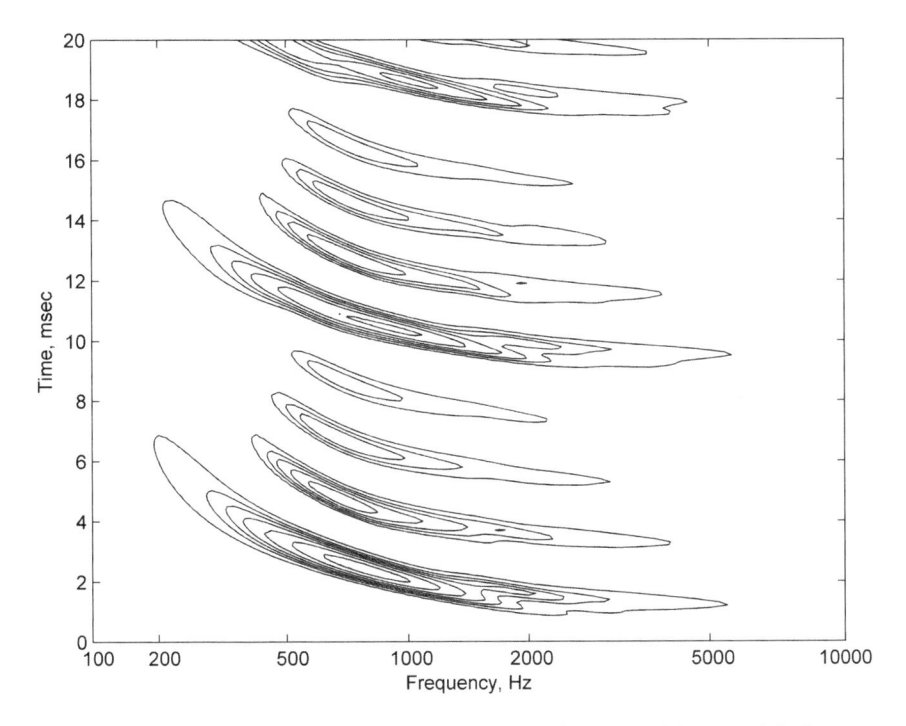

Figure 11-3. Neural firing patterns from the output from a cochlear model of a damaged ear with total outer hair cell loss for the synthesized syllable /da/.

auditory filter shapes in the good and impaired ears of subjects having unilateral cochlear hearing losses. The results for five subjects are plotted in Figure 11-4 for a center frequency of 1 kHz. The filters in the impaired ears are much broader than those in the normal ears, especially on the low-frequency side of the response that could be affected by a hypersensitive tail. The filters for the impaired ears also show much more variability than for the normal ears, which would be expected given the range of tuning curves shown in Figure 11-1.

Many other researchers have also found broader tuning curves in listeners having cochlear impairment (Festen & Plomp, 1983; Stelmachowitz et al., 1985; ter Keurs et al., 1993; Zwicker & Fastl, 1999). Some of the differences between the normal and impaired ears may be due to the higher levels of presentation needed for the impaired ears as the auditory filters in normal ears become broader as the level of excitation is increased (Nelson, 1991). But a hearing aid amplifies the signal,

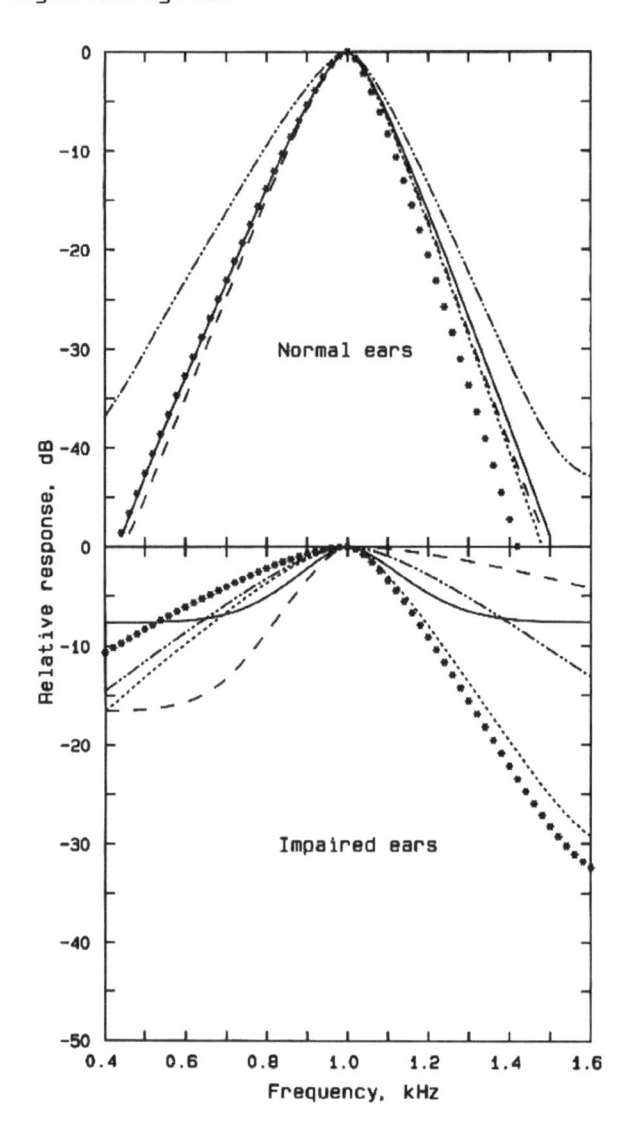

Figure 11-4. Comparison of psychophysical tuning curves for subjects having a unilateral hearing loss. The tuning curves for the normal ears are presented in the upper panel, and the tuning curves for the impaired ears in the lower panel. The test frequency was 1 kHz (from Glasberg & Moore, 1986, as redrawn in Moore, 2003).

so a hearing-impaired listener using a hearing aid will have broader auditory filters, and it is irrelevant whether the broader filters are caused by the hearing loss or result from the amplification.

The short-time spectrum is an important cue in identifying speech sounds, and the broader auditory filters in the impaired ear will make it more difficult to resolve spectral peaks and valleys. Whether the broader filters reduce speech intelligibility will depend in part on the spectral resolution remaining in the impaired ear compared to that needed to understand speech. Zahorian and Rothenberg (1981) found that speech synthesized using the first four principal components gave intelligibility for normal-hearing subjects of about 95% for words within a sentence context, and 80% accuracy in discriminating rhyming word pairs. The highest principal component used in this experiment had a period in the frequency domain of about 1000 Hz (on a linear frequency scale), so very little spectral resolution is needed to resolve the principal components. For example, ter Keurs et al. (1993) looked at how much smearing of the spectrum could be tolerated before intelligibility was reduced, and found that smearing over more than an octave was needed before there was a noticeable loss in intelligibility for sentences in noise for both normal-hearing and hearing-impaired listeners. Henry et al. (2005) found that hearing-impaired listeners had poorer spectral resolution than normal-hearing listeners when detecting ripple-noise spectra, but found only a weak correlation between the spectral resolution threshold and the hearing-impaired subjects' accuracy in recognizing isolated vowels or consonants.

It is still possible that increasing the spectral contrast may improve speech recognition performance. For example, Sidwell and Summerfield (1985) found that representing vowel-like spectra using narrow spectral peaks improved detection performance over that for broad peaks for both normal-hearing and hearing-impaired listeners, but the benefits were small and were less for the hearing-impaired than for the normal-hearing subjects. Leek et al. (1987) varied the peak-to-valley ratio for synthesized vowels in a background of harmonic tones, and found that hearing-impaired listeners needed a greater peak-to-valley ratio than normal-hearing subjects to achieve comparable performance. Both groups of subjects appeared to reach thresholds (2 dB for the normal and 6 dB for the impaired ears) beyond which performance no longer improved. DiGiovanni et al. (2005) conducted experiments on the detection of a narrowband noise embedded in a broadband noise. Both normal-hearing and hearing-impaired subjects showed an improved ability to detect and discriminate increments in the narrowband signal level when notches surrounding the frequency of the narrowband noise were placed in the broadband background noise.

Another aspect of hearing loss is increased upward spread of masking, in which a low-frequency sound interferes with the detection of a sound at a higher frequency. The increased upward spread of masking is related to the tip-to-tail ratio of the damaged auditory filters, as a poorer ratio would allow more low-frequency energy into an auditory filter tuned to a higher center frequency. For example, Gagné (1988) found 12 to 15 dB excess upward spread of masking in impaired ears compared to normal ears, and also found a correlation between the amount of excess masking and the degree of hearing loss.

PROCESSING STRATEGIES

Several different signal-processing strategies have been proposed for spectral contrast enhancement, depending on the aspect of the cochlear damage being considered. The broader auditory filters and reduced tip-to-tail ratio will lead to reduced signal-to-noise ratios (SNRs) in the impaired ear, and one strategy designed to overcome this problem is to suppress valleys in the speech spectrum assumed to be noise and thus improve the SNR. The broader auditory filters will lead to reduced spectral contrast in the impaired ear, and several strategies, such as raising the spectrum to a power greater than one or filtering the spectrum to increase local spectral contrast, are intended to increase the spectral contrast. The reduced tip-to-tail ratio in the impaired ear can lead to increased upward spread of masking, and a proposed strategy is to modify the spectrum to remove the excess signal power from each auditory frequency band. The reduced tip-to-tail ratio also allows the neural firing patterns for vowels to be captured by the first formant even in regions tuned to the second or third formants, and a strategy designed to overcome this problem is to provide additional amplification for the second formant to restore the neural firing patterns.

Spectral Valley Suppression

The reduced tip-to-tail ratio and broader auditory filters in the impaired ear will lead to a poorer SNR in the auditory filter outputs as compared to a normal ear. One hypothesis, therefore, is that removing some of the interfering noise will lead to an improvement in speech intelligibility for hearing-impaired listeners. A strategy to accomplish this end is to reduce the gain in the valleys of the short-time speech spectrum while leaving the peaks intact, the assumption being that the peaks represent the desired speech information whereas the valleys represent noise.

Kates (1994) investigated this strategy by reproducing speech using a sinusoidal signal-processing model. In sinusoidal modeling (McAulay & Quatieri, 1986; Quatieri & McAulay, 1986), the speech signal is represented by a limited number of sinusoidal components. The signal is divided into overlapping windowed segments, and an FFT is computed for each segment. The peaks of the FFT are identified, and the frequency, magnitude, and phase of each peak is saved. The output is then synthesized by generating one sinusoid for each selected peak using the measured frequency, magnitude, and phase values. If the sinusoid is close to the frequency of one generated for the previous segment, the frequency, magnitude, and phase are interpolated across the output segment duration to produce a sinusoid that smoothly varies in amplitude and phase. A frequency component that does not have a match from the previous segment is weighted with a rising ramp to provide a smooth onset transition, and a frequency component that was present in the previous segment but not in the current segment is weighted with a decaying ramp to provide a smooth transition to zero amplitude.

Quatieri and McAulay (1986) used a 10-kHz sampling rate with new speech segments acquired every 5 msec, and found that 40 to 60 sinusoids gave speech that was essentially indistinguishable from the original. Kates (1994) used a 20-kHz sampling rate with windowed segments 25.6 msec in length (512 samples). A new segment was acquired every 9.6 msec (192 samples). Kates found that reproduction using 32 sinusoids for these sampling parameters produced speech very close to the original in quality.

The spectral enhancement (Kates, 1994) was provided by reducing the number of sinusoids used to reproduce the speech so that fewer than 32 were used. Sinusoids corresponding to the speech peaks were kept, but sinusoids corresponding to the assumed noisy spectral valleys were discarded. An example is shown in Figure 11-5 for a section of the vowel /a/ from the speech token "ka." The speech magnitude spectrum is indicated on an arbitrary dB scale, and the 16 selected peaks are indicated by the vertical bars below the spectrum. The selected peaks include the domi-

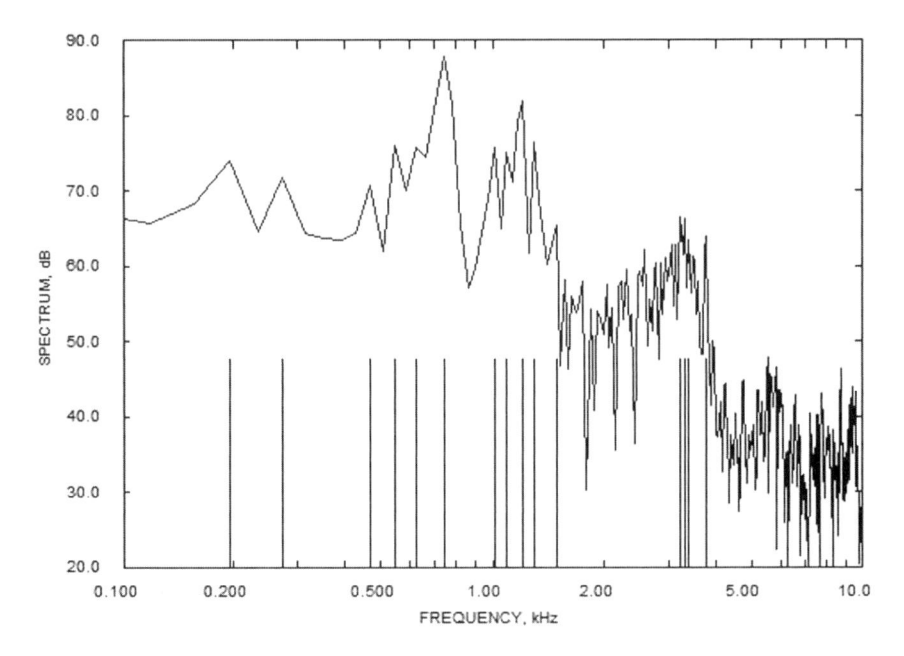

Figure 11-5. Spectrum for the vowel /a/ in "ka" indicated by the solid curve, with peaks selected for reproduction using 16 sinusoids indicated by the vertical bars (from Kates, 1994).

nant spectral components and modulation sidebands from the first three formants of the vowel, plus some additional low-frequency components in the vicinity of 100 to 300 Hz. Sinusoids in between the dominant spectral regions tend to be ignored by the selection procedure, leading to an increase in spectral contrast and a reduction in background noise.

The processing was evaluated using five normal-hearing subjects. The speech stimuli were isolated consonant-vowel and vowel-consonant tokens, presented in multitalker babble at a 25-dB or 5-dB SNR. The consonant recognition test results showed no benefit for the speech reproduced using 16 or 8 sinusoids as compared with the original speech at either SNR. Further analysis indicated that reducing the number of sinusoids used to reproduce the speech gave results similar to increasing the background noise level; halving the number of sinusoids was equivalent to reducing the SNR by 8 to 10 dB. These results lead to the conclusion that the low-level spectrum includes information useful for speech recognition, and that this information can be extracted by normal-hearing listeners even at a poor SNR. Related experiments (Kates, 1991b) led to similar conclusions for hearing-impaired listeners.

Spectral Contrast Modification

Several different procedures have been proposed to increase spectral contrast. The goal in all of these procedures is to increase the ratio of the peaks to the valleys of the power spectrum. Two basic approaches have been tried. The first is to raise the short-time magnitude spectrum to a power greater than one, and the second is to apply a frequency-domain filter to the magnitude spectrum to increase the local contrast.

RAISE SPECTRUM TO A POWER

One procedure to enhance the speech spectrum is to raise the magnitude spectrum to a power greater than one, thus exaggerating the spectral contrast as the high-level regions of the spectrum will receive more gain than the low-level regions. A block diagram for this processing system is presented in Figure 11-6. The incoming signal is divided into segments and windowed. The segment size is generally in the range of 10 to 30 msec. The FFT is computed for the windowed segment and the phase is saved. The magnitude spectrum is raise to a power greater than 1 and recombined with the original phase to produce the enhanced spectrum. The time-domain output is then produced by taking the inverse transform of the modified spectrum and combining the waveform with the previous output segments via overlap-add. Let the enhancement factor be denoted by μ. The modified magnitude spectrum is given by:

$$|\hat{S}(f)| = |S(f)|^{(1+\mu)} \quad \text{Equation (11.1)}$$

where $|S(f)|$ is the magnitude spectrum of the original signal and $\mu > 0$. If the spectrum is expressed in dB, the modification becomes:

$$|\hat{S}(f)| = (1+\mu)|S(f)|, dB \quad \text{Equation (11.2)}$$

332 Digital Hearing Aids

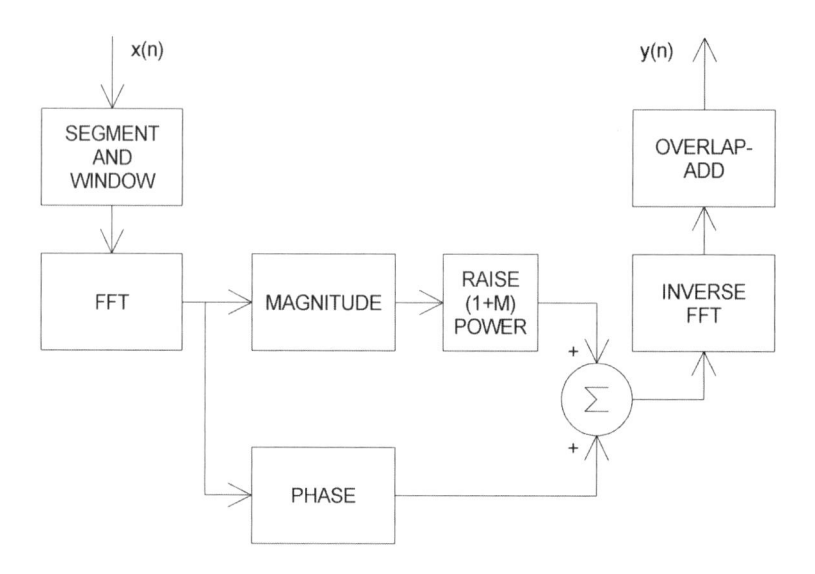

Figure 11-6. Block diagram for spectral enhancement based on raising the magnitude spectrum to a power greater than 1.

The processing of Eq. (11.2) can also be described as sending the short-time spectrum through a filter having a frequency response given by $\mu|S(f)|$ in dB. The speech spectrum is filtered by a scaled version of itself; the spectral peaks, which have a greater amplitude than the valleys, will receive proportionately greater amplification. Boers (1980) implemented this system with $\mu = 1$, thus squaring the magnitude spectrum. He found that the increased spectral contrast for speech in noise led to reduced speech-recognition scores for both normal-hearing and hearing-impaired listeners.

Bunnell (1990) implemented a modification of the processing given by Eq. (11.2). In his system the enhancement is given by:

$$|\hat{S}(f)| = C\big[|S(f)| - |\overline{S}(f)|\big] + |\overline{S}(f)|, \; dB \quad \text{Equation (11.3)}$$

where C is a frequency-dependent scale factor equal to $(1+\mu)$ at approximately 2.5 kHz and tapered toward 1 at lower and higher frequencies. The overbar term $|\overline{S}(f)|$ in Eq. (11.3) refers to the long-term average magnitude spectrum for the test utterance. If $\mu = 0$, then $C = 1$ at all frequencies and the processing reverts to reproducing the short-time magnitude spectrum for each speech segment. If $\mu = 1$, the processing squares the deviation of the segment short-time spectrum from the long-term average spectrum at 2.5 kHz while leaving the short-time spectrum unchanged at very low and very high frequencies. Yang et al. (2002) have proposed a similar system, but with the FFT bins first combined into auditory filter bandwidths prior to computing the enhancement gain as a function of frequency.

An example of the processing proposed by Bunnell (1990) is presented in Figure 11-7. The original magnitude spectrum for a vowel is presented in the upper panel (A), whereas the processed spectrum is presented in the lower panel (B). The first formant is at about 550 Hz, and the second and third formants are at about 1800 and 2400 Hz, respectively. The processing has reduced the magnitude of the valley between the first and second formants and attenuated the speech energy above the third formant. Note that the processing has also reduced the amplitude of the first formant and elevated the magnitude of the second and third formants. The processing thus combines an increase in the spectral contrast with a slight emphasis of the higher formant frequencies relative to that of the first formant. In evaluating the processing with a group of hearing-impaired subjects, Bunnell (1990) found that increasing the spectral contrast ($\mu = 1$) resulted in a slight increase in the performance for a consonant-identification task, whereas reducing the spectral contrast ($\mu = -1$) caused a slight reduction in the consonant-recognition scores. However, one cannot separate the effects of the contrast enhancement in his results from the effects of increasing the relative amplitude of the higher formants.

Lyzenga et al. (2002) implemented the processing given by *Eq. (11.2)* but, similar to Bunnell (1990) in *Eq. (11.3)*, limited the contrast enhancement to the frequency region from 400 to 4500 Hz. The processing was adjusted so that spectral ripples at rates consistent with formant bandwidths were allowed to be amplified whereas ripples at lower and higher rates were left unaffected. They also combined the contrast enhancement with a high-frequency emphasis filter providing 6 dB or 12 dB of additional amplification in the frequency region around 3 kHz. The processing was tested on normal-hearing subjects using spectral smearing to simulate the loss of frequency resolution typical of hearing loss. They found that the combination of spectral contrast enhancement and high-frequency emphasis improved the SNR for speech recognition

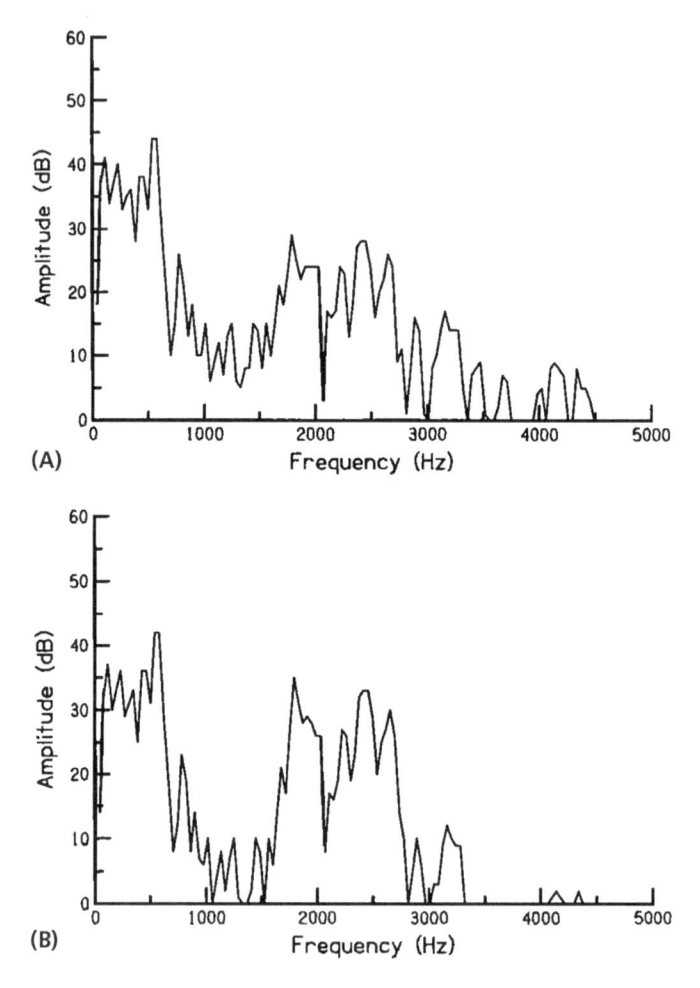

Figure 11-7. Spectral contrast enhancement showing the short-time spectrum of the original vowel (**A**) and the enhanced vowel (**B**) (from Bunnell, 1990).

in noise by about 1 dB, but that neither the contrast enhancement nor the high-frequency emphasis alone provided any benefit.

SPECTRAL FILTERING

A second approach to enhancing spectral contrast is to apply a frequency-domain filter to sharpen the spectral peaks. The goal is to make the spectral peaks narrower than normal so that when they are processed through the broader filters of the impaired auditory system the resultant neural excitation pattern will match that of the normal ear. Obviously there is a limitation to this processing approach. For example, if the input is a sinusoid, the excitation pattern in the impaired ear will be broader than in the normal ear but there is no way that the bandwidth of a single tone can possibly be reduced. However, if the bandwidth of the excitation is greater than that of the auditory filters in the impaired ear, then some reduction in the spread of excitation in the impaired ear may result from the processing.

The general approach (Cheng & O'Shaughnessy, 1991; Simpson et al, 1990) is similar to that shown in Figure 11-6 for raising the spectrum to a power greater than one. But instead of raising the spectrum to a power, the magnitude spectrum is convolved in the frequency domain with a sharpening function. The sharpened spectrum is recombined with the original phase and inverse transformed to produce the modified speech segment. The segments are then combined using overlap-add to produce the output signal.

The general form of the frequency-sharpening filter is illustrated in Figure 11-8. The filter has a peak at its center frequency, and then has regions of negative gain to either side of the peak. The modified spectrum produced by this filter will have high gain when the peak of the filter lies directly over a peak of the spectrum and reduced gain at other frequencies. For example, assume that the FFT spectrum has been summed across analysis bins to give a spectrum representative of auditory frequency analysis, with the auditory band index k running from 1 through K. A simple sharpening filter is given by:

$$|\hat{S}(k)| = |S(k)| - \mu|S(k-1)| - \mu\,S(k+1)|\quad \text{Equation (11.4)}$$

The modified spectrum in auditory band k is equal to the original spectrum minus μ times the amplitude of the auditory band amplitudes to either side. If the sharpening filter lies over a peak, then the magnitude of $S(k)$ will be high and the magnitudes of $S(k-1)$ and $S(k+1)$ will be low, and the modified spectrum will have a value nearly equal to that of the original spectrum. If the sharpening filter lies adjacent to a peak, then the magnitude of $S(k)$ will be low but the magnitude of either $S(k-1)$ or $S(k+1)$ will be high, and the magnitude of the modified spectrum will be much lower than that of the original spectrum. In a valley, the magnitude of S(k) will be lower than either the magnitude of S(k−1) or S(k+1); it is possible for this condition that the processing will return a negative value for the magnitude of the modified spectrum, which is normally replaced by zero. If the original spectrum is flat, the modified spectrum will have an amplitude equal to 1−2μ. For μ = 1/2, the filtering operation will completely cancel the flat spectrum and the modified spectrum given by Eq. (11.4) will be zero.

An example of a spectrum with increased spectral contrast is shown in Figure 11-9. The gain in the regions of the spectral peaks is only slightly reduced, but the gains in the spectral valleys are strongly attenuated as the valleys cause negative magnitudes in Eq. (11.4) and are replaced with zeros. Cheng and O'Shaughnessy (1991) showed that this general processing approach produced improvements in speech-quality metrics, such as segmental SNR, that were comparable to those produced by the spectral subtraction algorithm that they used for comparison. Stone and Moore (1992) implemented a similar system using an analog filter bank. They found no improvement in speech intelligibility, but they did find that some hearing-impaired subjects preferred the processed speech to the original.

Baer et al. (1993) compared several versions of the spectral contrast processing. They used the difference of a broad and a narrow Gaussian function to generate the spectral sharpening function shown schematically in Figure 11-8, and also used the difference between a wide and a narrow approximation to the shape of the human auditory filter. A modification to the processing that they investigated was to convert the spectral contrast enhancement given by Eq. (11.4) into a logarithmic enhancement gain function, expressed here in terms of the simple spectral-enhancement filter presented in Eq. (11.4):

$$D(k) = |S(k)| - \mu|S(k-1)| - \mu|S(k+1)| \quad \text{Equation (11.5a)}$$

$$Gain(k) = \begin{cases} 10^{\alpha D(k)}, & D(k) < 0 \\ 10 - (10-1)10^{-\alpha D(k)}, & D(k) \geq 0 \end{cases} \quad \text{Equation (11.5b)}$$

As the spectral contrast enhancement is used as an exponent, it removes the problem of zero or negative modified spectrum magnitudes

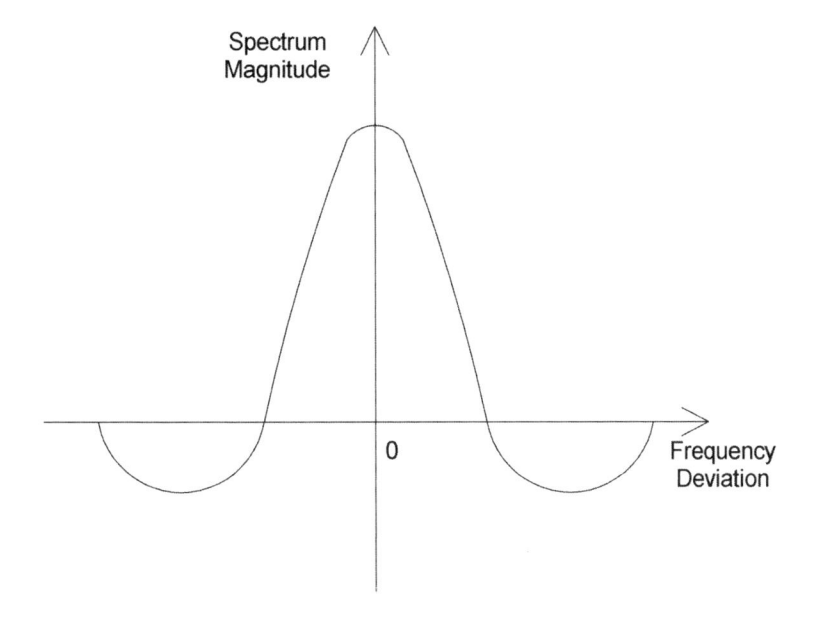

Figure 11-8. Schematic representation of a frequency-domain contrast-enhancement filter.

that arises from Eq. (11.4) for flat input spectra or spectral valleys. Eq. (11.5a) reproduces the spectral contrast enhancement formula of Eq. (11.4). However, the contrast enhancement is then transformed using Eq. (11.5b). A negative value for $D(k)$ resulting from a valley in the input spectrum is converted into an attenuation rather than zero gain. The form of spectral contrast enhancement given by Eq. (11.5b) provides unity gain for a flat spectrum and up to a maximum of 20 dB gain for a spectral peak.

An example of an enhanced spectrum for the Baer et al. (1993) processing approach using the difference between wide and narrow auditory filter shapes is presented in Figure 11-10. The upper panel is for the unprocessed condition, which corresponds to setting $\alpha = 0$ in Eq. (11.5b). The processed vowel is shown in the lower panel. The spectral contrast enhancement has reduced the bandwidth of the spectral peaks, increased the amplitude of the second and higher formants, and reduced the amplitude of the valleys in between the formant peaks. Experiments using hearing-impaired listeners show a very small improvement in the intelligibility of noisy speech for the spectral contrast enhancement, and

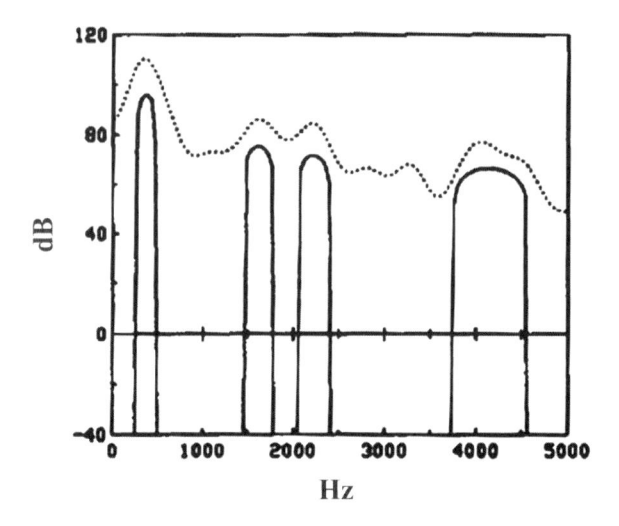

Figure 11-9. Spectral contrast enhancement using the approach given by *Eq. (11.4)* (from Cheng & O'Shaughnessy, 1991).

a small but statistically significant benefit for the spectral contrast enhancement combined with broadband dynamic-range compression; the net benefit was equal to an improvement in SNR of about 0.8 dB. Their experiments also showed a statistically significant reduction in reaction time in identifying words within sentences, suggesting that the subjects found that the spectral contrast enhancement reduced listening effort. However, an experiment using the same spectral-contrast enhancement processing (Franck et al., 1999) found no net benefit in improving the intelligibility of consonant-vowel-consonant (CVC) syllables for the spectral processing when used alone or in combination with dynamic-range compression; the small benefit found for vowels was more than offset by the loss in intelligibility for consonants.

One potential concern with the algorithms discussed in this section is that all of the implementations processed the signals in blocks ranging in duration from 12 to 32 msec. The signal processing is equivalent to filtering the speech through a filter that remains constant throughout the duration of the block even though the speech short-term spectrum may be dynamically changing. The filter duration is not a problem for a steady-state vowel, which has a relatively constant spectrum over a duration of 100 msec or longer. But speech transients, such as the onset

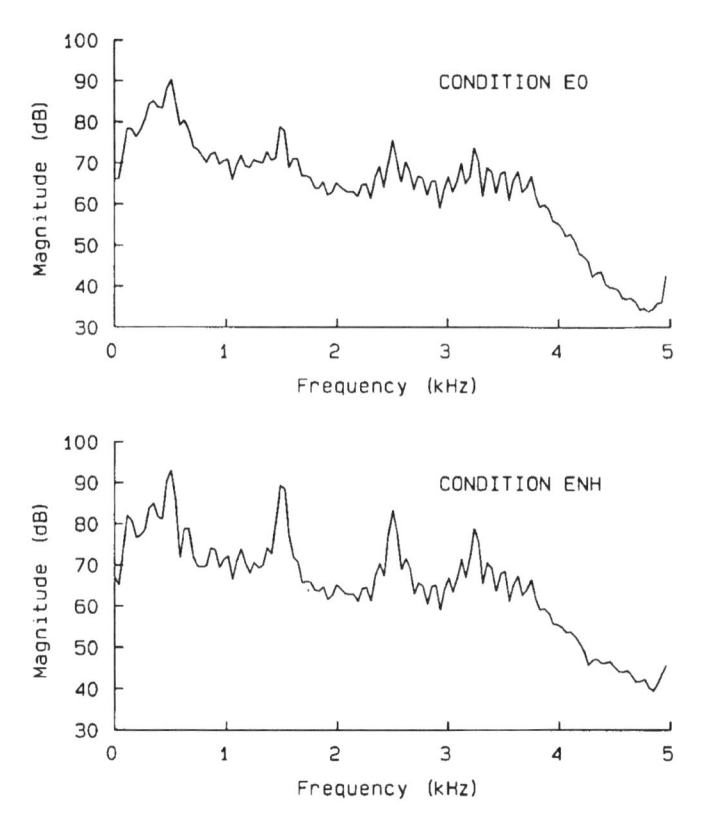

Figure 11-10. Spectral contrast enhancement using the approach of *Eq (11.5)* showing the average spectrum of a neutral vowel in noise for the control condition (E0, *upper panel*) and the enhanced condition (ENH, *lower panel*) (from Baer et al., 1993).

during a consonant burst or formant transitions, can occur on a much faster time scale. Filtering a descending formant transition, for example, through a filter based on the average formant frequency over the speech segment will impose unwanted amplitude modulations. The formant will be attenuated as it starts above the filter peak frequency, will reach a high gain at the filter peak, and then be attenuated again as it falls below the peak frequency. The interaction between block size and processing effectiveness would be an interesting question to investigate for noise-suppression and speech-enhancement algorithms.

Excess Upward Spread of Masking

One characteristic of auditory impairment is an increase in the upward spread of masking. A simple model for the increased upward spread of masking is to assume that a spectral smearing function has been applied to the signal power spectrum. The compensation for the excess upward spread of masking would then be the inverse of the smearing function.

Assume that the excess upward spread of masking can be approximated by adding to the power in each auditory filter band a decreasing fraction of the power in each of the lower frequency bands. The power in band k can thus be represented as the power in the band for the normal ear plus additional terms representing the excess masking:

$$|P(k)|^2 = |S(k)|^2 + \beta\, S(k-1)|^2 + \beta^2 |S(k-2)|^2 + \ldots + \beta^{k-1}|S(1)|^2$$

Equation (11.6)

where $|S(k)|^2$ is the signal power in auditory filter band k for a normal ear, $|P(k)|^2$ is the assumed power in the impaired ear, and $\beta < 1$. This relationship can be written for all of the auditory filter bands simultaneously using matrix notation:

$$|P|^2 = B|S|^2 \quad \text{Equation (11.7)}$$

Where B is the spectral smearing matrix given by:

$$B = \begin{bmatrix} 1 & 0 & 0 & 0 & \ldots \\ \beta & 1 & 0 & 0 & \\ \beta^2 & \beta & 1 & 0 & \\ \beta^3 & \beta^2 & \beta & 1 & \\ \ldots & & & & \end{bmatrix} \quad \text{Equation (11.8)}$$

S is the vector of spectrum samples in each normal auditory filter going from low frequencies to high:

$$S = [S(1), S(2), \ldots, S(K)] \quad \text{Equation (11.9)}$$

and P is the vector of spectrum samples in the impaired ear:

$$P = [P(1), P(2), \ldots, P(K)] \quad \text{Equation (11.10)}$$

The correction of the spectral smearing given by Eq. (11.6) is to sharpen the spectrum so that the output of the smearing operation in the impaired ear is an approximation to the original unsmeared spectrum. In matrix terms, the sharpening is provided by multiplying the input spectrum by a correction matrix given by the inverse of the smearing matrix B, resulting in:

$$|\tilde{S}|^2 = B^{-1}|S|^2 \quad \text{Equation (11.11)}$$

It turns out that the correction matrix B^{-1} has a particularly simple form:

$$B^{-1} = \begin{bmatrix} 1 & 0 & 0 & 0 & \cdots \\ -\beta & 1 & 0 & 0 \\ 0 & -\beta & 1 & 0 \\ 0 & 0 & -\beta & 1 \\ \cdots & & & & \end{bmatrix} \quad \text{Equation (11.12)}$$

Converting back from matrix notation to the individual power spectrum components yields:

$$|\tilde{S}(k)|^2 = |S(k)|^2 - \beta|S(k-1)|^2 \quad \text{Equation (11.13)}$$

The correction for excess upward spread of masking is just a one-sided version of the sharpening filter given by Eq. (11.4), but operating on the spectrum power rather than the spectrum magnitude. This form of processing has not been tested on listeners, but one would expect that its effectiveness would be similar to that of the spectral filtering described in the previous section.

F2/F1 Ratio

As shown in Figure 11-1, cochlear damage typically reduces the auditory filter gain in the vicinity of the tip of the tuning curve, whereas the gain in the tail remains unchanged or is even increased. The reduction in the tip-to-tail ratio allows much more out-of-band signal energy into the damaged auditory filter, thus reducing the effective ratio of desired signal power to interference within the filter. In particular, it is possible that the level of the first formant in a vowel will exceed that of the second formant in a damaged auditory filter tuned to the frequency of the second formant. Miller et al. (1999), in experiments on damaged cat cochleas, showed that the timing of the neural firing pattern in the vicinity of the vowel second formant could be captured by the periodicity of the first formant.

The correct timing of the neural firing patterns in the vicinity of the second formant can be restored by amplifying the second formant frequency region relative to that of the first formant (Bruce et al., 2003; Miller et al., 1999). An example of a modified spectrum is plotted in Figure 11-11. The line spectrum in the figure shows the unprocessed vowel spectrum, and the solid line shows the spectral envelope for the spectrum of the modified vowel. No amplification is provided for the first formant and 30-dB gain is provided for the second formant by the proposed contrast enhancement frequency shaping (CEFS) scheme. Bruce (2004) implemented this approach for running speech using a formant tracker to identify the frequency region associated with the second formant. Evaluation using a physiologic model showed that the CEFS second-formant boost can restore the desired timing behavior for the simulated neural spike patterns, and that combining the CEFS processing with multichannel compression did not reduce its effectiveness.

Processing Comparison

The differences between some of the spectral-contrast enhancement schemes are illustrated in Figures 11-12 through 11-16. The stimulus is the vowel /e/ from the word "the" spoken by a male talker. The speech was sampled at 44.1 kHz and down-sampled to 22.05 kHz. The frequency analysis was performed using frequency warping. The speech was sent through a cascade of 41 first-order all-pass filter sections having a filter coefficient of $a = 0.646$, followed by a 42-point FFT. The resulting warped frequency spectrum provides an auditory frequency analysis with filter spacing of approximately 1 Bark. (The warped frequency-analysis procedure is described in Chapter 8.)

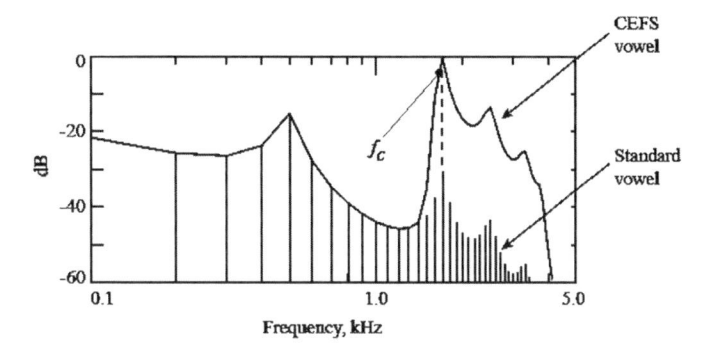

Figure 11-11. Power spectra of the standard and enhanced (CEFS) versions of the vowel / /. The line spectrum shows the spectral shape of the unprocessed vowel and the solid line shows the CEFS-modified spectral envelope (from Bruce et al., 2003).

The spectrum of the unprocessed speech is plotted in Figure 11-12. The spectrum has its strongest peak in band 5 (465 Hz), with additional peaks in bands 9 (1020 Hz) and 16 (2950 Hz). The enhancement gain for raising the spectrum to a power, given by Eq. (11.2), is plotted in Figure 11-13 for $\mu = 0.25$. The gain has been normalized so that its maximum value is 0 dB. The enhancement gain is proportional to the spectrum magnitude at all frequencies, so it is just a scaled version of the speech spectrum. The valleys between the spectral peaks have gains less than 0 dB, so they will be attenuated. As the higher frequency peaks in bands 9 and 16 are lower in amplitude than the low-frequency peak in band 5, the enhancement gain will attenuate these high-frequency peaks as well. Thus raising the spectrum to a power reduces the gain for the valleys, but also attenuates the amplitude of the second and third formants relative to that of the first formant.

The gain for the spectral contrast enhancement given by Eq. (11.4) is plotted in Figure 11-14 for a value of $\mu = 0.25$. The enhancement has high gain in the vicinity of the three peaks. The processing also provides high gain for bands 19 to 21 as a result of the shifts in the slope of the spectrum. The gain given by Eq. (11.4) goes negative in each of the valleys, so zero has been substituted for the signal amplitude in each of these regions. The gain for the compensation for upward spread of masking given by Eq. (11.13) is plotted in Figure 11-15, for $\beta = 0.25$. The result of the masking compensation is very similar to that shown in Figure 11-14. The major difference is that the filter passband regions

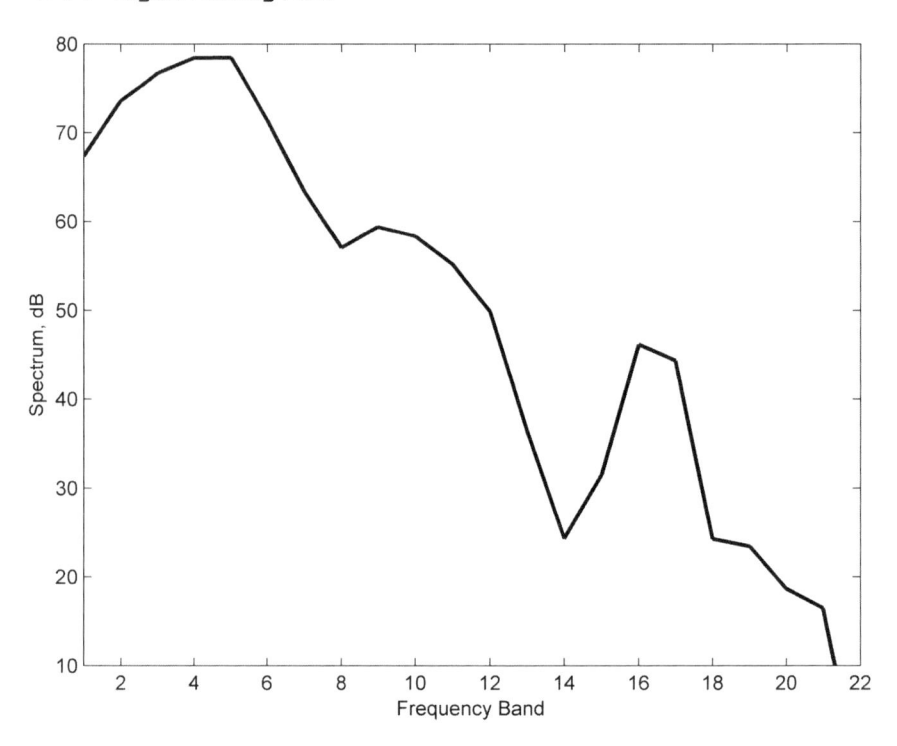

Figure 11-12. Spectrum for the vowel /e/ in the word "the." The spectrum is from a frequency-warped cascade of 41 all-pass filters with warping factor a = 0.646 followed by a 42-point FFT. The sampling rate is 22.05 kHz. Each frequency band is approximately 1 Bark wide.

around the three peaks are broader as the gain depends only on the difference between each band and the next-lower band.

The enhancement used by Baer et al. (1993) converts the absolute spectrum differences into logarithmic gain changes, and this effect can be seen in the plot of Figure 11-16. The enhancement processing is given by Eq. (11.5) with μ = 0.25 and α = 0.3. The processing gain has been normalized to give a maximum of 0 dB rather than the 20-dB maximum that results from applying Eq. (11.5) directly. The maximum gain provided by Eq. (11.5) is limited to a maximum of 20 dB, and this maximum is met in the vicinity of each of the spectral peaks. The logarithmic transformation also reduces the attenuation in the valleys, so the gain is now −10 dB relative to the peaks instead of the complete attenuation given by the other spectral filtering approaches.

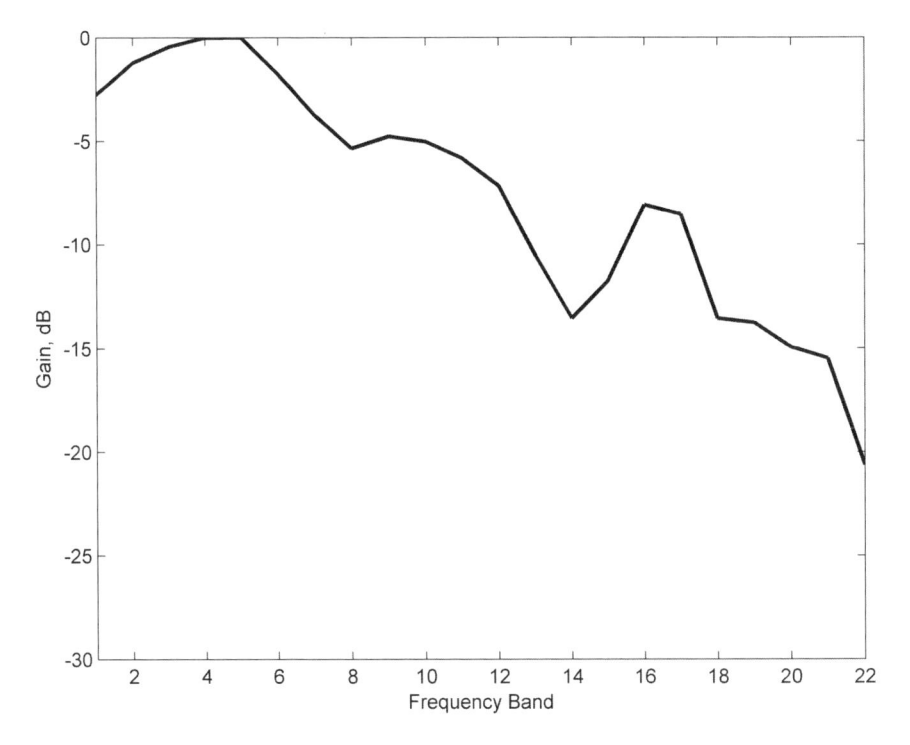

Figure 11-13. Spectral contrast enhancement gain provided by raising the spectrum to a power using $\mu = 0.25$ in *Eq. (11.2)*. The gain has been normalized so that the maximum gain is 0 dB.

Combining Spectral Enhancement With Compression

The different signal-processing strategies proposed for hearing aids are often considered in isolation because this gives the most direct procedure for designing and evaluating the processing. When different processing strategies are combined, however, the processing interactions may undo the desired effects. For example, multichannel dynamic-range compression undoes the effects of spectral contrast enhancement.

Assume that spectral contrast enhancement is used in cascade with multichannel dynamic-range compression. Let the spectral contrast enhancement be given by the system of *Eq. (11.2)*. The spectral contrast enhancement amplifies the high-level sounds more than the low-level sounds. Dynamic-range compression, on the other hand, amplifies the

346 Digital Hearing Aids

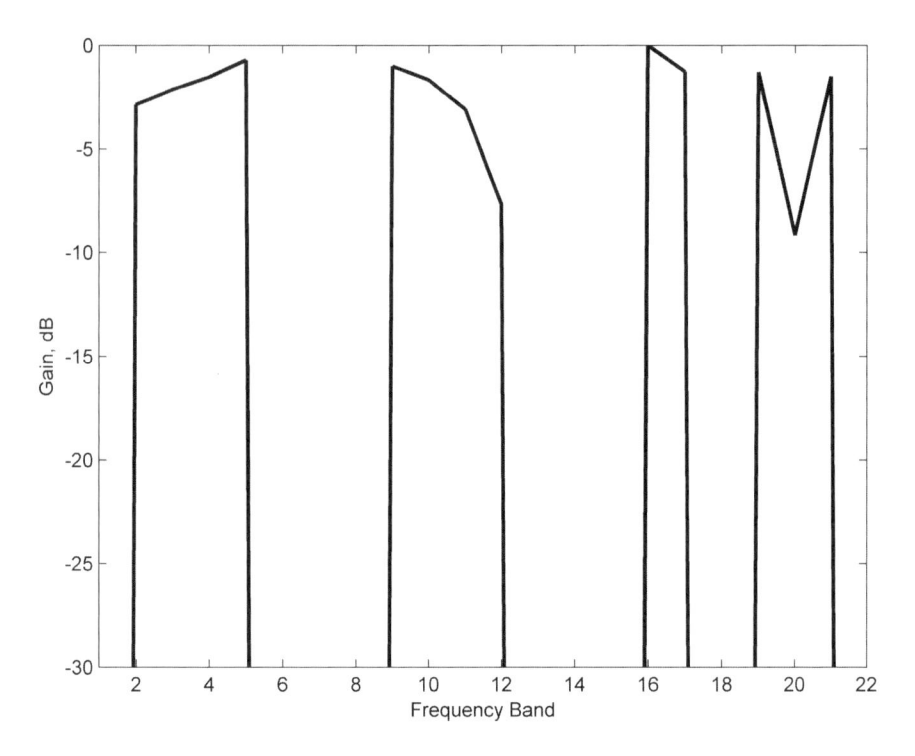

Figure 11-14. Spectral contrast enhancement gain provided by using *Eq. (11.4)* with μ = 0.25. The gain has been normalized so that the maximum gain is 0 dB.

low-level sounds more than the high-level sounds, and thus reduces the spectral contrast (Lyzenga et al., 2002). The system cascade is given by:

$$|\hat{S}(f)| = (1+\mu)|S(f)|, dB \quad \text{Equation (11.14a)}$$

$$|Y(f)| = (1-\delta)|\hat{S}(f)|, dB \quad \text{Equation (11.14b)}$$

where $|Y(f)|$ is the system output and $0 < \delta < 1$. Eq. (11.14a) is the spectral contrast enhancement, and Eq. (11.14b) is multichannel compression implemented in the frequency domain. The net change in the spectral contrast is given by $(1+\mu)(1-\delta)$. So if $(1-\delta) = 1/(1+\mu)$, the net effect is linear amplification. Linear processing can thus be considered to be spectral contrast enhancement combined with multichannel

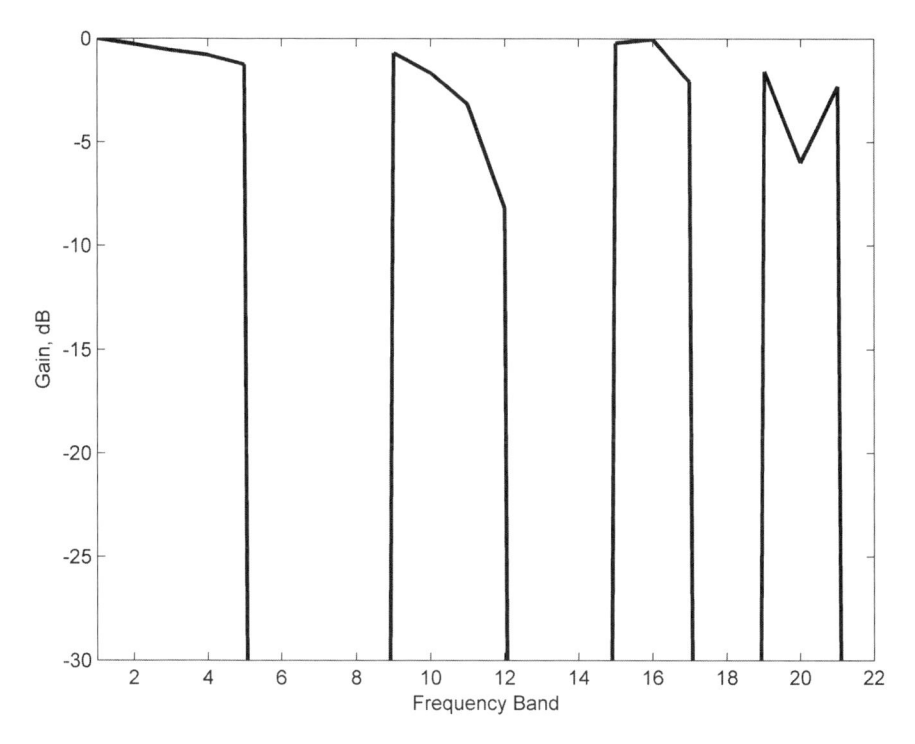

Figure 11-15. Spectral contrast enhancement gain provided by the compensation for upward spread of masking given by *Eq. (11.13)* with β = 0.25. The gain has been normalized so that the maximum gain is 0 dB.

compression, which may explain why linear processing or slow-acting compression is often more effective than more complicated processing schemes (Franck et al., 1999; Moore et al., 2004).

An alternative approach would be to design a compression system that preserves local spectral contrast. This objective can be accomplished by linking the compression gains across frequency bands rather than having independent compression in each band. Kates (1993b), for example, argued that two-tone suppression should be considered in designing a compression system along with auditory thresholds and auditory filter bandwidths. In two-tone suppression (Delgutte, 1990; Sachs & Kiang, 1968), a strong masking signal above or below the frequency of a probe tone will reduce the neural response to the probe. In the compression system proposed by Kates (1993b), the gain for each frequency band in a multichannel compressor is controlled by the strongest signal

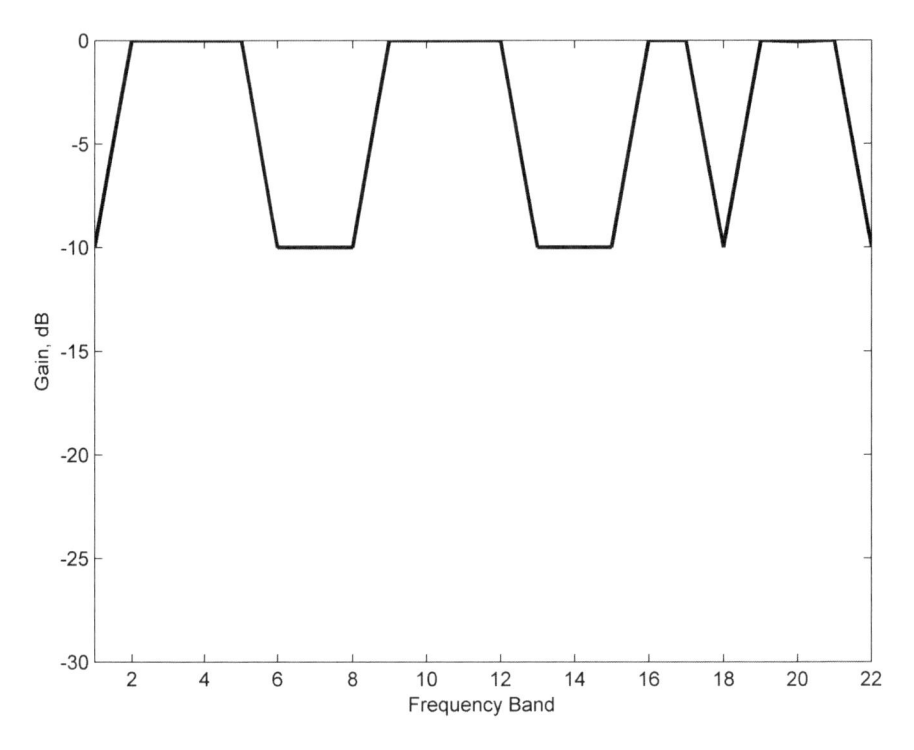

Figure 11-16. Spectral contrast enhancement gain provided by the procedure of Baer et al. (1993) given by *Eq. (11.5)* with µ = 0.25 and β = 0.3. The gain has been normalized so that the maximum gain is 0 dB.

found within a range of one-half octave below to one-half octave above the band frequency. As shown in Figure 11-17, the gain in the frequency bands surrounding a spectral peak is determined by the peak level and not the individual band levels. As a result, the gain in the region surrounding a peak is constant, preserving the local spectral contrast rather than reducing it as would happen in a conventional multichannel compression system.

Concluding Remarks

Spectral contrast enhancement refers to a family of algorithms that attempt to compensate for the changes in the auditory filter shapes caused by cochlear damage. The damage can cause broader auditory filter

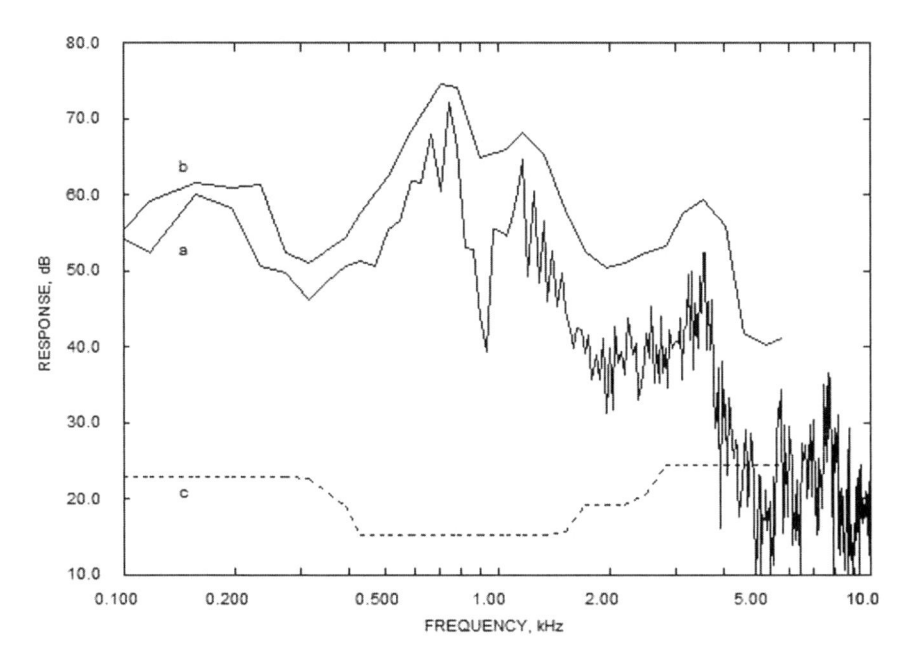

Figure 11-17. Spectrum for the sound /k/ in "ka": **a.** speech spectrum, **b.** spectrum in auditory analysis bands, and **c.** computed hearing-aid gain for a flat 60-dB hearing loss (from Kates, 1993b).

bandwidths and reduced tip-to-tail ratios. If we define the effective SNR as the ratio of the in-band signal to the sum of the in-band noise and out-of-band signal and noise, then the damaged cochlear filters will exhibit much lower effective SNRs than are found in the normal cochlea. The reduction in effective SNR can lead to changes in the neural firing patterns, in which the periodicity of the neural response is captured by strong low-frequency signal components instead of the signal component in the vicinity of the auditory filter center frequency.

Different signal-processing strategies have been proposed for spectral contrast enhancement, each emphasizing a different consequence of the cochlear damage. The processing includes spectral valley suppression, spectral sharpening filters, compensation for excess upward spread of masking, and amplification of the second formant region relative to that of the first formant to improve the capture of the second formant periodicity in the neural response. However, the benefit of the processing in improving speech intelligibility for hearing-impaired listeners, in those experiments where it has been tried on human subjects, has been small. The best results show that the processing is equivalent to about a 1-dB change in the SNR. An additional concern is that multichannel compression works in opposition to spectral contrast enhancement, and implementing both processing strategies in the same device may lead to mutual cancellation of the processing effects.

The conventional approach to designing signal processing for hearing aids is to focus on one aspect of the hearing problem and then create an algorithm that addresses that specific concern. But hearing loss appears to be more than a sum of separate processing issues that can be solved one at a time, and a more global approach may be needed. One such approach is to model the normal and impaired ears. The hearing-aid filtering is then adaptively adjusted so that the output from the model of the impaired ear, given the processed input, matches as closely as possible the output from the model of the normal ear (Bondy et al., 2004; Kates, 1993b). This approach simultaneously takes all factors of the peripheral hearing loss into account, and thus provides an inherent tradeoff between the different effects of cochlear damage.

References

Baer, T., Moore, B. C. J., & Gatehouse, S. (1993). Spectral contrast enhancement of speech in noise for listeners with sensorineural hearing impairment: Effects on intelligibility, quality, and response times. *Journal of Rehabilitation Research and Development, 30,* 49–72.

Boers, P. M. (1980). Formant enhancement of speech for listeners with sensorineural hearing loss. *IPO Annual Progress Report*, No. 15 (Institut voor Perceptie Onderzoek), pp. 21–28.

Bondy, J., Becker, S., Bruce, I., Trainor, L., & Haykin, S. (2004). A novel signal-processing strategy for hearing-aid design: Neurocompensation. *Speech Communication, 84,* 1239–1253.

Bruce, I. C. (2004). Physiological assessment of contrast-enhancing frequency shaping and multiband compression in hearing aids. *Physiological Measures, 25,* 945–956.

Bruce, I. C., Sachs, M. B., & Young, E. D. (2003). An auditory-periphery model of the effects of acoustic trauma on auditory nerve responses. *Journal of the Acoustical Society of America, 113,* 369–388.

Bunnell, H. T. (1990). On enhancement of spectral contrast in speech for hearing-impaired listeners. *Journal of the Acoustical Society of America*, 88, 2546–2556.

Cheng, Y. M., & O'Shaughnessy, D. (1991). Speech enhancement based conceptually on auditory evidence, *IEEE Transactions Signal Processing*, 39, 1943–1954.

Delgutte, B. (1990). Two-tone suppression in auditory nerve fibers: Dependence of suppressor frequency and level. *Hearing Resolutions*, 49, 225–246.

DiGiovanni, J. J., Nelson, P. B., & Schlauch, R. S. (2005). A psychophysical evaluation of spectral enhancement. *Journal of Speech, Language, and Hearing Research*, 48, 1121–1135.

Festen, J. M., & Plomp, R. (1983). Relations between auditory functions in impaired hearing. *Journal of the Acoustical Society America*, 73, 652–662.

Franck, B. A .M., Sidonne, C., van Kreveld-Bos, G. M., Dreschler, W. A., & Verschuure, H. (1999). Evaluation of spectral enhancement in hearing aids, combined with phonemic compression. *Journal of the Acoustical Society of America*, 106, 1452–1464.

Gagné, J-P. (1988). Excess masking among listeners with a sensorineural hearing loss. *Journal of the Acoustical Society of America*, 83, 2311–2321.

Glasberg, B. R., & Moore, B. C. J. (1986). Auditory filter shapes in subjects with unilateral and bilateral cochlear impairments. *Journal of the Acoustical Society of America*, 79, 1020–1033.

Henry, B. A., Turner, C. W., & Behrens, A. (2005). Spectral peak resolution and speech recognition in quiet: Normal hearing, hearing impaired, and cochlear implant listeners. *Journal of the Acoustical Society of America*, 118, 1111–1121.

Kates, J. M. (1991a). A time-domain digital cochlear model. *IEEE Transactions on Signal Processing*, 39, 2573–2592.

Kates, J. M. (1991b). A simplified representation of speech for the hearing impaired, *Journal of the Acoustical Society of America*, 89 (Pt. 2), 1961.

Kates, J. M. (1993a). Accurate tuning curves in a cochlear model. *IEEE Transactions on Speech and Audio Processing*, 1, 453–462.

Kates, J. M. (1993b). Toward a theory of optimal hearing aid processing. *Journal of Rehabilitation Research and Development*, 30, 39–48.

Kates, J. M. (1994). Speech enhancement based on a sinusoidal model. *Journal of Speech and Hearing Research*, 37, 449–464.

Kates, J. M. (2002). Hearing-aid benefits and limitations: Predictions from a cochlear model. *Proceedings of the 7th International Conference on Spoken Language Processing* (pp. 413-416), Denver, Sept 16–20, 2002.

Leek, M. R., Dorman, M. F., & Summerfield, Q. (1987). Minimum spectral contrast for vowel identification by normal-hearing and hearing-impaired listeners. *Journal of the Acoustical Society of America, 81,* 148–154.

Liberman, M. C., & Dodds, L. W. (1984). Single neuron labeling and chronic cochlear pathology. III. Stereocilia damage and alterations of threshold tuning curves. *Hearing Research, 16,* 55–74.

Lyzenga, J., Festen, J. M., & Houtgast, T. (2002). A speech enhancement scheme incorporating spectral expansion evaluated with simulated loss of frequency selectivity. *Journal of the Acoustical Society of America, 112,* 1145–1157.

McAulay, R. J., & Quatieri, T. F. (1986). Speech analysis/synthesis based on a sinusoidal representation. *IEEE Transactions on Acoustics, Speech, and Signal Processing, ASSP-34,* 744–754.

Miller, R. L., Calhoun, B. M., & Young, E. D. (1999). Contrast enhancement improves the representation of /ɛ/-like vowels in the hearing-impaired auditory nerve. *Journal of the Acoustical Society of America, 106,* 2693–2708.

Miller, R. L., Schilling, J. R., Franck, K. R., & Young, E. D. (1997). Effects of acoustic trauma on the representation of the vowel /ɛ/ in cat auditory nerve filters. *Journal of the Acoustical Society of America, 101,* 3602–3616.

Moore, B. C. J. (2003). *An introduction to the psychology of hearing* (5th ed.), San Diego, CA: Academic Press.

Moore, B. C. J., Stainsby, T. H., Alcántara, J. I., & Kühnel, V. (2004). The effect on speech intelligibility of varying compression time constants in a digital hearing aid. *International Journal of Audiology, 43,* 399–409.

Nelson, D. A. (1991). High-level psychophysical tuning curves: Forward masking in normal-hearing and hearing-impaired listeners. *Journal of Speech and Hearing Research, 34,* 1233-1249.

Quatieri, T. F., & McAulay, R. J. (1986). Speech transformations based on a sinusoidal model. *IEEE Transactions on Acoustics, Speech, and Signal Processing, ASSP-34,* 1449–1464.

Sachs, M. B., & Kiang, N. Y-S. (1968). Two-tone inhibition in auditory-nerve fibers. *Journal of the Acoustical Society of America, 43,* 1120–1128.

Sidwell, A., & Summerfield, Q. (1985). The effect of enhanced spectral contrast on the interal representation of vowel-shaped noise. *Journal of the Acoustical Society of America, 78,* 495–506.

Simpson, A. M., Moore, B. C. J., & Glasberg, B. R. (1990). Spectral enhancement to improve the intelligibility of speech in noise for hearing-impaired listeners. *Acta Otolarygolica.* (Suppl. 469), 101–107.

Stelmachowicz, P. G., Jesteadt, W., Gorga, M. P., & Mott, J. (1985). Speech perception ability and psychophysical tuning curves in hearing-impaired listeners. *Journal of the Acoustical Society of America, 77,* 620–627.

Stone, M. A., & Moore, B. C. J. (1992). Spectral enhancement for people with sensorineural hearing impairment: Effects on speech intelligibility and quality. *Journal of Rehabilitation Research and Development, 29*, 39–56.

ter Keurs, M., Festen, J. M., & Plomp, R. (1993). Limited resolution of spectral contrast and hearing loss for speech in noise. *Journal of the Acoustical Society of America, 94*, 1307–1314.

Versnel, H., Prijs, V. F., & Schoonhoven, R. (1997). Auditory-nerve filter responses to clicks in guinea pigs with a damaged cochlea. *Journal of the Acoustical Society of America, 101*, 993–1009.

Yang, J., Luo, F -L., & Nehorai, A. (2002). Spectral contrast enhancement: Algorithms and comparisons. *Speech Communications, 39*, 33–46.

Zahorian, S. A., & Rothenberg, M. (1981). Principal-components analysis for low-redundancy encoding of speech. *Journal of the Acoustical Society of America, 69*, 832–845.

Zwicker, E., & Fastl, H. (1999). *Psychoacoustics: Facts and models* (2nd ed.). New York: Springer.

12

Sound Classification

SOUND CLASSIFICATION IN HEARING AIDS is an application of a more general set of procedures that has been developed for pattern classification or pattern recognition. Pattern classification is something that humans do quite easily, as when we identify someone from seeing a photograph or hearing a voice over the telephone. The objective in using a machine for pattern classification is to find patterns or structure in a set of data, and to use these patterns to identify the source of the data. Pattern classification generally proceeds in three steps: (1) extract a meaningful set of features from the data, (2) find the class that has the highest probability of having generated the observed features, and (3) make a decision based on the identified class.

Sound classification is used in hearing aids to identify different listening situations. The underlying assumption is that optimum speech intelligibility or sound quality for different classes of sounds will be achieved using different settings of the hearing-aid processing parameters. The chapter therefore begins with a review of some evidence that different processing parameters may be preferred under different signal conditions.

Sound classification does not modify the hearing-aid output directly, but rather provides a means for controlling the other processing algorithms implemented in the device. A block diagram of a hearing aid using sound classification is presented in Figure 12-1. The incoming signal

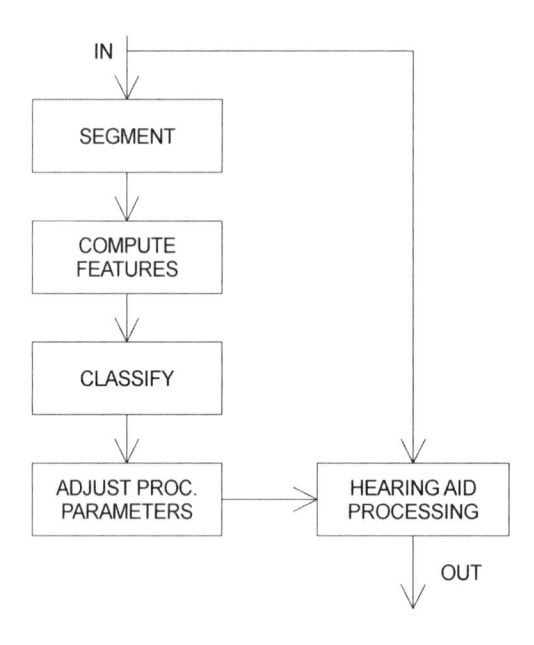

Figure 12-1. Block diagram showing sound classification used to adjust the processing parameters in a hearing aid in response to the properties of the incoming signal.

is divided into segments and the signal in the segment is described using a set of extracted signal features. The features are processed to find the relevant signal class, and the hearing-aid processing parameters are then adjusted to give the best performance for the selected class.

The accuracy of the classifier depends on the ability to find reliable differences between different signal classes. Our understanding of the relationship between the signal behavior and the source of the sound is embedded in the features used for the classification. A wide variety of features has been proposed for sound classification, and representative features and a procedure for selecting the most useful ones are described in the chapter. The features form the input to the classifier, which is a procedure for determining the most probable sound class given the set of features. Again, many classifier algorithms can be used, and some of the most appropriate for hearing aids are described. The chapter concludes with an example of a classifier showing how the selection of features and the signal conditions can affect the classifier performance.

The Rationale for Classification

The assumption behind sound classification is that different hearing-aid processing parameters will be preferred when listening under different conditions or to different classes of sounds. Consider wide-dynamic-range compression. For speech in quiet, fast-acting compression will amplify low-intensity speech sounds and can improve their audibility. For speech presented in noise or competing speech, however, the compression will modulate the background signal along with the desired speech, and this unwanted modulation can lead to a reduction in intelligibility (Stone & Moore, 2003). A sound classifier could be used to control a compressor by identifying listening conditions, such as speech in quiet, speech in babble, and speech in noise, where different compression parameters may be desired.

The compression ratios and time constants preferred in dynamic range compression when listening to speech have been found to depend on the amount and type of background noise. In one set of experiments, Neuman et al. (1995) used an attack time of 5 msec and investigated the effects of three release times of 60, 200, and 1000 msec in a digital broadband (single-channel) compression system. The compression ratios were 1.5:1, 2:1, and 3:1. The SNR was varied by choosing one of three types of noise: ventilation system noise at 50 dB SPL, apartment background noise at 59 dB SPL, and multitalker babble at 71 dB SPL. The speech was always input to the system at 85 dB SPL, with the noise added to the speech prior to compression and the compressed signal presented using the NAL-R amplifier gain-versus-frequency response calculated for each of the 20 hearing-impaired listeners. The results were that there was no preference between the three release times for the ventilation noise, a slight but not statistically significant preference for the two longer release times in the apartment noise, and a statistically significant preference for the longer release times in the babble. The 1000-msec release time was preferred most often for the babble. Thus, tying the compressor release time to the amount and type of background noise could lead to user judgments of improved sound quality.

Neuman et al. (1994) also investigated the effects of varying the compression ratio under the same speech and noise conditions. The compressor attack time was set to 5 msec and the release time was set to 200 msec. Hearing-impaired subjects having a residual dynamic range of less than 30 dB preferred the linear system (compression ratio of 1:1) for the cafeteria noise, but preferred a compression ratio of 1.5:1 for the apartment noise and preferred compression ratios of 1.5:1 or 2:1 for the ventilation noise. The linear system was preferred in all three noises by those listeners having a residual dynamic range greater than 30 dB. Humes et al. (1999) compared analog linear to two-channel wide dynamic-range-compression aids in a study using 55 hearing-impaired subjects. The results were that the compression instrument gave better speech intelligibility for sentence test materials at 50 or 60 dB SPL in quiet, but that the linear instrument gave better intelligibility for the materials at 75 dB SPL in babble at an SNR of 10 or 5 dB. Listening effort showed the same trend, with the compression instrument preferred at low levels in quiet and the linear instrument preferred at high levels in babble. The results of these two studies indicate that as the noise level is increased, listeners prefer reduced amounts of compression, and the preferred compression ratio may also depend on the type of background noise as well as its intensity.

Another distinction that could affect compression preferences is the type of signal being processed, for example, speech or music. Hansen (2002) use six normal-hearing and six hearing-impaired subjects. A 15-channel compression system was used, with identical settings in each channel. In one experiment the compression ratio was set to 2.1:1 and the compression threshold to 20 dB SPL whereas the attack and release times were varied. The normal hearing subjects preferred the sound quality produced by the hearing aid having a 1-msec attack time and a 4-sec release time when listening to speech, but preferred a 100-msec attack time when listening to music. The hearing-impaired subjects, however, showed no changes in hearing-aid preference between the music and speech signals. In a second experiment, the normal-hearing subjects preferred a hearing aid having a 40-msec release time and a 50 dB SPL threshold over a hearing aid having a 4-sec release time and a 20 dB SPL threshold for music, but the preferences were reversed for speech. Again, the hearing-impaired subjects showed no changes in hearing-aid preference between the music and speech signals. These results suggest that some listeners may prefer different compressor parameter settings depending on the type of signal and degree of hearing loss.

Signal Features

Many signal features have been proposed for classifying sounds. Typically, a combination of features is used as the input to the classification algorithm. The general problem in a hearing aid is to separate speech from nonspeech acoustic inputs. The features most useful for a given classification problem, such as separating speech from music, may not be the same as those most useful for a different task, such as separating speech from traffic noise. Some features that have been proposed for distinguishing speech from music are listed in Table 12-1, and similar features have also been proposed for distinguishing speech from other nonspeech signals such as traffic noise or babble. Signal processing that can be used to extract most of these features is described in Appendix 12-A.

The first two features are based on temporal characteristics of the signal. The mean-squared signal power (Allamanche et al., 2001; Liu et al., 1997; Peltonen et al., 2002; Pfeiffer et al., 1996; Srinivasan et al., 1999; Zhang & Kuo, 2001;) measures the energy in each group of blocks. The fluctuation of the energy from group to group is represented by the standard deviation of the signal envelope, which is related to the variance of the block energy used by several researchers (Liu et al., 1997; Pfeiffer et al., 1996; Srinivasan et al., 1999). The silence ratio, which is the fraction of the signal blocks that lie below a threshold level, has also been proposed as a classification feature (Aarts & Dekkers, 1999; Liu et al.,1997; Lu et al., 2001; Rizvi et al., 2002; Saunders, 1996; Scheirer & Slaney, 1997 Tzanetakis & Cook, 2000; Zhang & Kuo, 2001;).

The shape of the spectrum is described by the mel cepstral coefficients (Carey et al., 1999; Chou & Gu, 2001; Nordqvist & Leijon, 2004; Peltonen et al., 2002). The cepstrum is the inverse Fourier transform of the logarithm of the power spectrum. The first coefficient gives the average of the log power spectrum, the second coefficient gives an indication of the slope of the log power spectrum, and the third coefficient indicates the degree to which the log power spectrum is concentrated toward the center or the edges of the spectrum. The mel cepstrum is the cepstrum computed on an auditory frequency scale. The fluctuations of the short-time power spectrum from group to group are given by the delta cepstral coefficients (Carey et al., 1999; Chou & Gu, 2001; Takeuchi et al., 2001). The delta cepstral coefficients are computed as the first difference of the mel cepstral coefficients.

TABLE 12-1.
Representative Signal Features That Have Been Proposed for Sound Classification

Number	Feature	Abbreviation
1	Mean-Squared Signal Power	Pow
2	Standard Deviation of the Signal Envelope	σ Env
3	Mel Cepstrum Coefficient 1	Cep1
4	Mel Cepstrum Coefficient 2	Cep2
5	Mel Cepstrum Coefficient 3	Cep3
6	Mel Cepstrum Coefficient 4	Cep4
7	Delta Cepstrum Coefficient 1	Δ Cep1
8	Delta Cepstrum Coefficient 2	Δ Cep2
9	Delta Cepstrum Coefficient 3	Δ Cep3
10	Delta Cepstrum Coefficient 4	Δ Cep4
11	Power Spectrum Centroid	Cent
12	Delta Centroid	Δ Cent
13	Standard Deviation of the Centroid	σ Cent
14	Zero Crossing Rate (ZCR)	ZCR
15	ZCR of the Signal 1st Difference	ZCR1
16	Standard Deviation of the ZCR	σ ZCR
17	Power Spectrum Entropy	Ent
18	Broadband Envelope Correlation Lag	BLag
19	Broadband Envelope Correlation Peak	BPk
20	Four-Band Envelope Correlation Lag	4Lag
21	Four-Band Envelope Correlation Peak	4Pk

The abbreviations are used in Table 12-2 and in Figure 12-2.

Another indication of the shape of the power spectrum is the power spectrum centroid (Büchler et al., 2005; Kates, 1995; Liu et al., 1997; Peltonen et al., 2002; Scheirer and Slaney, 1997; Tzanetakis & Cook, 2000). The centroid is the first moment of the power spectrum, and indicates where the power is concentrated in frequency. Changes in the shape of the power spectrum give rise to fluctuations of the centroid. These fluctuations are indicated by the standard deviation of the centroid (Tzanetakis & Cook, 2000) and the first difference of the centroid (Büchler et al., 2005).

The zero crossing rate (ZCR) counts the number of times the signal changes sign in the segment, and it tends to reflect the frequency of the strongest component in the spectrum. The ZCR will also be higher for noise than for a low-frequency tone such as the first formant in speech (Carey et al., 1999; El-Malah et al., 2000; Peltonen et al., 2002; Saunders, 1996; Scheirer & Slaney, 1997; Srinivasan et al., 1999; Zhang & Kuo, 2001). Changes in the spectrum and shifts from tonal sounds to noise will cause changes in the ZCR, and these fluctuations are reflected in the standard deviation of the ZCR (Lu et al., 2001; Saunders, 1996; Srinivasan et al., 1999). Most of the power of a speech signal is concentrated in the first formant; taking the first difference of the signal results in low-frequency attenuation and the ZCR of the signal first difference thus tracks the tonal characteristics of the high-frequency part of the signal.

Another potentially useful cue is the whether the spectrum is flat or has a peak. Spectral flatness (Allemanche et al., 2001), the spectral crest factor (Allemanche et al., 2001; Rizvi et al., 2002), and tonality indicators (Büchler et al., 2005) are all attempts to characterize the overall spectral shape as being flat or peaked. Another spectral-shape indicator is the power spectral entropy, which will be high for a flat spectrum and low for a spectrum having one or more dominant peaks.

An additional class of features proposed for separating speech from music is based on detecting the rhythmic pulse present in many music selections (Lu et al., 2001; Scheirer & Slaney, 1997; Takeuchi et al., 2001). If a rhythmic pulse is present, it is assumed that there will be periodic peaks in the signal envelope which will cause a stable peak in the normalized envelope autocorrelation function. The location of the peak is given by the broadband envelope correlation lag, and the amplitude of the peak is given by the broadband envelope correlation peak. The rhythmic pulse should be present at all frequencies, so a multiband procedure can be implemented in which the power spectrum is divided into four frequency regions (e.g., 340–700, 900–1360, 1640–2360, and 2840–4240 Hz). The envelope autocorrelation function is computed separately in each frequency region, the normalized autocorrelation functions summed across the four bands, and the location and amplitude of the peak then found for the summed functions.

Feature Selection

Table 12-1 lists more features than can be implemented in a practical hearing-aid sound-classification system. Somewhere between four and eight features can probably be implemented in a practical system; computational limitations make more than eight features unlikely in the near future. Therefore an important problem is to find the best set of features for a given classification algorithm. It would be even more useful to find a procedure for identifying the best features for use with any classification algorithm.

One approach to feature selection is to identify those features that convey the maximum amount of information about the signal classes while at the same time minimizing the duplication of information provided by the other features in the set. The mutual information between the features and the signal classes, and between the features and each other, provides a tool that has been used to develop algorithms for feature selection (Battiti, 1994; Kwak & Choi, 1999; Yang & Moody, 1999; Yang et al., 2000). Feature selection based on joint mutual information (Yang & Moody, 1999; Yang et al., 2000) and on simplified algorithms that estimate the joint mutual information using pair-wise calculations (Battiti, 1994; Kwak & Choi, 1999) have all been shown to perform better than random selection of feature sets for neural network classifiers. Mutual information and the feature-selection algorithms are discussed next.

MUTUAL INFORMATION

The mutual information between two random variables x and y is given by the entropies $H(x)$, $H(y)$, and $H(x,y)$:

$$I(x;y) = H(x) + H(y) - H(x,y) \quad \text{Equation (12.1)}$$

The entropy measures the uncertainty or randomness of a random variable in bits, and is given by

$$H(x) = -\sum_{x} P(x) \log_2 P(x) \quad \text{Equation (12.2)}$$

where $P(x)$ is the probability density function for x and the summation is over all observed values of x. A variable that has a wide range, with a large number of possible states and a low probability of being in any one of them, will have a large entropy. Conversely, a variable that never changes will have an entropy of zero. The mutual information can also be written as:

$$I(x;y) = \sum_{x}\sum_{y} P(x,y) \log_2 \frac{P(x,y)}{P(x)P(y)} \quad \text{Equation (12.3)}$$

The mutual information gives the degree to which one variable is related to another. The higher the mutual information, the greater the ability of measurements of one variable to accurately predict the other. The mutual information is unity for variables that are linearly related, such as the output and input of a filter, and is zero for independent variables, such as two independent Gaussian noise sequences.

Mutual information is a more general concept than correlation. A high degree of correlation requires that the two waveforms being correlated duplicate each other. A nonlinear relationship between two variables will always reduce the correlation because the waveforms will no longer match exactly. Mutual information, however, only requires that knowledge of one waveform be sufficient to reproduce the other waveform. Nonlinear operations do not necessarily reduce the mutual information. Thus mutual information can describe nonlinear dependencies between variables that correlation may miss.

The random variables for which the mutual information is computed are not necessarily jointly Gaussian. Thus, a nonparametric estimation procedure is often be used. The joint probability distribution of the variables x and y in Eq. (12.3) can be estimated using a two-dimensional histogram (Tourassi et al., 2001). The x and y bin widths for the histogram are computed using Scott's (1979) rule:

$$h = 3.5 \sigma n^{-1/3} \quad \text{Equation (12.4)}$$

where h is the histogram bin width, σ the sample standard deviation, and n the number of samples in the population. The number of histogram bins is then chosen to span the range of each variable. For each histogram bin, the joint probability distribution $P(x,y)$ is then estimated by counting the number of times that the inputs fall into a particular bin and dividing by the total number of cases. The same technique can also be applied to the marginal distributions $P(x)$ and $P(y)$. The mutual information is then computed using Eq. (12.3) for all histogram bins having non-zero values.

The mutual information between each feature computed from a selection of sound samples and the four sound classes of speech, multitalker babble, music, and traffic noise is plotted in Figure 12-2. A high amount of mutual information indicates that the feature is effective in determining the sound class from which it comes, and a low level of mutual information indicates that the feature conveys very little information about the underlying sound class. The features having the greatest mutual information with the sound classes are Features 5 (mel cepstrum 3), 13 (standard deviation of the centroid), and 17 (power spectrum entropy). Features 3 (mel cepstrum 1), 6 (mel cepstrum 4), and 12 (delta centroid) also provide high amounts of mutual information with the sound classes. The lowest values of mutual information are for Features 1 (mean-squared signal power), 15 (ZCR of the signal first difference), and 10 (delta cepstrum 4). Features 4 (mel cepstrum 2), 8 (delta cepstrum 2), and 9 (delta cepstrum 3) also provide low amounts of mutual information with the sound classes. Overall, the mel cepstrum features provide more mutual information with the sound classes than the delta cepstrum features, and the centroid features also appear to be useful.

The mutual information between pairs of features is plotted in Figure 12-3. The diagonal entries represent the entropy of each feature, and the off-diagonal entries give the mutual information between any pair of features. Features 11 (power spectrum centroid), 14 (ZCR), and 17 (power spectrum entropy) have high amounts of mutual information, which indicates that these features describe related attributes of the signal. The lowest amounts of mutual information are for Features 7 through 10 (delta cepstrum coefficients 1–4), which indicates that the delta cepstrum coefficients do not duplicate information provided by any other features; however the plot of Figure 12-2 indicates that the delta cepstrum coefficients also provide very little information about the signal classes.

FEATURE SELECTION USING MUTUAL INFORMATION

The feature selection algorithms operate by choosing the features sequentially. The objective is to find a new feature that provides a high degree of mutual information with the sound classes while avoiding duplication of the information provided by the features previously selected. It would be preferable to find the new feature that maximizes the amount of new information contributed to the classification problem, but this would involve computing the joint information between the candidate feature and all of the features previously selected, a process which would quickly become computationally untenable as the number of selected features grows.

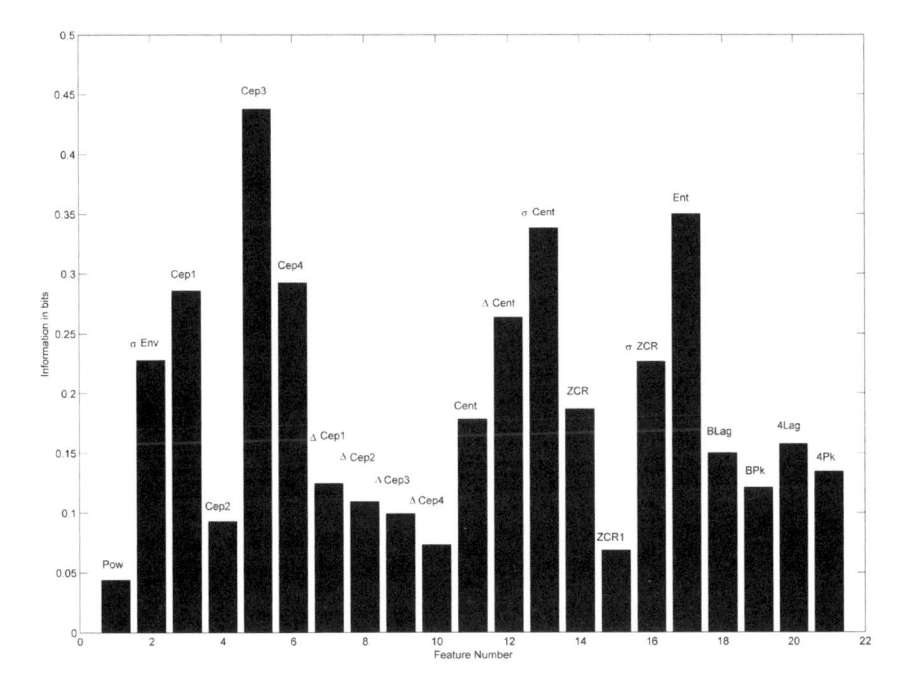

Figure 12-2. Mutual information between each signal feature listed in Table 12-1 and the sound classes of speech, multitalker babble, music, and traffic noise. The mutual information is averaged over the four classes.

Battiti (1994) proposed solving the feature selection problem by using only the mutual information between features, and Kwak and Choi (1999) improved on the calculation used to estimate the additional information contributed by each new feature as it is selected. These algorithms replace the joint mutual information between the new feature and the entire set of previously selected features with the weighted sum of the mutual information between the new feature and each of the previously-selected features. A parameter β controls the amount of mutual information between features that is included in the calculation. If $\beta = 0$, the calculation uses only the mutual information between the features and the signal classes. As β grows, the selection process favors features that have reduced amounts of mutual information with those already selected at the expense of features that have high mutual information with the signal classes.

The features selected using the Kwak and Choi (1999) algorithm are

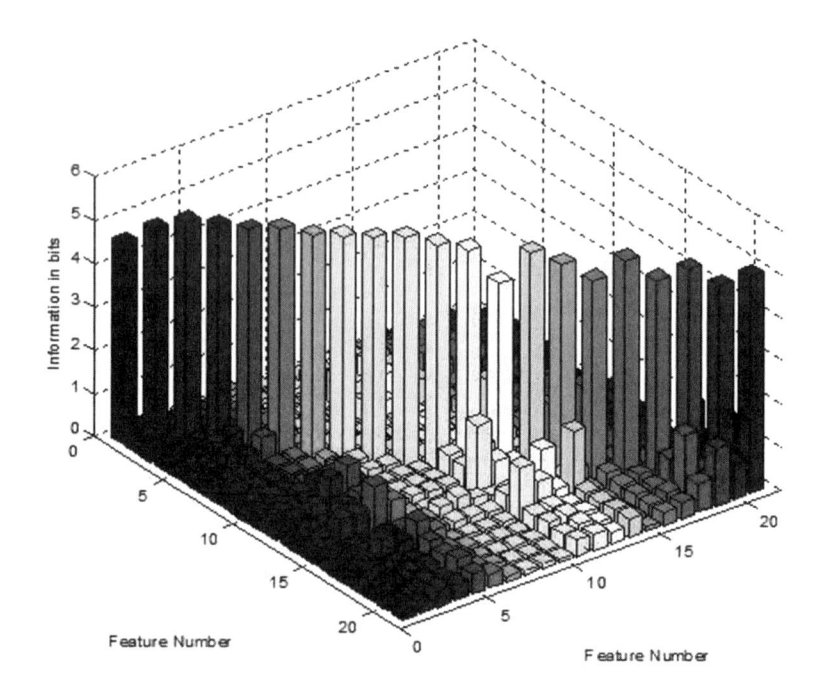

Figure 12-3. Mutual information between pairs of features.

shown in Figure 12-4. The left column is for the algorithm with $\beta = 0$, which gives a ranking based purely on the mutual information between the features and the four signal classes. The results for the algorithm with $\beta = 0.5$ are shown in the middle column, and the results for $\beta = 1$ are shown in the right column. The mel cepstrum coefficients describe the shape of the log spectrum, and coefficients 1, 3, and 4 are ranked at the top of all three lists. The spectrum entropy, which also gives information about the spectral shape, and the standard deviation of the zero crossing rate (ZCR) complete the best five features, which are the same independent of the value of β.

As one moves farther down the lists, the influence of the relative importance placed on providing new information as opposed to duplicating information already acquired becomes more apparent. Certain features, such as the standard deviation of the envelope and the delta cepstrum coefficients, increase in value as β increases. These features may contribute a relatively small amount of new information, but the information

Sound Classification

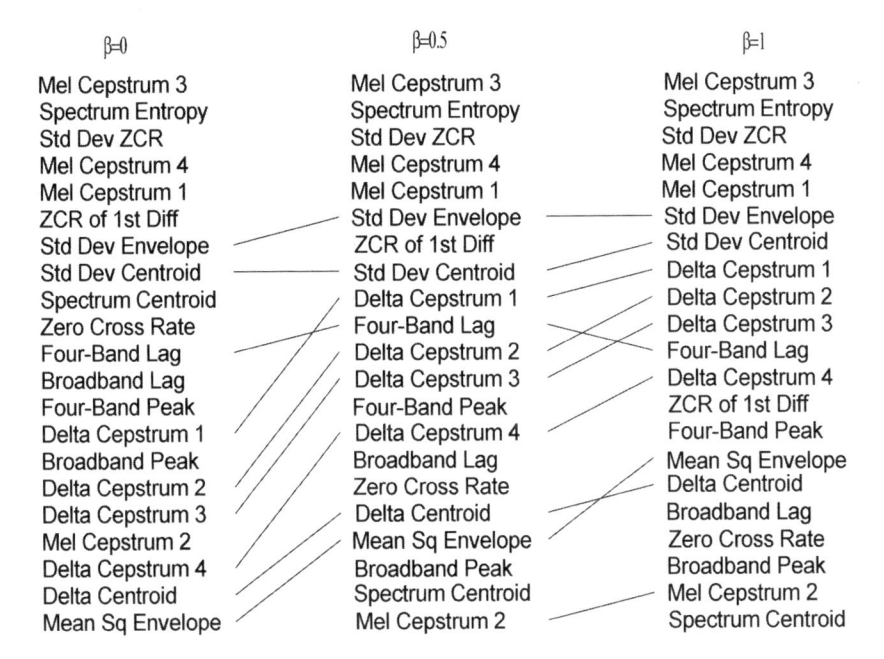

β=0	β=0.5	β=1
Mel Cepstrum 3	Mel Cepstrum 3	Mel Cepstrum 3
Spectrum Entropy	Spectrum Entropy	Spectrum Entropy
Std Dev ZCR	Std Dev ZCR	Std Dev ZCR
Mel Cepstrum 4	Mel Cepstrum 4	Mel Cepstrum 4
Mel Cepstrum 1	Mel Cepstrum 1	Mel Cepstrum 1
ZCR of 1st Diff	Std Dev Envelope	Std Dev Envelope
Std Dev Envelope	ZCR of 1st Diff	Std Dev Centroid
Std Dev Centroid	Std Dev Centroid	Delta Cepstrum 1
Spectrum Centroid	Delta Cepstrum 1	Delta Cepstrum 2
Zero Cross Rate	Four-Band Lag	Delta Cepstrum 3
Four-Band Lag	Delta Cepstrum 2	Four-Band Lag
Broadband Lag	Delta Cepstrum 3	Delta Cepstrum 4
Four-Band Peak	Four-Band Peak	ZCR of 1st Diff
Delta Cepstrum 1	Delta Cepstrum 4	Four-Band Peak
Broadband Peak	Broadband Lag	Mean Sq Envelope
Delta Cepstrum 2	Zero Cross Rate	Delta Centroid
Delta Cepstrum 3	Delta Centroid	Broadband Lag
Mel Cepstrum 2	Mean Sq Envelope	Zero Cross Rate
Delta Cepstrum 4	Broadband Peak	Broadband Peak
Delta Centroid	Spectrum Centroid	Mel Cepstrum 2
Mean Sq Envelope	Mel Cepstrum 2	Spectrum Centroid

Figure 12-4. Features ranked from most useful (*top*) to least (*bottom*) according to the Kwak and Choi (1999) mutual information algorithm. The value of β indicates the relative importance of mutual information between the feature and the signal classes (β = 0) and as opposed to reducing the redundancy between the new feature and the previously selected features (β = 1). The lines connect those features that change in rank as is increased.

that they do contribute is not duplicated by any of the features already selected. Other features, such as the spectrum centroid, decrease in value as β increases. These features contribute information that duplicates the information already provided by the features selected before them.

Classifier Algorithms

The input to the classifier is a set of features, termed a feature vector, and the output is the assignment of the sound to one or more classes. The classifier strives to answer one of two closely related questions: (1) "What is the most probable sound class given the observed signal features?" or (2) "What is the probability that the signal features have come from each of the available classes?" Many different classifier algorithms have been developed, and several of them have been applied to the problem of classifying sounds. In the next section, several different classification approaches are briefly described. The reader is referred to one of the many texts on pattern classification or pattern recognition (Bishop, 2006; Duda et al., 2001; Fukunaga, 1995) for the mathematical details and theoretical underpinnings of the algorithms.

TRAINING THE CLASSIFIER

In general, the type of classifier is chosen at the beginning of a problem, and the classifier parameters are then adjusted to give optimum performance. Training refers to the process of using the feature vectors to determine the parameters of the classifier. A large number of signal segments are generated for each of the desired classes, and feature vectors are extracted from the segments. The feature vectors and their associated classes form the training set.

In supervised classification, the classifier is presented with each feature vector and its associated class label from the training set, and the classifier is adjusted to minimize the classification error. The goal is to give the most accurate performance in the real world, where situations not included in the training set can be expected to occur. The ability to deal with these unanticipated situations is called generalization, and the goal in training the classifier is thus to produce accurate generalized results. A classifier is usually tested using a data set different from the one used to train it in order to assess both the classifier accuracy and its degree of generalization.

Often the supervised learning is iterative. The classifier is presented with a training vector and its associated class, and a classification output that differs from the correct answer generates an error signal that is used to modify the classifier parameters. For example, if a weighted combination of the features is being used in the classifier, the error signal would be used to adjust the weights. A large number of feature vectors (e.g., 10,000 to 100,000) is typically used, with each feature vector making a small contribution to the overall solution. The amount of adjustment with each feature vector is correspondingly small, and the training set may be re-used several times to ensure convergence of the classifier parameters.

In unsupervised classification, the classifier organizes the feature vectors into groups that occur "naturally," without reference to the assigned classes. The classifier searches for feature vectors that tend to form related clusters. One can specify the number of clusters at the beginning of unsupervised learning, but the labels are not known a priori. Techniques that rely on unsupervised learning are often used for exploratory data analysis, in which the main question is "How many classes are there?" rather than "What is the best way to assign sounds to classes that have already been identified?"

In summary, the goal in training a classifier is to design a system that generalizes to all situations of interest. But the training set has to be limited to a manageable number of feature vectors, so not every possible situation can be included. Thus, there is always the risk that the classifier will learn the unique characteristics of the training data rather than the general feature properties that define the signal classes. Such a classifier is said to be overfitted to the data. If the classifier is tested with the same features as are used for the training, it will be not be clear whether the classifier has learned general signal properties or simply memorized some peculiarities of the training data. The proper test of a classifier, therefore, is to test it with different data than used to train it.

TYPES OF CLASSIFIERS

Classifiers can be divided into two general types of algorithms (Rubinstein & Hastie, 1997). One type, termed discriminative, determines the boundaries between classes without modeling the probabilities directly. Examples of this type of classifier include the linear discriminant, Support Vector Machine, and Neural Networks. Training these algorithms can be difficult because it involves consideration of all of the classes at the same time and often involves iterative algorithms not guaranteed to converge to a useful result. Discriminative classifiers can be effective when there is enough sufficiently varied data to train the classifier, and can work even in those situations where the underlying probability distributions for the features are unknown.

The other type, termed generative (or informative), models the probability distributions for the features that arise from each sound class. Classification is performed by determining the probability that each class produced the observed set of features, and selecting the class that has the highest probability. Examples of this type of classifier include Hidden Markov Models and Bayes Classifiers. These are relatively easy to train because the probability distributions for the features can be determined separately for each class. Generative classifiers can be effective if the underlying probability distributions for the features can be accurately estimated, or if a priori knowledge is available that can help determine what the distributions should look like.

CLUSTERING

Clustering refers to a group of unsupervised procedures that group feature vectors based on their measured similarity (Duda et al., 2001). Feature vectors that are close together are assigned to the same cluster. A Euclidean distance metric, computed as the sum of the squares of the differences between two feature vectors, is commonly used, but other distance metrics can also be used. Each cluster can be identified by its centroid, which is a feature vector that defines the center of the cluster. If a new feature vector is obtained, the vector is assigned to the cluster having the closest centroid using the distance metric.

In hierarchical clustering, the set of feature vectors is first divided into two clusters so that the distance between them is maximized. Each cluster is then subdivided to form two clusters which again are maximally separated, and so until the desired number of clusters is obtained. In *k-means* clustering, the desired number of clusters is chosen at the beginning of the analysis and the initial cluster centroids are feature vectors chosen at random. The feature vectors are then each assigned to the closest centroid, and the centroid locations are updated by averaging over the assigned feature vectors. This process is iterated until no further reduction in the error is observed. An example of clustering is shown in Figure 12-5 for three classes and feature vectors comprising two features. The ellipses denote the approximate boundaries of each cluster. The left-hand cluster consists of all of the feature vectors for the class denoted by the crosses, whereas the two right-hand clusters both contain some errors as the distributions of the feature vectors from the two remaining signal classes overlap the cluster boundaries.

One of the first attempts to classify sounds for hearing aids used clustering. Kates (1995) classified 11 different noises using hierarchical clustering. The features chosen were the variance of the envelope modulation, the spectrum centroid, the low-frequency slope of the spectrum in dB/octave, and the high-frequency slope of the spectrum in dB/octave. Eleven different sounds were used in the experiment. The sounds could be assigned to eleven clusters, in which case the feature vectors from each sound form a single cluster, or to a reduced number of clusters, in which case the feature vectors from related sounds were grouped together into a single cluster. The classification accuracy,

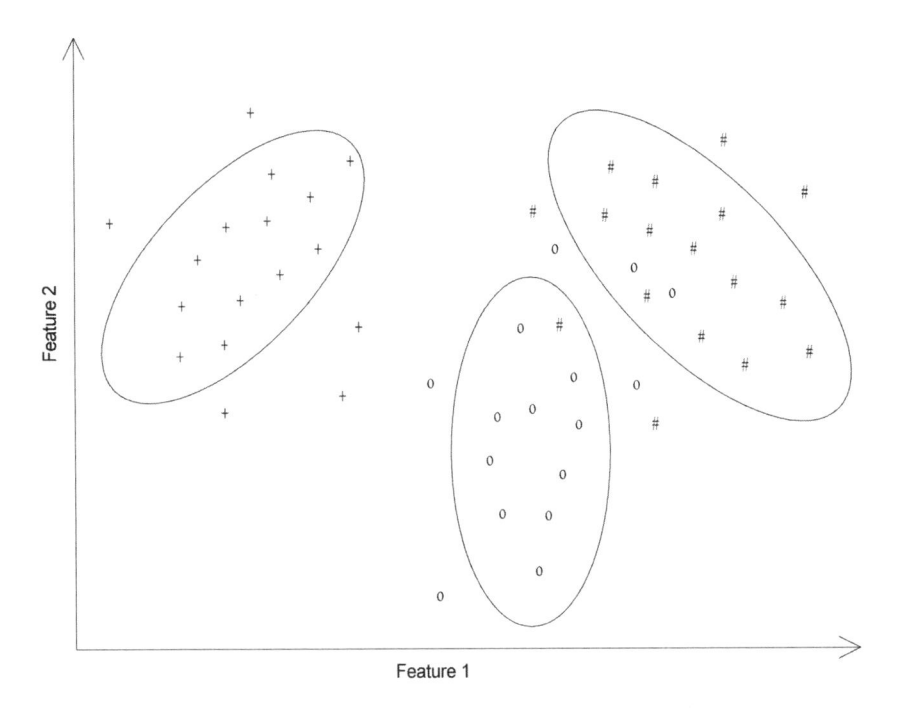

Figure 12-5. Clusters formed for three classes of sounds. The feature vector vectors from the three classes are denoted by crosses (+), circles (o), and hash marks (#), respectively.

when the classifier was tested on the same data used for training, was about 88% when all 11 clusters were used. The errors were assigning a feature vector from one sound, typically far from the centroid for that sound cluster, to the cluster associated with the feature vectors a different sound. When the number of clusters was reduced, the feature vectors for related sounds were assigned to the same cluster and a feature vector that might have been on the edge of a smaller cluster could end up nearer the center of the combined cluster. As a result the performance improved as the number of clusters was reduced, and improved to about 93% when six clusters were used.

LINEAR DISCRIMINANT

Imagine that we want to separate two classes of sounds by building a brick wall between the feature vectors for one class of sounds and the feature vectors for the other. This is a supervised learning problem as the correct class must be known for each feature vector before the wall can be constructed. If the feature vectors only consist of two features, then each feature vector is a point in a two-dimensional plane and the wall is just a straight line that separates them. The linear discriminant function (Duda et al., 2001) will position the line in the plane so as to minimize the mean squared distance for the feature vectors that fall on the wrong side of the line. If there are three signal classes, as shown in Figure 12-6, then lines will be produced to divide the plane into three regions, one region for each signal class. Each region of the feature space is identified by a "label" computed as a weighted average of the feature vectors within that region. The linear discriminant attempts to maximize the distance between these labels while simultaneously minimizing the scatter of the feature vectors included with each region. In general the feature vectors consist of more than two features, so the lines dividing each class get replaced by hyperplanes that separate regions of the feature hyperspace.

SUPPORT VECTOR MACHINE

The support vector machine (SVM) (Burgess, 1998; Cortes & Vapnik, 1995; Gunn, 1998) is a variation on the basic idea of the linear discriminant function. The goal is to find the hyperplane that has the largest possible distance (e.g., maximum margin) from the feature vectors that lie near the edges of the signal classes. These edge vectors are termed the support vectors. The optimum separating hyperplane is again found as a linear combination of the features, but the weights are determined by comparing the feature vectors with the support vectors. Maximizing the separation at the margins has the effect of promoting good generalization of the classifier. Not every set of features can be effectively separated using a linear discriminant, but a nonlinear transformation of the feature vectors to a sufficiently high dimension will yield a problem that can be solved using a linear discriminant (Cortes & Vapnik, 1995). The features can be raised to a power, formed into a polynomial, exponentiated, used as the argument of a hyperbolic tangent, and so on. The optimal hyperplane is then found for the transformed data. The resultant higher dimension hyperplanes, when inscribed on the original data, permit curved boundaries between the classes and thus give a more general solution to the classification problem than possible with linear discriminant functions while still maintaining good generalization.

In a preliminary study of support vector machines for hearing-aid ap-

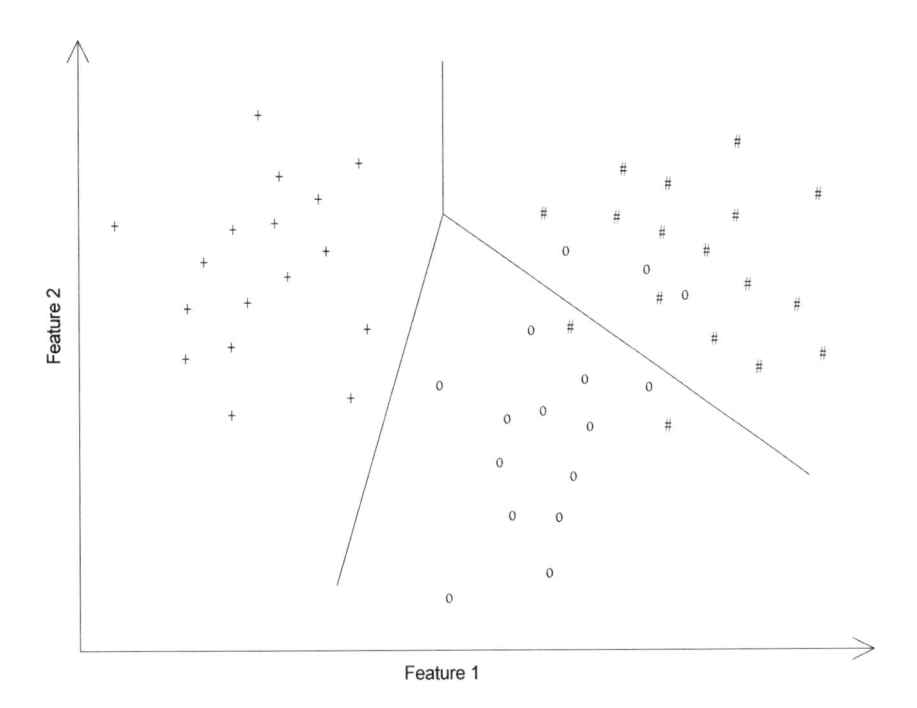

Figure 12-6. Decision boundaries produced by a linear discriminant function for a three-class problem. The feature vector vectors from the three classes are denoted by crosses (+), circles (o), and hash marks (#), respectively.

plications, Kates (2003) found that the error rate was less than 1.5% for separating speech from classical music for a small set of signals using a feature vector comprising six features. Mesgarani et al. (2004) found an accuracy of about 94% correct for a task of separating speech from music using an SVM with a feature vector consisting of 13 features. The amount of computation needed to establish the class boundaries in the transformed feature space can be very large, however, especially if a large number of support vectors are used. But this part of the problem is solved when the classifier is trained, where the amount of processing time is not a critical limitation. Once trained, the SVN classifier requires that the weighted nonlinear combination be computed and assigned to the nearest class. If the number of support vectors can be reduced while still giving accurate classification, then the SVM could be implemented in a hearing aid.

One approach to reducing the number of support vectors is the relevance vector machine (RVM) (Tipping, 2001). The goal in the RVM is to select the nonlinear transformations to use in the classifier at the same time that the classifier is being trained. Instead of selecting the features and nonlinear transformations in one step and then using those transformed features in a classifier in the second step, the RVM combines the two operations to identify the most effective set of transformed features to use in a SVM classifier. During training, those support vectors that do not contribute to the classifier accuracy are eliminated. The accuracy of the resultant classifier is similar to that of the SVM, but the computational requirements for the final implementation, as in a hearing aid, are greatly reduced.

NEURAL NETWORK

The original motivation for neural networks (Demuth et al., 2006; Hagan et al., 1996; Haykin, 1998) is the neural structure of the brain. Many layers of neurons exist in the brain, with the outputs from several neurons in one layer forming the inputs to a neuron at the next level. The neuron inputs interact, and one input may inhibit neural firing whereas another may increase the firing rate. The inputs may also undergo nonlinear transformations such as saturation, in which the output firing rate is limited to a maximum value whenever the sum of the inputs exceeds a threshold.

In mathematical terms neural networks are related to linear discriminants. However, the nonlinear transformations embedded in neural networks allow the formation of arbitrary boundaries between the signal classes. The boundaries that segregate the different classes can be complex curves in hyperspace as well as the linear boundaries that result from linear discriminants. One advantage of neural networks is that the algorithms for training the networks are fairly simple and the forms of the nonlinearities can be learned from the training data. However, ensuring good generalization can often be a challenge. The training can also require a large amount of computer processing time, but once trained the classification algorithms are efficient enough to be implemented in a hearing aid.

A neural network consists of layers of neurons that are combined in a feed-forward network in which the outputs from one layer form the inputs to the next. An example of a neural network is presented in Figure 12-7. This particular network consists of an input layer, one hidden layer, and an output layer. More than one hidden layer can be used, although additional hidden layers generally add more to the system complexity than they add to the accuracy of the classifier. The network has as many inputs as there are features being used for the classification; this example shows three inputs but there can be as many as desired. There is one output for each sound class.

The hidden layer combines the inputs and then sends the sum through a nonlinear transformation. This operation is shown in the inset in Figure 12-7 for the kth neuron in the hidden layer. The input to the neuron is a weighted sum of the outputs from the previous layer. For the first hidden layer, the inputs would therefore be a weighted sum of the input feature values. In addition, a bias term indicated by b_k is added; the bias can shift the weighted sum toward or away from the saturation point of the nonlinear transformation. The output can be expressed as:

$$y_k(m) = F_{Nonlin}\left[b_k + \sum_{j=1}^{J} w_{jk} x_j(m)\right] \quad \text{Equation (12.5)}$$

where m is the segment index, b_k is the bias for neuron k, w_{kj} are the weights applied to the J outputs $x_j(m)$ from the previous layer, and F is the nonlinear transformation function.

A typical transformation, also termed the activation function, is also shown in the inset. The nature of the nonlinearity affects the boundaries between the classes created by the neural network, and one often tries several different nonlinearities when designing the network to see which one gives the best results. The output layer neurons have a structure that is the same as the neurons in the hidden layer. The number of neurons in the hidden layer does not have to match the number of inputs or the number of outputs, but instead is chosen to provide the needed level of model complexity. Too few neurons in the hidden layer and the neural network will be unable to accurately extract the class information from the feature vectors, whereas too many neurons can cause the network to memorize the details of the specific training set rather than generate a general solution.

The neural network is trained by providing the features at the inputs and the associated class at the outputs. If a feature vector belongs to a given class, then the desired classifier output is 1 for that class and 0 for all of the other classes. A neural network is also capable of producing continuously valued outputs, and can be used for approximating a func-

376 Digital Hearing Aids

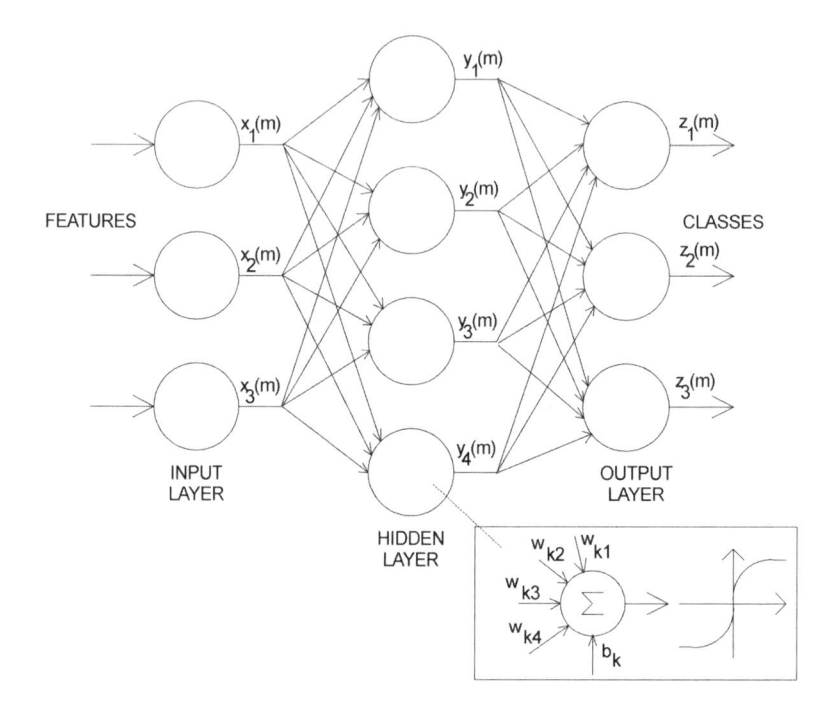

Figure 12-7. Neural network for sound classification showing the input layer, one hidden layer, and the output layer.

tional relationship. For example, instead of providing a 1 for the correct class and a 0 for the other classes, the network could be trained to provide the amount of signal power present in each of the classes when speech is presented in a background of music or noise. The weights and the bias for each neuron are adjusted during training to minimize the error in assigning the features to the output class or power levels.

At the beginning of the training the weights are generally small random numbers. The initial behavior of the neural network is thus approximately linear. As the training progresses the weights grow, and the behavior of the neural network becomes more nonlinear. The stronger nonlinear transformations increase the ability to separate the classes based on the features, but also increase the probability of overfitting. The tradeoff between accuracy and overfitting is sometimes controlled by slowly decaying the weights back toward zero unless the weight is consistently pulled toward a large value by the data.

HIDDEN MARKOV MODEL

A Markov model describes a system that has a discrete number of states. The Markov model gives the probability of remaining in a state and the probabilities of moving from that state to any of the other states possible in the system. Consider the example of tossing a coin. Each toss of the coin is assumed to be independent of the previous or following tosses. If the previous result was *Heads*, then the probability that the next result will be *Heads* is given by $P(Heads)$, and the probability that it will be *Tails* is given by $P(Tails) = 1 - P(Heads)$.

The Markov model for this example is diagrammed in Figure 12-8. The result of a coin toss is either *Heads* or *Tails*, so each of these possible results is a state of the system: state s_1 for a result of heads and state s_2 for a result of tails. The transition probabilities are shown in the diagram by arrows that link the state s_1 to itself, giving the probability that the system will be in state s_1 after the next toss given that it was in state s_1 after the previous toss, and link state s_1 to s_2, giving the probability that the system will be in state s_2 given that it was in state s_1 after the previous toss. The same probabilities hold if the previous result was *Tails*, with transitions shown from state s_2 to s_2 and from state s_2 to s_1.

In the above example the outcome of the coin toss is clear; we can see if the result of a toss was *Heads* or *Tails*. In classifying sounds, however, a set of measured features is available, but we never know for certain what kind of sound produced those features. The sound class has to be inferred from the measurements. A Markov model may still be appropriate to describe the sequence of states, but the model is hidden because only the features and not the underlying states of the model can be observed.

An example of a hidden Markov model (HMM) (Rabiner, 1989) for classifying sounds is shown in Figure 12-9. The continuous sound signal is modeled as the output of a system that randomly moves between sound-generation states that represent the different sound classes. In this example there are three states: s_1 for speech, s_2 for music, and s_3 for noise. Assume that at a given instant in time the system is in state s_j, where $j = 1$, 2, or 3 for speech, music, or noise. At the end of the next segment the system will be in state s_k, where again $k = 1$, 2, or 3 for speech, music, or noise. The transition probability of going from state j to state k is a_{jk}, and the system can either stay in the same state with probability a_{jj} or go to a new state with probability a_{jk}, where $k \neq j$.

The possible feature outputs in this example are $f_1, f_2,$ and f_3. These

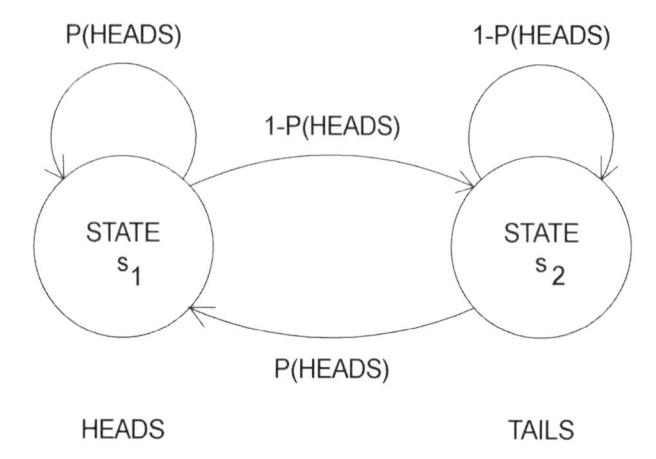

Figure 12-8. Markov model for a coin toss. The model has two states: s_1 for heads and s_2 for tails.

feature values could be, for example, three different zero-crossing rates. The probability of producing ZCR f_l when in state s_j is given by b_{jl}. The three zero-crossing rates are assumed to occur in sequence patterns that are unique for each sound class. For example, let the three ZCR values be denoted by A, B, and C. Then the pattern AAABBBCCC. . . might be observed for speech, ABCABCABC. . . observed for music, and AABAA-CAAB. . . observed for noise. The sequence of ZCR values observed over a number of signal segments can then be used to determine the state with the highest probability of having produced them, and hence the most likely sound class.

Implementing an HMM for sound classification involves two stages. First, the HMM needs to trained on sequences of feature vectors and their associated sound classes. The training establishes the values of a_{jk} and b_{jl}, as well the initial distribution of state probabilities to be used when the classifier is turned on. Once the HMM is trained, a different algorithm (Viterbi, 1967) is used to find the most probable sound class given the observed sequence of feature vectors. The training of an HMM can be very time consuming, but the sound classification algorithm, once the system is trained, is efficient enough to be implemented in a hearing aid (Büchler et al., 2005; Nordqvist & Leijon, 2004). Nordqvist & Leijon (2004), for example, started with a vector of four delta cepstrum coefficients that were grouped into clusters; the features input to

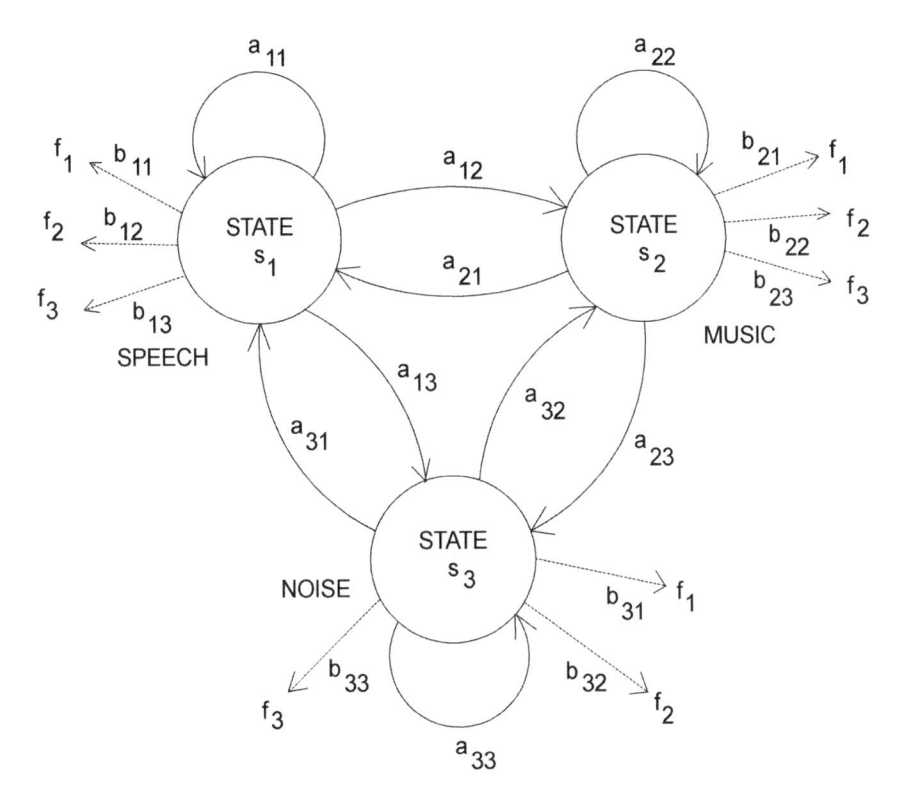

Figure 12-9. Hidden Markov model (HMM) for sound classification. The model has three states: s_1 for speech, s_2 for music, and s_3 for noise.

the HMM were then the sequence of cluster centroids closest to each of the delta cepstrum vectors. Classification accuracy for the three classes of clear speech, speech in babble, and speech in traffic noise at SNRs ranging from 0 to 5 dB was approximately 98.6%. Büchler et al. (2005), using a vector of six features, achieved an average accuracy of 88% for an HMM classifier for test data representing clean speech, speech in a variety of noises, the noises alone, and music.

BAYES CLASSIFIER

A Bayes classifier starts with a feature vector, and estimates the probability that the observed features come from each class (Duda et al., 2001). The class having the highest probability is then selected. To perform this calculation, the classifier needs probability distributions for the feature vectors and the classes. The training of the Bayes classifier consists of determining the probability distributions for the feature vectors associated with each class, and determining the probability of occurrence for each class.

Segments are first generated for a sound class, and the feature vectors computed for the segments. One way of estimating the distributions is to use histograms. If there are K features in the feature vector, then the histogram will be generated in a K-dimensional space. The range of each feature is measured, and bins established along each of the K dimensions using the bin spacing given, for example, by Eq. (12.4). Each feature vector is then assigned to the corresponding bin in the K-dimensional feature space and the total in that bin is incremented. The probability that a feature vector arises from a given sound class is then estimated as the count in each histogram bin divided by the total number of feature vectors generated for the class. This procedure is repeated for each sound class, so each class has its own multidimensional normalized histogram distribution.

The probability that a certain class generated the feature vector came is computed using the Bayes equation below (Sivia, 1996):

$$P(class_j | f_{1-K}) = \frac{P(f_{1-K} | class_j)P(class_j)}{\sum_{j=1}^{J} P(f_{1-K} | class_j)P(class_j)} \quad \text{Equation (12.6)}$$

where there are J sound classes and there are K features in the feature vector f. The class having the highest probability is then chosen as the best estimate for the observed features. The denominator in the right-hand side of Eq. (12.6) sums the probabilities overall of the classes, and serves to normalize the total probability that the feature vector came from one of the classes to 1.

The term $P(f_{1-K} | class_j)$ is computed by finding the histogram bin for the feature vector for the given class and extracting the normalized histogram contents for that bin. In addition, the classifier needs to be given the a priori probability of each class. Classes that are rarely seen are given a lower overall probability than classes that are more often seen even if the probability of the feature vector occurring for that class is high. For example, the feature vector for a hair dryer would be expected to very different from that for speech or traffic noise. A good match between a feature vector and one for a hair dryer could give a high value of $P(f_{1-K} | class_j)$ for the hair-dryer class. However, if the hearing-aid user is someone who doesn't own a hair dryer, then $P(class_j)$ for the hair-dryer class would be nearly zero and the overall value of $P(class_j | f_{1-K})$ for the hair-dryer class would also be very small.

The Bayes classifier as described above requires computing the joint probability distribution of the features for each sound class. A simpler approach, termed the Naïve Bayes Classifier, is to assume that the probability distributions of the features are independent. That is, a value for one feature tells us nothing about the values of the other features measured at the same time. This independence assumption means that the distribution for each feature can be determined separately. If histograms are used to estimate the probability distributions, for example, then a separate histogram would be generated for each feature for each sound class. The Bayes equation then becomes:

$$P(class_j | f_{1-K}) = \frac{[P(f_1 | class_j)P(f_2 | class_j) ... P(f_K | class_j)]P(class_j)}{\sum_{j=1}^{J}[P(f_1 | class_j)P(f_2 | class_j) ... P(f_K | class_j)]P(class_j)}.$$

Equation (12.7)

Because of the assumed independence of the features, the joint probability distribution is just the product of the separate distributions for each feature. Calculating the probability that a sound belongs to a specific class requires forming the product of the probabilities that each feature in the feature vector came from that class, times the probability of that class being present. The Naïve Bayes Classifier can greatly reduce the computational requirements compared to the Bayes Classifier, and often the classifier accuracy is not substantially compromised (Rubinstein & Hastie, 1997).

PERSONALIZING THE CLASSIFIER

As the above hair-dryer example illustrates, the best performance for the Bayes classifier is obtained for the most accurate probability distributions and a priori assumptions. In the ideal world, the classifier would be trained on segments obtained from the hearing-aid user's listening situations, and the probability of each of these situations occurring would also be obtained. The classifier could then be trained for that individual's specific listening problems. In a practical implementation, however, the classifier must be trained in advance, with histograms obtained for the anticipated range of listening situations. A degree of personal adjustment is still possible; the probability of occurrence for the different listening situations could be obtained for each hearing-aid user via a short questionnaire, and $P(class_j)$ personalized using the questionnaire results during the hearing-aid fitting.

Other types of classifiers can also be personalized, but not as easily. In a neural network, for example, the probability of occurrence for each class can be indirectly inserted into the training by making the number of feature vectors from each class in the training set proportional to the probability that the class will be encountered. A small number of neural networks trained on different proportions of everyday sounds could then be used for listeners with different lifestyles, such as factory worker, office worker, or a retiree spending most of the time at home.

A second problem is that the classifier may correctly identify the listening situation, but that the processing parameters in the hearing aid may not reflect the listener's preferences for that situation. Listeners with different degrees of hearing loss, for example, may have different preferences in the same listening situation; in the first section of the chapter differences in the preferred compression parameters were shown to be related to the audiogram. Given individual differences, one would like to train the hearing aid, as it is being used, to adapt to the preferences of the user. One approach is to provide feedback to the hearing aid every time the classifier identifies a new listening environment and changes the processing parameters. The feedback indicates if the user likes or dislikes the new settings. Over time, using an adaptive Bayes approach, the processing parameters can be adjusted to more accurately reflect the user's processing preferences (de Vries et al., 2006; Ypma et al., 2006).

Classification Examples

The accuracy of a classifier depends on the features selected and the training and test conditions. These effects are illustrated in this section for a neural network classifier. The results for other approaches, such as the support vector machine, HMM, and Bayes classifiers, would differ in detail but show similar trends.

NUMBER OF FEATURES

The neural network was implemented using the MATLAB Neural Network Toolbox (Demuth et al., 2006). The set of selected features forms the input to the neural network. The inputs connect to the hidden layer, which contains the same number of neurons as there are inputs for up to eight inputs, and is limited to eight neurons for more than eight inputs. The neurons in the hidden layer connect to the four neurons in the output layer. The log-sigmoid transfer function was used for both the hidden and output layers. The training used the resilient back propagation algorithm (Demuth et al., 2006). For each signal class, the target outputs were defined as 1 for the indicated signal class and 0 at the other three outputs.

The classification system was tested using four classes of signals: speech, multitalker babble, traffic noise, and classical music. The feature vectors were computed once every group of eight 24-sample blocks, which gives a sampling period of 12 msec (192 samples at the 16-kHz sampling rate). A total of 10,000 feature vectors were extracted for each of the speech, babble, and music classes, and 8282 feature vectors for the traffic.

The neural network was trained by randomizing the order of the 38,282 feature vectors. Because the order of the inputs is different for each training sun, the neural network will produce slightly different results each time. Each feature vector was applied to the neural network inputs, and the corresponding sound class output was set to 1 with the other three outputs set to 0. A total of 100 iterations of the resilient back propagation algorithm were used for the training. After the training was completed, the system was evaluated by applying the set of input feature vectors and computing the neural network output for each one. The output having the greatest amplitude was chosen as the signal class.

The neural network classifier was tested using different combinations of features as shown in Table 12-2. The number of features ranged from four to 21. The evaluation started with an ad hoc set of four features. These features, the first three delta cepstrum coefficients and the zero crossing rate, are often chosen for speech and music classifiers. The classifier results are poor. Although the it does a reasonably good job with babble, its accuracy is very bad for traffic noise. The overall accuracy, averaged over the four sound classes, is just 64.0% correct. Replacing the four ad hoc features with four best features shown in Figure 12-4 using the mutual information criterion (Kwak & Choi, 1999) with $\beta = 0.5$ greatly improves the classifier accuracy. Babble is still classified the most accurately, with 96.8% correct, and music is the poorest at 85.4% correct. The overall accuracy has improved to 90.3% correct, which shows that choosing a good set of features can greatly improve the classifier performance even when only a small set of features is used.

Increasing the number of features from four to six improves the classifier accuracy. The six ad hoc features add the variance of the ZCR and the spectrum centroid to the four ad hoc features previously chosen, and the overall performance improves from 64.0 to 91.1% correct. The high error rate in classifying traffic noise has been eliminated by adding the additional features. However, the best six features from Figure 12-4 give even better performance, with an average accuracy of 94.3%. Not only is the average accuracy better for the features selected using the mutual information criterion than for the ad hoc selection, but the classifier performance is better for each of the four separate classes. Increasing the number of features from six to eight gives a small improvement in performance to 96.6% correct, which comes close to the accuracy when all 21 features are used. Using all 21 of the features from Table 12-1 or Figure 12-4 results in excellent performance, with an average of 99.6 of the segments classified correctly, but such a large number of features would not be practical in a hearing aid with its limited computational and memory resources. Furthermore, such high accuracy could not be

TABLE 12-2. Neural Network Classifier Performance as the Number of Features Selected from Table 12-1 Is Varied

Features	Percent Correct				
	Speech	Babble	Traffic	Music	Average
ΔCep1, ΔCep2, ΔCep3, ZCR	70.8	88.3	27.2	69.6	64.0
Best 4, $\beta = 0.5$	88.8	96.8	90.0	85.4	90.3
ΔCep1, ΔCep2, ΔCep3, ZCR, σZCR, Cent	94.7	95.9	92.6	81.3	91.1
Best 6, $\beta = 0.5$	95.0	96.8	94.9	90.5	94.3
Best 8, $\beta = 0.5$	98.3	97.7	97.6	92.7	96.6
All 21 from Table 12-1	99.7	99.8	99.6	99.5	99.6

Features selected according to the Kwak and Choi (1999) mutual-information criterion are indicated by $\beta = 0.5$ and are taken in order from the center column of Figure 12-4. The results are the average of 10 runs for each test case.

expected in the real world with its wide variety of signals, including many that were not included in the training set.

ISOLATED SIGNALS VS. MIXTURES

The results of Table 12-2 indicate that a system using eight features is both practical and accurate. But there still remains the question of how accuracy under ideal laboratory conditions relates to the accuracy to be expected in the real world. A second experiment was conducted to investigate this question.

A neural network, similar to that used for the data of Table 12-2, was used as the classifier. Features were computed for three classes of signals: speech, classical music, and noise. The noise class combined the babble and traffic noise classes into a single class, along with some miscellaneous noises such as a hair dryer, keyboard typing, and water running from a faucet. Eight features, chosen using the mutual information criterion (Kwak & Choi, 1999) from an expanded set of 28 possible features, were used as inputs to the neural network.

For one training condition, a file was chosen at random from the classes of speech, music, or noise, and the neural network was trained to identity the selected class. The output for the selected class was set to 1 and the other outputs were set to 0. For the second training condition, composite sound files were created by combining speech, music, and noise sequences. A signal from one class was chosen at random and given a gain of 1. A second class from chosen from the remaining two classes and the associated signal given a random gain between 0 and −40 dB re: 1. The gain for the remaining class was set to 0. The neural network was then trained using an output of 1 for the class of the first (stronger) signal, a gain between 0.01 and 1 for the second (weaker) signal, and a gain of 0 for the signal not selected for the mixture.

A total of 100,000 feature vectors (20 minutes of data) were extracted for training the neural network, with 250 vectors computed from each random combination of signal classes before a new combination was formed, the processing reinitialized, and 250 new feature vectors obtained. Thus, features were computed for a total of 4000 different random combinations of the sound classes. A separate random selection of 100,000 files was used to generate the test features. Both the neural network initialization and the order of the training inputs are governed by sequences of random numbers, so the neural network will produce slightly different results each time; the tabulated results were therefore taken as the average of 10 runs.

One important test of a sound classifier is the ability to accurately identify the signal class or the component of the signal mixture having the largest gain. This task corresponds to the standard problem of determining the class when the signal is assumed a priori to represent one class alone. The standard problem consists of training the neural network using features for the signal taken from one class at a time, and then testing the network using data also corresponding to the signal taken from one class at a time. The results for the standard problem are shown in the first row of Table 12-3. The eight best features for separate signal classes were used. The neural network has an average accuracy of 98.2%, and is slightly more accurate in classifying speech and less accurate in classifying noise. The large number of potential noise signals, ranging from passing traffic to crumpling paper or a hair dryer, may explain the poorer performance for the noise class.

Training the neural network using two-signal mixtures and then testing using the separate classes produces the next row of Table 12-3. The discrimination performance is reduced compared to both training and testing with separate classes because the test data do not correspond to the training data. The performance is still quite good, however, with an average of 95.6% correct. Again the performance for speech is the best of the three classes and noise the poorest.

A more difficult test is identifying the dominant component of a two-signal mixture. The test feature vectors for this task are all computed with signals from two classes present at the same time, so the test features reflect the signal mixtures. When the neural network is trained on the separate classes but tested using the two-signal mixtures, the performance degrades substantially. The average identification accuracy is reduced to 86.9%. The music class now has the best results, and the speech and noise classes have each been reduced in accuracy by about 15%. This performance loss is indicative of what will happen when a system trained on ideal data is put to work in the real world.

The identification performance for the two-signal mixtures improves when the neural network is trained on the mixtures instead of separate classes. The training data now match the test data. The average percent correct is 88.6%, which is about 1.7% better than for the system trained on separate classes but still 9.5% worse than the system trained and tested on separate classes. The performance thus reflects the difficulty of the mixture classification task, but also shows that the classifier per-

TABLE 12-3.
Neural Network Classifier Performance as the Training and Test Protocols Are Varied

Training Protocol	Test Protocol	Percent Correct			
		Speech	Music	Noise	Avg.
Separate Classes	Separate Classes	99.4	98.2	96.9	98.2
2-Signal Mixture	Separate Classes	98.7	95.1	93.1	95.6
Separate Classes	2-Signal Mixture	84.8	93.3	82.6	86.9
2-Signal Mixture	2-Signal Mixture	86.6	90.8	88.4	88.6

The neural network classifier used the eight best features chosen from an extended set of 28 features using the Kwak and Choi (1999) mutual-information criterion.

formance is improved when the system is trained for the more realistic test conditions.

Concluding Remarks

The problem of sound classification can be divided into two parts. The first part is generating the features to be used by the classifier. The features embody our knowledge of speech and hearing. The objective is to choose features that reflect the differences between the different signal classes, but it is often hard to predict which features will be the most useful. As a result, many features have been proposed for sound classification. These features include spectral shape, changes in spectral shape, zero crossing rate, rhythm extraction, and many others. The limited computational and memory resources in a hearing aid limit the number of features that can be implemented in a classifier. Selecting those features that maximize the mutual information between the features and the sound classes appears to lead to more accurate classifier performance than choosing features at random or by intuition. A classifier using eight features selected using the mutual information criterion gives accuracy close to that from a classifier using all available features while needing only a fraction of the computational resources.

The second part of the classifier problem is the classifier itself. The selection of the classifier is most likely less important than the selection of the features. However, there are subtle differences between classifier designs that make one approach more suitable to a given problem than another approach. For example, an HMM can encode the temporal aspects of a pattern, whereas a neural network can give continuously valued outputs that may be more useful in evaluating mixtures of signals, and a Bayes classifier may be easier to personalize to individual listening situations. The choice of which classifier approach to use is not a simple decision and the optimal strategy for hearing aids is not obvious.

It is easy to design a classifier that gives very good results in the laboratory, or to design test and evaluation conditions that will yield performance that looks wonderful in an advertisement. The real challenge is to design a system that will be accurate in the real world when presented with signals that weren't present during the training, or when presented with the mixtures of signal types that often occur when listening under realistic conditions. The classifier boundaries that separate the feature vectors into the different classes need to be general enough, or capable of being adapted during the use of the hearing aid, so that they will work for new sounds and new combinations of sounds. This is a difficult design objective because it requires that the system function properly under unknown conditions.

And finally, even if we design the perfect classifier, there is the question of what to do with it. There is some evidence that selecting different hearing-aid processing parameters under different listening conditions can lead to improved user satisfaction. An example would be the compression ratios and time constants used in dynamic-range compression. A modern hearing aid, however, has several processing algorithms running at the same time. The challenge now becomes to determine when and how the entire set of processing parameters within the hearing aid should be adjusted to optimize intelligibility or sound quality, and how to do this in response to each user's individual hearing loss and listening preferences. The solution may be to combine sound classification with adaptive learning of the user's processing preferences for the classes.

APPENDIX 12-A

SIGNAL FEATURES

A total of 21 features are listed in Table 12-1. The features described in this appendix are listed in the numerical order given in Table 12-1. The signal sampling rate is set to 16 kHz. The features are assumed to be computed using a block size of 24 samples, which gives a block sampling rate of 667 Hz. The classification decisions do not need to be made at this rapid an update rate, so the values computed for each block can be combined across blocks. For example, the block outputs can be combined into groups of eight blocks, which results in a feature sampling period of 12 msec and a corresponding classification update rate of 83 Hz.

Feature I. Mean-Squared Signal Power

The input signal sequence is $x(n)$. Define N as the number of samples in a block (N = 24 in these examples) and L as the number of blocks in a group (L = 8). The mean-squared signal power for group m is the average of the square of the input signal summed across all of the blocks that make up the group:

$$p(m) = \frac{1}{NL} \sum_{j=0}^{NL-1} x^2(n-j) \quad \text{Equation (A.1)}$$

Feature 2. Standard Deviation of the Signal Envelope

The signal envelope is the square root of the mean-squared signal power and is given by:

$$s(m) = [p(m)]^{1/2} \quad \text{Equation (A.2)}$$

The long-term signal power and the long-term signal envelope are smoothed versions of the values calculated for each signal block. The smoothing can be implemented using a one-pole low-pass filter having a time constant, for example, of 200 msec, giving:

$$\hat{p}(m) = \alpha \hat{p}(m-1) + (1-\alpha) p(m)$$
$$\hat{s}(m) = \alpha \hat{s}(m-1) + (1-\alpha) s(m) \quad \text{Equation (A.3)}$$

The standard deviation of the signal envelope is then given by:

$$\sigma(m) = [\hat{p}(m) - \hat{s}^2(m)]^{1/2} \quad \text{Equation (A.4)}$$

Features 3-6. Mel Cepstrum Coefficients 1 Through 4

Let $X(k,l)$ be the spectrum in auditory analysis bands for band k, $1 \leq k \leq K$, and signal block l. The spectrum can be the output of a warped FFT, or it can be from a conventional FFT with the FFT bins combined into auditory bands. The signal power for group m is then given by the sum over the blocks in the group:

$$P(k,m) = \frac{1}{L}\sum_{l=1}^{L}|X(k,l)|^2 \quad \text{Equation (A.5)}$$

The mel cepstrum is the cepstrum computed on an auditory frequency scale, so computing the cepstrum using the auditory-spaced FFT outputs automatically produces the mel cepstrum. The mel cepstrum coefficients are low-pass filtered using a one-pole low-pass filter having a time constant of 200 msec. The jth mel cepstrum coefficient for group m is thus given by:

$$cep_j(m) = \alpha cep_j(m-1) + (1-\alpha)\sum_{k=1}^{K}\log[P(k,m)]c_j(k)$$
$$\text{Equation (A.6)}$$

where $c_j(k)$ is the jth weighting function, $1 \leq j \leq 4$, given by:

$$c_j(k) = \cos[(j-1)(k-1)\pi/(K-1)] \quad \text{Equation (A.7)}$$

The weighting functions are then normalized. The weighting functions, after normalization, are plotted in Figure 12-A1.

Features 7-10. Delta Cepstrum Coefficients 1 Through 4

The delta cepstrum coefficients are the first differences of the mel cepstrum coefficients computed using Eq. (A.6). The delta cepstrum coefficients are thus given by:

$$\Delta cep_j(m) = cep_j(m) - cep_j(m-1) \quad \text{Equation (A.8)}$$

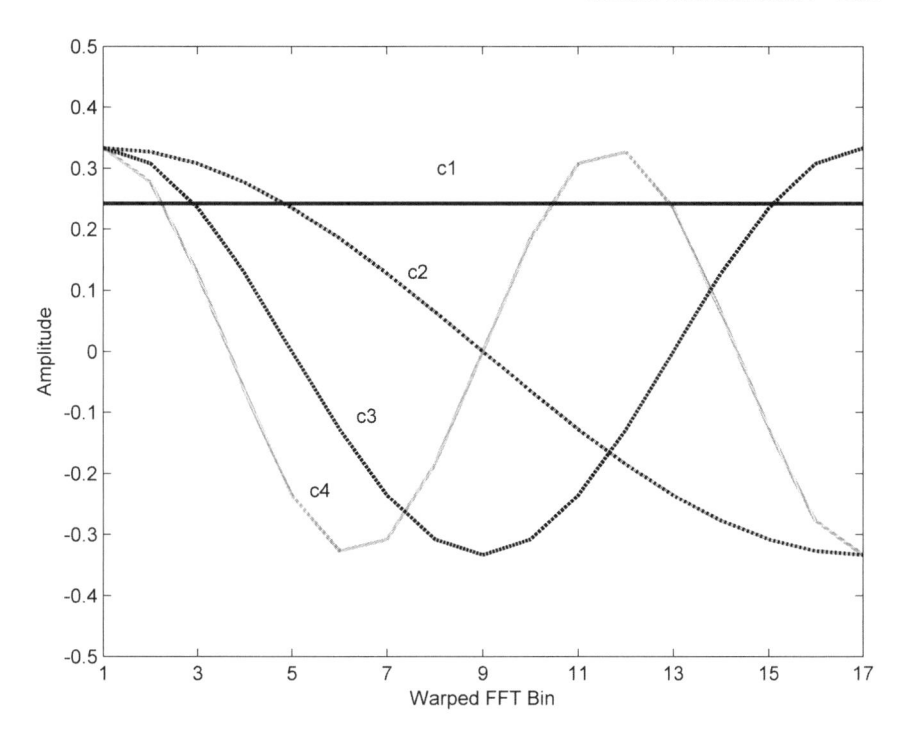

Figure 12-A1. Mel cepstrum frequency weighting functions for the first four cepstral coefficients.

Features 11-13. Zero-Crossing Rate (ZCR), ZCR of Signal First Difference, and Standard Deviation of the ZCR

The zero-crossing rate (ZCR) for the mth group of blocks is defined as:

$$ZCR(m) = \sum_{n=0}^{NL-1} \left| sign[x(n)] - sign[x(n-1)] \right| \quad \text{Equation (A.9)}$$

where NL is the total number of samples in the group. The ZCR is low-pass filtered using a one-pole filter having a time constant of 200 msec, giving the feature:

$$z(m) = \alpha z(m-1) + (1-\alpha)ZCR(m) \quad \text{Equation (A.10)}$$

The ZCR of the first difference is computed using Eqs. (A.9) and (A.10), but with the first difference of the signal $y(n) = x(n) - x(n-1)$ replacing the signal $x(n)$.

The standard deviation of the ZCR is computed using the same procedure as is used for the signal envelope. The average of the square of the ZCR is given by:

$$v(m) = \alpha v(m-1) + (1-\alpha) ZCR^2(m) \quad \text{Equation (A.11)}$$

The standard deviation of the ZCR is then estimated using:

$$\zeta(m) = \left[v(m) - z^2(m)\right]^{1/2} \quad \text{Equation (A.12)}$$

Features 14-16. Power Spectrum Centroid, Delta Centroid, and Standard Deviation of the Centroid

The power spectrum centroid is the first moment of the power spectrum. It is given by:

$$centroid(m) = \sum_{k=1}^{K} kP(k,m) / \sum_{k=1}^{K} P(k,m) \quad \text{Equation (A.13)}$$

The centroid feature is the low-pass filtered centroid, using a one-pole low-pass filter having a time constant of 200 msec, given by:

$$f(m) = \alpha f(m-1) + (1-\alpha) centroid(m) \quad \text{Equation (A.14)}$$

The delta centroid feature is then given by the first difference of the centroid:

$$\Delta f(m) = f(m) - f(m-1) \quad \text{Equation (A.15)}$$

The standard deviation of the centroid uses the average of the square of the centroid, given by:

$$u(m) = \alpha u(m-1) + (1-\alpha) centroid^2(m) \quad \text{Equation (A.16)}$$

with the standard deviation then given by:

$$\upsilon(m) = \left[u(m) - f^2(m)\right]^{1/2} \quad \text{Equation (A.17)}$$

Feature 17. Power Spectrum Entropy

The power spectrum entropy is an indication of the smoothness of the spectrum. First compute the fraction of the total power in each auditory frequency band:

$$\rho(k,m) = P(k,m) / \sum_{k=1}^{K} P(k,m) \quad \text{Equation (A.18)}$$

The entropy in bits for the group of blocks is then computed and low-pass filtered (200-msec time constant) to give the signal feature:

$$e(m) = \alpha e(m-1) + (1-\alpha)\sum_{k=1}^{K}\rho(k,m)\log_2\left[\rho(k,m)\right] \quad \text{Equation (A.19)}$$

Features 18-19. Broadband Envelope Correlation Lag and Peak Level

The broadband signal envelope uses the middle of the spectrum. Assume, for example, that there are 17 auditory bands. The broadband envelope would then be computed as:

$$b(m) = \sum_{k=3}^{14} \left[P(k,m)\right]^{1/2} \quad \text{Equation (A.20)}$$

where the 17 bands cover the frequencies from 0 to π. The signal envelope is low-pass filtered using a time constant of 500 msec to estimate the signal mean:

$$\mu(m) = \beta\mu(m-1) + (1-\beta)b(m) \quad \text{Equation (A.21)}$$

The signal envelope is then converted to a zero-mean signal:

$$a(m) = b(m) - \mu(m) \quad \text{Equation (A.22)}$$

The zero-mean signal is center clipped:

$$\hat{a}(m) = \begin{cases} a(m), & |a(m)| \geq 0.25\mu(m) \\ 0, & |a(m)| < 0.25\mu(m) \end{cases} \quad \text{Equation (A.23)}$$

The envelope autocorrelation is then computed over the desired number of lags (each lag represents one group of blocks, or 12 msec) and low-pass filtered using a time constant of 1.5 sec:

$$R(j,m) = \gamma R(j,m-1) + (1-\gamma)\hat{a}(m)\hat{a}(m-j) \quad \text{Equation (A.24)}$$

where j is the lag.

The envelope autocorrelation function is then normalized to have a maximum value of 1 by forming:

$$r(j,m) = R(j,m) / R(0,m) \quad \text{Equation (A.25)}$$

The maximum of the normalized autocorrelation is then found over the range of 8 to 48 lags (96 to 576 msec). The location of the maximum in lags is the lag feature, and the amplitude of the maximum is the peak level feature.

Features 20–21. Four-Band Envelope Correlation Lag and Peak Level

The four-band envelope correlation divides the power spectrum into four nonoverlapping frequency regions. The signal envelope in each region, again assuming 17 auditory frequency bands, is given by:

$$b_1(m) = \sum_{k=3}^{5}[P(k,m)]^{1/2}$$

$$b_2(m) = \sum_{k=6}^{8}[P(k,m)]^{1/2}$$

$$b_3(m) = \sum_{k=9}^{11}[P(k,m)]^{1/2} \quad \text{Equation (A.26)}$$

$$b_4(m) = \sum_{k=12}^{14}[P(k,m)]^{1/2}$$

The normalized autocorrelation function is computed for each band using the procedure given by *Eqs. (A.21)* through *(A.25)*. The normalized autocorrelation functions are then averaged to produce the four-band autocorrelation function:

$$\hat{r}(j,m) = \frac{1}{4}[r_1(j,m) + r_2(j,m) + r_3(j,m) + r_4(j,m)] \quad \text{Equation (A.27)}$$

The maximum of the four-band autocorrelation is then found over the range of 8 to 48 lags. The location of the maximum in lags is the lag feature, and the amplitude of the maximum is the peak level feature.

References

Aarts, R. M., & Dekkers, R. T. (1999). A real-time speech-music discriminator. *Journal of the Audio Engineering Society*, 47, 720–725.

Allamanche, E., Herre, J., Hellmuth, O., Fröba, B., Kastner, T., & Cremer, M. (2001). Content-based identification of audio material using MPEG-7 low level description. In J. S. Downie & D. Bainbridge, Ismir (Eds.), *Proceedings of the Second Annual International Symposium on Music Information Retrieval* (pp. 197–204).

Battiti, R. (1994). Using mutual information for selecting features in supervised neural net learning. *IEEE Transactions on Neural Networks*, 5, 537–550.

Bishop, C. (2006). *Pattern recognition and machine learning*. New York: Springer.

Büchler, M., Allegro, S., Launer, S., & Dillier, N. (2005). Sound classification in hearing aids inspired by auditory scene analysis. *EURASIP Journal of Applied Signal Processing*, 18, 2991–3002.

Burgess, C. J. C. (1998). A tutorial on support vector machines for pattern recognition. *Data Mining and Knowledge Discovery*, 2, 121–167.

Carey, M. J., Parris, E. S., & Lloyd-Thomas, H. (1999). A comparison of features for speech, music discrimination (paper 1432). *Proceedings of the ICASSP*; Phoenix, AZ.

Chou, W., & Gu, L. (2001). Robust singing detection in speech/music discriminator design. *Proceedings of the ICASSP 2001* (paper Speech-P9.4), Salt Lake City, Utah.

Cortes, C., & Vapnik, V. (1995). Support vector networks. *Machine Learning*, 20, 273–297.

Demuth, H., Beale, M., & Hagan, M. (2006). *Neural network toolbox for use with MATLAB: Users' guide Version 5*. Natick, MA: The MathWorks, Inc. Available at http://www.mathworks.com/access/helpdesk/help/pdf_doc/nnet/nnet.pdf

Duda, R., Hart, P., & Stork, D. (2001). *Pattern classification* (2nd ed.). New York: John Wiley and Sons.

El-Maleh, K., Klein, M., Petrucci, G., & Kabal, P. (2000). Speech/music discrimination for multimedia applications. *Proceedings of the ICASSP*, Vol. IV (pp. 2445–2448), Istanbul.

Fukunaga, K. (1995). *Introduction to statistical pattern recognition* (2nd ed.), New York: Academic Press.

Gunn, S. (1998). *Support vector machines for classification and regression*. ISIS Technical Report, University of Southampton, May 10, 1998.

Hagan, M., Demuth, H., & Beale, M. (1996). *Neural network design*. University of Colorado at Boulder, Campus Publication Service.

Hansen, M. (2002). Effects of multi-channel compression time constants on subjectively perceived sound quality and speech intelligibility. *Ear and Hearing*, 23, 369–380.

Haykin, S. (1998). *Neural networks: A comprehensive foundation* (2nd ed.). Englewood Cliffs, NJ: Prentice-Hall.

Humes, L. E., Christensen, L., Thomas, T., Bess, F. H., Hedley-Williams, A., & Bentler, R. (1999). A comparison of the aided performance and benefit provided by a linear and a two-channel wide dynamic range compression hearing aid. *Journal of Speech Language and Hearing Research*, 42, 65–79.

Kates, J. M. (1995). Classification of background noises for hearing-aid applications. *Journal of the Acoustical Society of America*, 97, 461–470.

Kates, M. A. (2003). *Speech/music classifier using support vector machines*. Research Project Report to GN ReSound, May 2003.

Kwak, N., & Choi, C.-H (1999). Improved mutual information feature selector for neural networks in supervised learning. *Proceedings of the 1999 International Joint Conference on Neural Networks*, Vol. 2 (pp. 1313–1318); Washington, D.C. Vol. 2.

Liu, Z., Huang, J., Wang, Y., & Chen, T. (1997). Audio feature extraction and analysis for scene classification. *Proceedings of the IEEE 1st Multimedia Workshop*; Princeton, NJ, June 23–25, 1997.

Lu, L., Jiang, H., & Zhang, H. (2001). A robust audio classification and segmentation method. *Proceedings of the 9th ACM International Conference on Multimedia* (pp. 203–211); Ottawa, Canada.

Mesgarani, N., Shamma, S., & Slaney, M. (2004). Speech discrimination based on multiscale spectro-temporal modulations. *Proceedings of the IEEE International Conference on Acoustics, Speech, and Signal Processing* (pp. I:601–I:604.); Monteal, May 17–21, 2004.

Neuman, A. C., Bakke, M. H., Hellman, S., & Levitt, H. (1994). Effect of compression ratio in a slow-acting compression hearing aid: Paired-comparison judgments of quality. *Journal of the Acoustical Society of America, 96*, 1471–1478.

Neuman, A. C., Bakke, M. H., Mackersie, C., & Hellman, S. (1995). Effect of release time in compression hearing aids: Paired-comparison judgments of quality. *Journal of the Acoustical Society of America, 98*, 3182–3187.

Nordqvist, P., & Leijon, A. (2004). An efficient robust sound classification algorithm for hearing aids. *Journal of the Acoustical Society of America, 115*, 3033–3041.

Peltonen, V., Tuomi, J., Klapuri, A., Huopaniemi, J., & Sorsa, T. (2002). Computational auditory scene recognition. *Proceedings of the ICASSP 2002*, Vol. II (pp. 1941–1944). Orlando, FL.

Pfeiffer, S., Fischer, S., & Effelsberg, W. (1996). *Automatic audio content analysis*. Technical Report TR-96-008, Department of Math and Computer Science, University of Mannheim, Germany.

Rabiner, L., (1989). A tutorial on hidden Markov models and selected applications to speech recognition. *Proceedings of the IEEE, 77*, 257–286.

Rizvi, S. J., Chen, L., & Özsu, T. (2002). *MADClassifier: Content-based continuous classification of mixed audio data.* Technical Report CS-2002–34, School of Computer Science, University of Waterloo, Ontario, Canada.

Rubinstein, Y. D., & Hastie, T. (1997). Discriminative vs. informative learning. In D. Heckerman, H. Mannila, & D. Pregibon (Eds.), *Proceedings of the Third International Conference on Knowledge Discovery and Data Mining* (pp 49–53). Menlo Park, CA: AAAI Press.

Saunders, J. (1996). Real-time discrimination of broadcast speech/music. *Proceedings of the ICASSP 1996* (pp. 993–996), Atlanta, GA.

Scheirer, E., & Slaney, M. (1997). Construction and evaluation of a robust multifeature speech/music discriminator. Proceedings of the ICASSP 1997 (pp. 1331–1334); Munich.

Scott, D. W. (1979). On optimal and data-based histograms. *Biometrika, 66,* 605-610.

Sivia, D. S. (1996). *Data analysis: A Bayesian tutorial.* New York: Oxford University Press.

Srinivasan, S., Petkovic, D., & Ponceleon, D. (1999). Towards robust features for classifying audio in the CueVideo system. *Proceedings of the 7th ACM Conference on Multimedia* (pp. 393–400).

Stone, M. A., & Moore, B. C. J. (2003). Effect of the speed of a single-channel dynamic range compressor on intelligibility in a competing speech task. *Journal of the Acoustical Society of America, 114,* 1023–1034.

Takeuchi, S., Yamashita, M., Uchida, T., & Sugiyama, M. (2001). Optimization of voice/music detection in sound data. *Proceedings of the CRAC.* Aalborg, Denmark, Sept. 2, 2001.

Tipping, M. E. (2001). Sparse Bayesian learning and the relevance vector machine. *Journal of Machine Learning Research, 1,* 211–244.

Tourassi, G., Frederick, E, Markey, M., & Floyd, C., Jr. (2001). Application of the mutual information criterion for feature selection in computer-aided diagnosis. *Medical Physics, 28,* 2394–2402.

Tzanetakis, G., & Cook, P. (2000). Sound analysis using MPEG compressed audio. *Proceedings of the ICASSP 2000,* Vol. II (pp. 761–764); Istanbul.

Viterbi, A. (1967). Error bounds for convolutional codes and an asymptotically optimal decoding algorithm. *IEEE Transactions on Information Theory, IT-13,* 260–269.

de Vries, B., Ypma, A., Dijkstra, T., & Heskes, T. M. (2006). Bayesian incremental utility elicitation with application to hearing aids personalization. *Proceedings of the ISBA 8th World Meeting on Bayesian Statistics,* June 2006, Benidorm, Spain.

Yang, H., & Moody, J. (1999). Feature selection based on joint mutual information. In *Advances in Intelligent Data Analysis (AIDA), Computational Intelligence Methods and Applications (CIMA).* Rochester, NY: International Computer Science Conventions.

Yang, H., Van Vuuren, S., Sharma, S., & Hermansky, H. (2000). Relevance of time-frequency features for phonetic and speaker-channel classification. *Speech Communication, 31,* 35–50.

Ypma, A., de Vries, B., & Geurts, J. (2006). Robust volume control personalization from on-line preference feedback. *Proceedings of the IEEE International Workshop on Machine Learning for Signal Processing*, Maynooth, Ireland, Sept. 6–8, 2006.

Zhang, T., & Kuo, C.-C. (2001). Audio content analysis for online audiovisual data segmentation and classification. *IEEE Transactions on Speech and Audio Processing, 9*, 441–457.

13

Binaural Signal Processing

THE SIGNAL PROCESSING that has been considered thus far can be implemented in one hearing aid. When hearing aids are used on both ears, termed a binaural fitting, the hearing-aid processing still operates independently at each ear. In the binaural signal processing discussed in this chapter, however, the processing works in tandem at the two ears. The binaural algorithms compare the signals at the two ears, and the processing parameters at each ear depend on both the signal at that (ipsilateral) ear and at the opposite (contralateral) ear.

The motivation for binaural hearing-aid processing is binaural auditory processing. Two ears are better than one, and there are many situations where binaural listening provides substantial benefits over using just one ear. There are several ways in which the binaural auditory system responds to speech and noise that differ from the response when just one ear is used. For example, there are physiologic links between the neural outputs of the two cochleas, and augmenting the effects of these links provides one approach to binaural signal processing. Signals that are uncorrelated at the two ears are perceived differently from signals that are highly correlated, and another binaural signal processing approach is to emphasize correlated signals and suppress uncorrelated signals. Signals presented to the two ears can also merge to form a single percept despite occupying nonoverlapping frequency bands, and this behavior can be exploited to compensate for cochlear hearing damage while preserving the perceived integrity of the speech.

This chapter begins with a brief review of the benefits of binaural listening in noise and interference. This material summarizes some of the factors that can aid binaural signal detection that are unavailable in monaural listening. Three binaural signal processing techniques are then described. The first, binaural compression, is motivated by neural connections between the two ears that can affect the amount of amplification provided by the cochlea. Next is binaural noise suppression, based on the amount of correlation between the signals at the two ears or on models of sound localization. The third technique is complementary comb filters, intended to compensate for the increase in auditory filter bandwidth in the impaired cochlea. These approaches are all quite different from each other, and show the range of signal processing that is possible when binaural hearing is considered.

The "Cocktail Party" Problem

Microphone arrays improve speech intelligibility in noise by reducing the gain for interference coming from directions other than that of the desired speech. The human auditory system also has the ability to exploit the spatial and other signal characteristics of speech and noise. The ability to attend to a single voice from among many competing voices, as when carrying out a conversation at a noisy party, is termed the "cocktail party problem" (Cherry, 1953). Many factors are assumed to influence the ability to track a desired talker among several competing voices, including the location of the desired and competing sources, visual cues, the spectral and temporal properties of the desired and competing signals, and linguistic information (Bronkhorst, 2000; Cherry, 1953; Ebata, 2003; Haykin & Chen, 2005).

An important factor in separating the desired from the competing sources is the interaural level difference (ILD), and interaural time difference (ITD) observed for the signals arriving at the two ears from different azimuths. The magnitude of the sound pressure at the eardrum is strongly affected by the angle to the sound source, and interaural differences of up to 20 dB as a function of incident angle occur at high frequencies (Shaw, 1974; Shaw & Vaillancourt, 1985). Interaural time differences are also a function of the angle of incidence, and range from 0 msec for sounds coming from straight ahead to 0.8 msec for a sound coming from the side at low frequencies (Kuhn, 1977). The effects of azimuth are discussed in more detail in Chapter 3.

A second factor that has been studied under laboratory conditions is the phase of the interference relative to that of the noise. The change in SNR for binaural as opposed to monaural or diotic (same signal at both ears) listening for the detection of a signal in noise is termed the binaural masking level difference (BMLD), and the change in SNR that yields equal speech intelligibility gives the binaural intelligibility level difference (BILD). The phase dependence of the BMLD has been investigated by varying the interaural phase of the signal and/or noise presented at the two ears. Using signal and interference both in phase at the two ears (SoNo) as the reference condition, Levitt and Rabiner (1967a) found that signal anti-phase and interference in-phase (SπNo) resulted in a BMLD of 13 dB when the signal and interference were both Gaussian noise band limited to below 4800 Hz. They found a BILD of 6 dB when speech was used as the anti-phase signal and the Gaussian noise as the in-phase interference. The opposite condition, in which the signal is in-phase at the two ears and the noise anti-phase (SoNπ), results in a slightly reduced BMLD of about 13 dB (van de Par & Kohlrausch, 1999).

Binaural listening has been shown to give better speech intelligibility than monaural listening in noise when the speech and noise originate from different directions (Carhart, 1965; Dirks & Wilson, 1969a). Speech intelligibility for noise and speech both coming from directly in front of a normal-hearing subject requires a 10-dB higher SNR for the same level of recognition accuracy than required when the noise is coming from 90 degrees to one side (Bronkhorst & Plomp, 1988). Furthermore, the improvement in speech intelligibility for the separated speech and noise sources is not just due to the improvement in SNR at the ear opposite the noise source. For speech coming from 45 degrees to one side of the listener and noise from 45 degrees on the opposite side of the head, the head shadow provides approximately 6 dB improvement in SNR and binaural release from masking an additional 3 dB improvement in effective SNR (Markides, 1977). For speech coming from the side of the subject and the interference from the front, binaural listening again gives a 3-dB advantage over monaural listening using as the reference the ear on the same side of the head as the speech loudspeaker

(Dirks & Wilson, 1969b). The type of interference also has an effect. In an experiment using up to three interfering sources of sound, the binaural advantage was found to be about 2 to 4 dB for stationary speech-shaped noise and speech-modulated noise, but increased to 6 to 7 dB for speech and time-reversed speech (Hawley et al., 2004).

The binaural advantages for aided hearing-impaired listeners appear overall to be similar to those observed for normal-hearing subjects even if the absolute level of performance is not as good (Bronkhorst & Plomp, 1992; Dirks & Wilson, 1969b). The benefit from interaural time differences for aided hearing-impaired listeners appears to be close to that found for normal-hearing listeners, although the benefit from interaural intensity differences may be significantly reduced if there is substantial high-frequency hearing loss (Bronkhorst & Plomp, 1989). If amplification is provided so that most of the speech and noise is audible at both ears, the binaural advantage for hearing-impaired subjects is very close to that for normal-hearing listeners (Markides, 1977). However, the binaural advantage for hearing-impaired listeners appears to be reduced relative to that for normal-hearing listeners at poor SNR values (Arsenault & Punch, 1999). Even in those situations where the differences in speech intelligibility between monaural and binaural hearing aid use are small, there can still be significant preferences for binaural hearing aid use (McKenzie & Rice, 1990), with the clarity of the speech the most important factor (Balfour & Hawkins, 1992).

Signal Transmission

Binaural signal processing requires the ability to get the acoustic signal from one side of the head to the other. The simple solution is to connect the two hearing aids with a wire. However, the cosmetic concerns associated with a visible wire have discouraged this simple solution. So before it is possible to have hearing aids incorporating binaural algorithms, we must have hearing aids that contain wireless binaural links.

A wireless link is a radio system that transmits the signal acquired at one hearing aid to a receiver located in the hearing aid at the contralateral ear. As it is expected that data will be sent both ways, each hearing aid must house both a transmitter and a receiver. The problems with a wireless link are that the transmitter and antenna require additional space within each hearing aid, it takes power to transmit data from one side of the head to the other, and the processing necessary for the signal transmission and reception introduce a time delay.

Many digital hearing aids use 16-bit words to encode the audio signal, and sample the signal at 16 kHz. The data rate is then 16 bits/sample x 16,000 samples/sec = 256 kbits/sec. Data rates this high are difficult to achieve in a circuit having low power consumption, so the interaural data rate must be reduced. Some form of data compression is needed to reduce the data rate in bits/sec (note that data rate compression is not the same as dynamic range compression). The problem is similar to streaming audio over the Internet; bandwidth is the limitation for streaming audio rather than power consumption, but the solution is the same in that the data rate must be reduced in order to have a practical system. One solution for hearing aids, as on the Internet, would be to use a data-encoding scheme such as MP3 to represent the signal with fewer bits/sec. Even with data compression, however, the current drain may still be too high. For example, digital transmission or reception at 128 kb/sec using a recent integrated circuit design (Gennum, 2006) would draw approximately 2.5 mA from the battery, which is about double the current drain needed for everything else in the hearing aid.

An additional concern for sending the audio signal from one side of the head to the other is the transmission latency, which is the time delay needed to prepare the signal for transmission and to convert the transmitted digital signal back into audio at the other end. The signal may be processed using MP3 or a related scheme to reduce the data rate. Error-protection coding (requiring extra bits) is added to ensure that the transmission is not corrupted by noise or reflections. The encoded digital audio must then be converted into a sequence of transmitted pulses. The signal is transmitted in blocks, which require additional header information to identify the source of the signal, the data rate, and the encoding parameters so that the signal can be properly decoded by the receiver. At the receiver, the header information must be decoded, the error protection stripped away to restore the original bit stream, and the bits converted back into the audio signal.

All of these operations require processing time, and thus delay the transmitted signal. The hearing-aid designer now has a problem. If the latency were 10 msec, for example, then a processing algorithm that requires both the left and right signals to be present at the same time would have to delay the ipsilateral signal by 10 msec in order to synchronize it with the contralateral signal being transmitted from the other ear.

This delay would be added to the delay already present in the hearing aid for its other processing functions such as dynamic-range compression. So if the hearing aid has a 6-msec delay when used monaurally, the delay will be closer to 16 msec for a linked binaural system. Thus, the latency in the binaural link could push the overall hearing-aid processing delay from acceptable to unacceptable (see Chapter 8 on Processing Delay). Not every algorithm requires that the left and right signals be exactly synchronized, however; often the gain adjustments provided by the signal processing can lag behind the audio signal with only a small decrement in sound quality.

The power consumption can be substantially reduced by not transmitting the audio signal but instead sending processing parameters from one hearing aid to the other. The goal in this case is not to process the left and right audio signals in each hearing aid, but rather to synchronize the algorithm gain settings and processing parameters. Reducing the data rate to 500 bits/sec in the Gennum circuit referenced above, for example, reduces the current drain to approximately 0.5 mA, which is much more acceptable.

Binaural Compression

In a typical binaural hearing aid fitting, the signal processing at each ear operates independently from the processing at the contralateral ear. There are some binaural effects, however, in which the presentation of signals at both ears changes the perceptual or physiologic response in comparison to a stimulus presented to only one ear. Binaural compression systems have been proposed to exploit some of these differences between monaural and binaural signal presentation. Differences in loudness perception are considered in a compression system that uses binaural loudness summation to adjust the compression gains, and the effects of the auditory efferent neural system in controlling the gain of the cochlear amplifier are considered in the second compression system.

COMPRESSION USING BINAURAL LOUDNESS SUMMATION

When a stimulus is presented to both ears, the perceived loudness is greater than when the same stimulus is presented to one ear alone. This effect is termed binaural loudness summation. If the two signals are of equal intensity, the loudness of the binaural presentation is about the same as a monaurally presented signal having an intensity 6 to 8 dB greater than the left- or right-ear signal (Zwicker & Zwicker, 1991). For soft sounds, the loudness of the binaural presentation is about double that of monaural presentation, whereas for loud sounds the binaural presentation is about 1.4 times as loud as the monaural presentation. The summation effect is strongest when the signals at the two ears are of equal intensity, and decreases as the interaural level difference becomes greater. Binaural summation of loudness in hearing-impaired listeners appears to be similar to that for normal-hearing listeners (Hawkins et al., 1987).

One theory in designing a compression system is that the amplification should match the loudness of the signal presented to the impaired ear to the loudness of the same signal presented to a normal ear. The loudness will be greater for binaural presentation than for monaural amplification, so the compression gain should be designed to take the change in loudness into account. Kollmeier et al. (1993) have designed a binaural compression system in which the compression gain is based on the sum of the signal powers at the two ears. This approach reduces the gain compared to a monaural compression system as the signal power used to set the gain at each ear is the combined power at both ears, which will always be greater than the power at either ear alone.

A block diagram of the Kollmeier et al. (1993) system is presented in Figure 13-1. The system sampling rate is 30 kHz. Successive short-term spectra are computed in the left and right channels using a 512-point (17 msec) FFT for Hamming-windowed data segments of 408 samples (13.6-msec duration). The data segments have a 50% overlap, so a new segment is processed every 6.8 msec. The FFT bins are then grouped into auditory critical bands by summing the energy in the FFT bins constituting each band. Upward spread of masking is implemented as a linear ramp on a dB scale having a slope of 10 dB/Bark, and downward spread of masking is implemented using a slope of −25 dB/Bark. The effective signal level in each auditory band is taken as the maximum of either the signal level originating in that band or the masking component in that band projected from any of the other bands. The power level for controlling the compressor is then computed as the sum of the effective energy values from the left and right channels.

The binaural compression system was fitted to six hearing-impaired listeners using a loudness-scaling procedure (Kollmeier et al., 1993).

408 Digital Hearing Aids

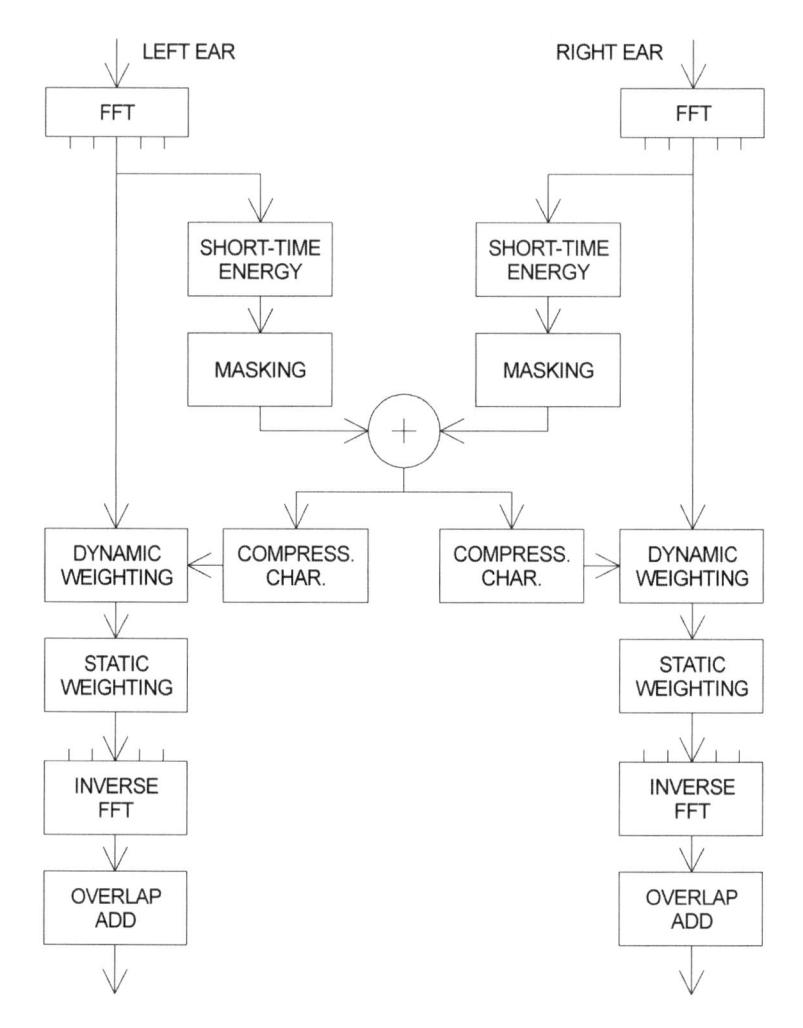

Figure 13-1. Block diagram of a binaural compression system in which the summed signal power from the two ears is used to control the compression gain (after Kollmeier et al., 1993).

Speech intelligibility was measured using sentence materials in cafeteria babble. Two of the subjects showed an improvement in intelligibility for the binaural compression compared to linear frequency shaping, whereas one subject showed no significant change and three subjects performed worse with the compressed stimuli. Speech quality judgments showed that the unprocessed stimuli were preferred over the linear frequency shaping, and the binaural compression was in general preferred over the linear system.

AUDITORY EFFERENTS

Auditory physiology can also be used as an argument for the design of a binaural compression system. Afferent neural fibers carry stimulus signals from the periphery to the brain, and efferent fibers carry control signals from the brain back to the periphery (Pickles, 1988). In the auditory system, the efferent fibers provide a binaural auditory link; a stimulus to one ear acts via the efferent fibers to reduce the neural response to a signal in the contralateral ear. Because the efferents operate via synaptic connections to the outer hair cells (Liberman & Kujawa, 1999), it is likely that the efferent effects are reduced in impaired ears due to outer hair-cell damage. The efferent fibers consist of the olivocochlear bundle (OCB), which connects the superior olive to the cochlea. The OCB connection is bilateral, with the uncrossed OCB providing a pathway for sensory inputs to cause changes in the behavior of the cochlea on the same side of the head, and the crossed OCB (COCB) providing a pathway for neural signals from one ear to modify the behavior of the cochlea in the contralateral ear. Stimulating the COCB, either electrically or by contralateral sound, causes a reduction in the sensitivity to sounds presented to the ipsilateral ear.

Experiments using human subjects have typically used a noise masker in one ear while monitoring the level of distortion products induced in the contralateral ear. A reduced level of distortion products indicates a reduction in the activity of the cochlear amplification provided by the outer hair cells. A contralateral noise masker has been shown to reduce the level of transient-evoked otoacoustic emissions (TEOAE) in humans (Berlin et al., 1995; Hood et al., 1996) and distortion-product otoacoustic emissions (DPOAE) in both humans (Chéry-Croze et al., 1993) and in animals (Puel & Rebillard, 1990). Other contralateral masking signals, such as clicks, tones, and narrow-band noise, have also been shown to cause suppression of otoacoustic emissions (Berlin et al., 1993; Maison et al., 1998).

Several experiments (Berlin et al., 1993; Hood et al., 1996; Puel & Rebillard, 1990) have measured the distortion-product amplitude as a function of the level of the contralateral masker. There appears to be a threshold for the COCB inhibition, as masking noise below about 30 to 40 dB SPL does not significantly reduce the distortion product amplitude in the contralateral ear. For maskers above this threshold, the amount of distortion-product suppression in dB appears to be proportional to the masker intensity in dB above threshold for masker intensities from about 30 to 100 dB SPL.

The time course of the TEOAE suppression in humans can be inferred from the data of Berlin et al. (1995). They measured the distortion-product amplitude at several different time delays after the cessation of the contralateral masking noise. The temporal nature of the series of four clicks used to measure the distortion products makes a clear determination of the time constant difficult, but it appears that a time constant in the vicinity of 20 to 60 msec is appropriate for the release time constant of the assumed COCB effects in humans. The same time constant would also apply to the COCB attack time given the similarity of the attack and release times in the guinea pig data of Sridhar et al. (1995).

COMPRESSION USING AUDITORY EFFERENTS

A simple but effective model of the cochlea, and the model that forms basis of most dynamic-range compression systems, is a parallel filter bank with independent compression in each frequency band. The auditory efferents can be added to this model by providing additional attenuation linked to the contralateral outputs. One frequency band of such a multiband binaural cochlear model is shown in Figure 13-2. The left and right channels are identical. The overall system gain is the result of a combination of compression of the input signal in the ipsilateral channel combined with the efferent attenuation signal from the contralateral channel. Both sets of signals are first peak-detected to generate the control signals for the ipsilateral gain adjustment, and the time constants for this compressor operation would be chosen to reproduce monaural cochlear behavior. The ipsilateral compressors are then followed by a linked binaural system that duplicates the contralateral COCB function. The contralateral peak detectors would have time constants in the range of 20 to 60 msec to reproduce the temporal response of the efferent signal attenuation.

A binaural compression system that mimics the effects of the efferent neural connections has been proposed by Kates (2004a). A block diagram of the basic system is presented in Figure 13-3. The incoming signal at each ear is peak detected using syllabic time constants, with an attack time of 5 msec and a release time of 70 msec in each frequency band. The peak-detection output is then converted to its logarithm as a rough approximation to the auditory loudness scale. This peak-detected

Binaural Signal Processing 411

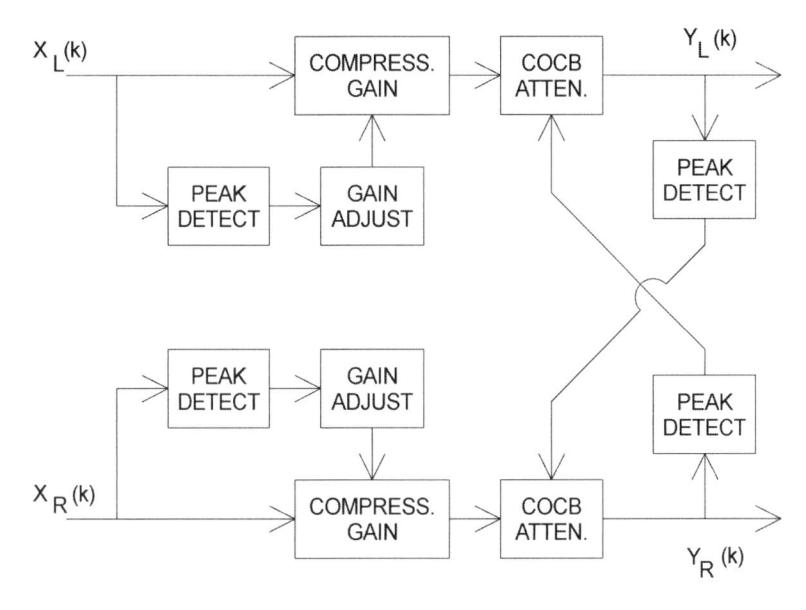

Figure 13-2. Block diagram of a signal processing model of a feed-forward binaural cochlear compression system with crossed COCB feedback linkages.

signal, in the absence of the contralateral links, would be the sole control of the compression input/out gain rule. In addition, the signal from the other ear is peak detected using 60-msec attack and release times and converted to its log value to approximate the COCB signal. The contralateral COCB signal is scaled by a factor a and added (in dB) to the ipsilateral control signal. The combined ipsilateral plus scaled contralateral signal then is used to set the ipsilateral compression gain.

The binaural compression system can suppress noise under some conditions. Assume that speech is present at a positive SNR in dB. If the speech is the stronger signal at one ear, and noise the signal at the other ear, then the compression gain at the speech ear will be set mostly by the speech signal. However, the gain at the noisy ear will be reduced by the cross-linked speech signal. A similar result can be achieved by taking the maximum of the left and right ear signals and using that value to control the compression gain at both ears. This latter approach results in the system of Figure 13-4. The maximum of the left- and right-ear signals is the input to the peak detector, and the output of the peak detector forms the control signal for the compressors at the two ears.

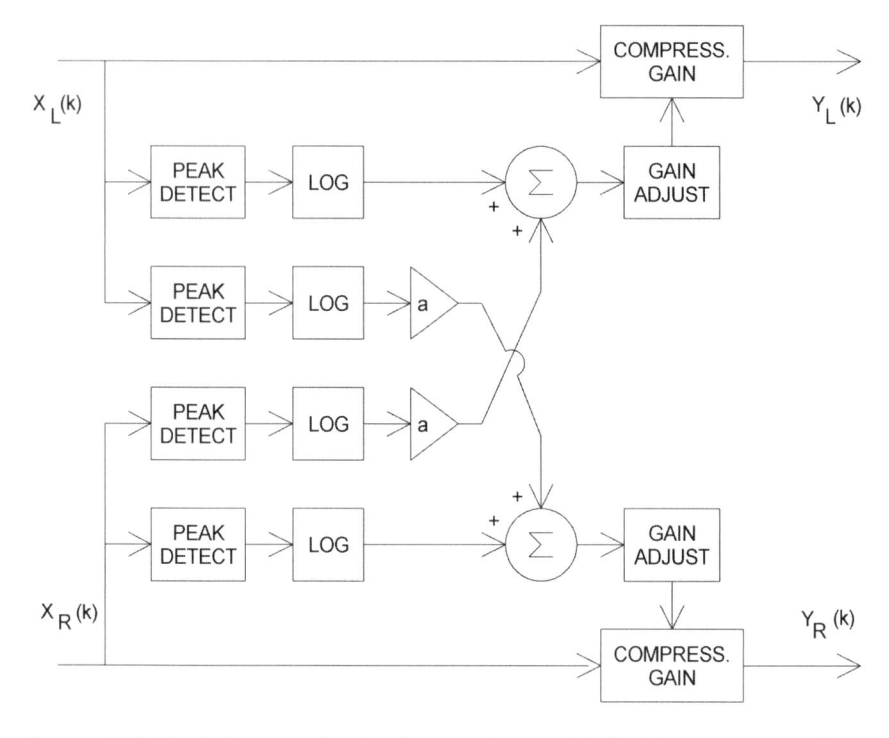

Figure 13-3. Block diagram of a signal processing model of a binaural compression system simulating the COCB efferent linkages and using the input signals to control the compressor gain.

By what degree does the binaural compression actually reduce the intensity of the noise? The binaural systems of Figures 13-3 and 13-4 were simulated in MATLAB using a 17-band frequency-warped compressor architecture (Kates & Arehart, 2005). The compressors used an attack time of 5 msec and a release time of 70 msec, the parameter $a=$ 0.2 for the system of Figure 13-3, and the compression ratio in each frequency band was set to 2:1. The test stimulus consisted of two signals. The desired signal was a segment of the "Rainbow Passage" read by a male talker and presented at an azimuth of 90 degrees to the right of a simulated head at a RMS level of 70 dB SPL. The interfering signal was speech-shaped noise presented at an azimuth of 90 degrees to the left ear of the simulated head at a RMS level of 60 dB SPL. The frequency-dependent interaural time and level differences were simulated using a

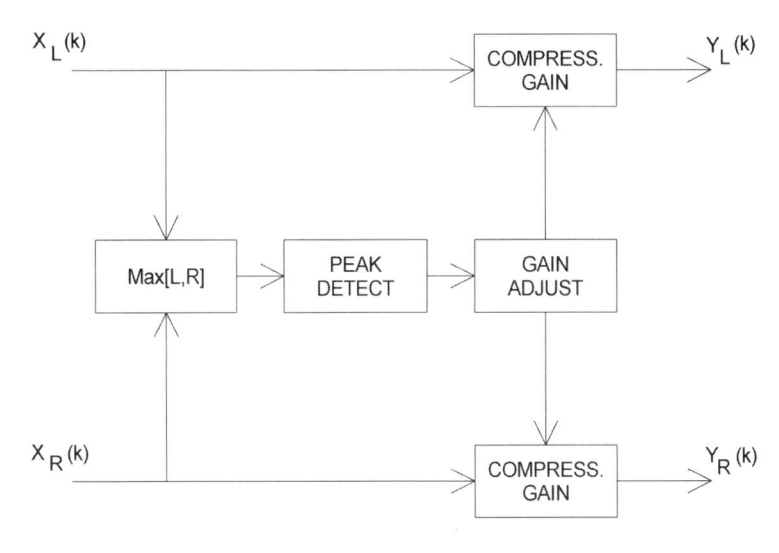

Figure 13-4. Block diagram of a signal processing model of a simplified binaural COCB compression system using the maximum of the left and right ear signals to control the compressor gain.

spherical head model (Brown, 1996; Brown & Duda, 1998) developed for binaural sound synthesis. The head model provided realistic signal leakage from one side of the head to the other, and the left and right ear signals were similar to those that would be obtained in dummy-head testing of a binaural behind-the-ear (BTE) system in an anechoic environment.

The evaluation criterion for the simulation was the amount of suppression of the left-ear noise signal caused by the right-ear speech signal. The envelope of the input speech signal is plotted in Figure 13-5. The reference condition is the system providing independent monaural compression for each ear. The difference in the compressed output signal envelopes between the independent monaural processing and the linked binaural processing for the left ear indicates the amount of noise suppression that would be expected in practice.

The left-ear envelope difference for the COCB compressor of Figure 13-3 is shown in Figure 13-6. During most of the speech the binaural COCB compressor provides about 1.25 dB of suppression. A pause in the speech occurs between 2.6 and 3.4 sec, during which the noise signal is more intense than the speech signal; during the pause the sup-

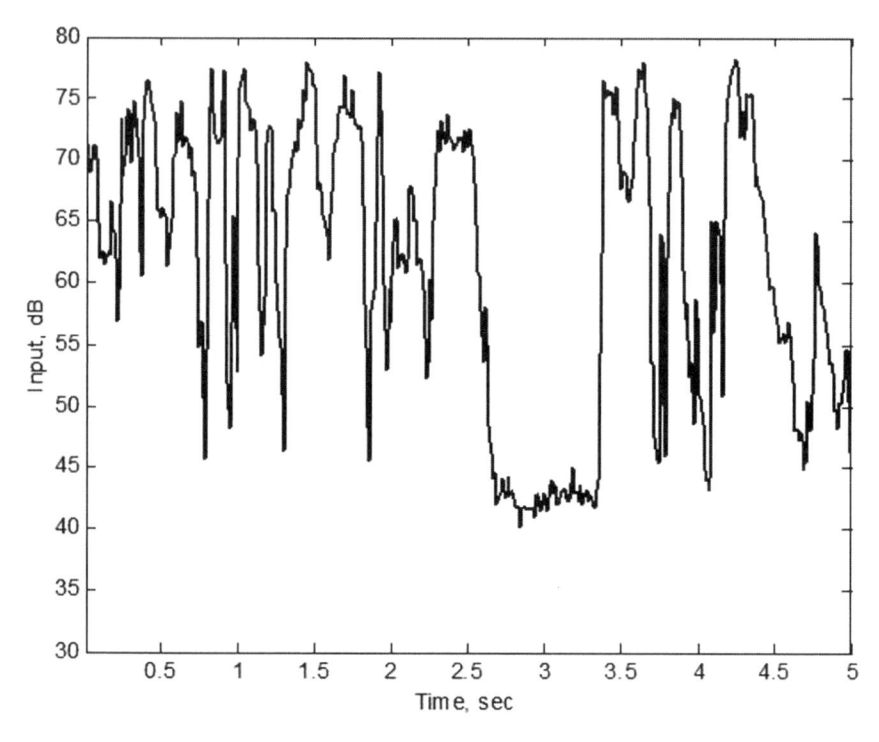

Figure 13-5. Envelope of the speech signal presented to the simulated head from the direction of the right ear.

pression is reduced to about 0.5 dB. The 60-msec time constant used for the contralateral signal detection results in relatively smooth suppression as a function of time. However, the difference between the ipsilateral and contralateral detection time constants causes a difference in the detected peak levels when the stimulus intensity changes, so there is some residual suppression even during the speech pause.

The left-ear envelope difference for the compressor of Figure 13-4 that uses the maximum of the left and right signals to control the compression gain for both ears is shown in Figure 13-7. The use of the detected signal peak results in stronger suppression behavior. The average suppression is about 1 dB, which is quite similar to that observed for the COCB systems, but the speech peaks cause short-term suppression effects of up to 3.5 dB. Also, there is essentially no suppression observed for the pause in the speech between 2.6 and 3.4 msec where the noise

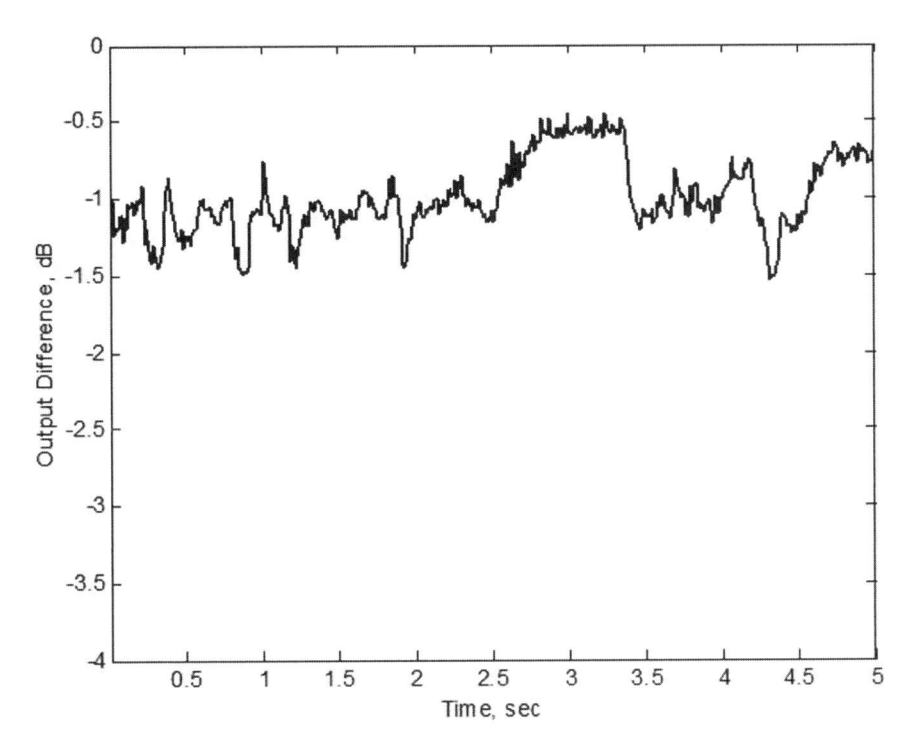

Figure 13-6. Difference in the left-channel output signal envelopes between the COCB cross-linked compressor of Figure 13-3 using separate ipsilateral and contralateral time constants and the independent monaural compression.

signal is the more intense of the inputs at the two ears. The modulation of the left ear noise signal by the speech at the right ear is much stronger for this system than for the COCB system. Given an improvement in SNR of about 1 dB under the most favorable conditions, one would not expect either the binaural compression system of Figure 13-3 or 13-4 to provide a measurable improvement in speech intelligibility in noise.

The listener preference for the binaural loudness summation system and the binaural scheme of Figure 13-3 were determined for 10 hearing-impaired listeners under a variety of everyday listening situations (Kollmeier et al., 2002). The listening conditions included conversation in a supermarket, walking from a busy store out to the street, a party, construction noise, and conversation in quiet. The binaural processing schemes were compared to each other and to independent compression

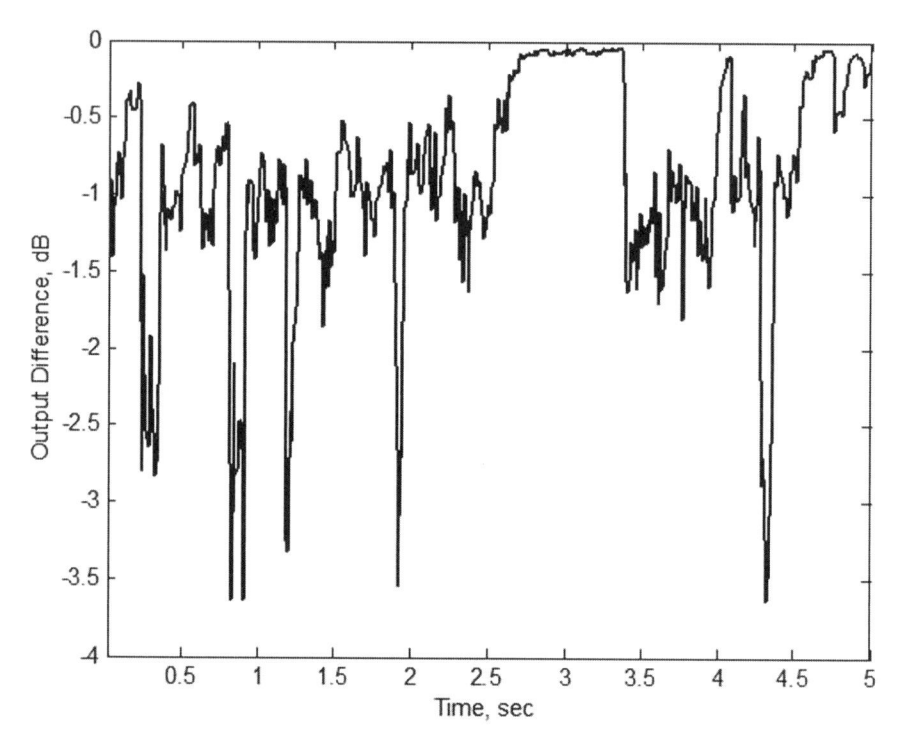

Figure 13-7. Difference in the left-channel output signal envelopes between the COCB cross-linked compressor of Figure 13-4 using the maximum of the ipsilateral and contralateral signals and the independent monaural compression.

in each ear. The subjects used a five-point rating scale. The test results indicated only small differences between the different algorithms, with no consistent pattern with regard to stimulus, subject, or listening property being evaluated. All of the compression systems provided natural sound, good localization, and acceptable listening effort. The conclusion of the report (Kollmeier et al., 2002) was that there was no clear advantage for any of the binaural compression systems.

Binaural Noise Suppression

As shown with the binaural compression algorithms above, any signal processing that exists independently in the left and right hearing aids can be converted into binaural processing by linking processing parameters such as the estimated signal and noise levels. But in addition to sharing parameters, there are also aspects of the spatially separated signals at the two ears that can be exploited to suppress the noise.

Figure 13-8 shows a desired source of sound in front of the listener and interfering sources of sound surrounding the listener. For the desired source, the signals at the two ears will be the same given the symmetry of the source location relative to the two ears. For noise sources surrounding the listener, however, the signals at the two ears will differ. In a diffuse noise field, the correlation between the pressure measured at two locations in space decreases with increasing separation, and becomes small for two points greater than one-half wavelength apart (Rafaely, 2000). The separation between the ears is about 15 cm in an adult, which is one-half wavelength at approximately 1100 Hz. So, at frequencies above 1 kHz the signals at the two ears will be essentially uncorrelated in a diffuse noise field.

Thus, if the desired source of sound in front of the listener is close

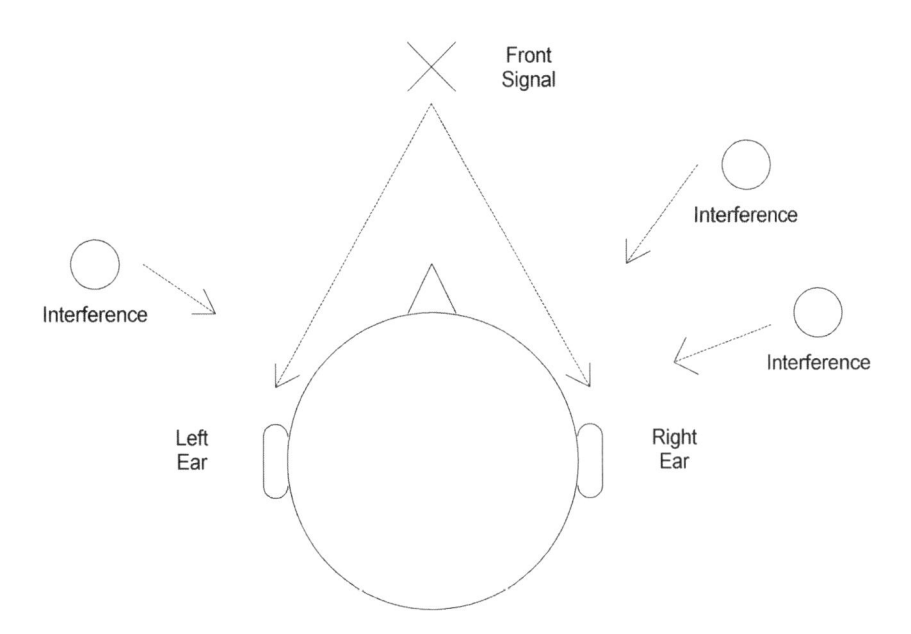

Figure 13-8. Centered front signal (X) and spatially separated sources of interference surrounding the listener.

enough (within the critical distance) not to be affected by room reverberation, but the noise sources are far enough away to be primarily diffuse sources when the room reflections are taken into account, then across a wide frequency range the desired signals at the two ears will be highly correlated with each other whereas the noise signals at the two ears will be uncorrelated. This property of high interaural correlation for the desired signal and low interaural correlation for the noise is the basis of the first three binaural algorithms described in this section.

Note that if the desired source of sound is beyond the critical distance there will be more signal power in the reverberant field than in the direct signal from the source. Under these conditions the interaural correlation will be low for the desired signal as well as for the interference. As the binaural signal-processing systems use the cross-correlation to indicate the presence of the desired signal, they will decrease the gain in a band having a low interaural correlation even if the frequency band contains a preponderance of speech.

The last two algorithms discussed below are based on models of auditory localization. These algorithms use localization cues such as the interaural level difference and the interaural timing difference that change with shifts in the source azimuth. The goal is to separate the interfering sound sources from the desired source, and then suppress the interfering sources.

INTERAURAL CROSS-CORRELATION

The first group of signal processing strategies described in this section sets the gain high for those frequency bands that have a high interaural correlation, and reduces the gain in those bands that have a low interaural correlation. A block diagram of the general system approach is shown in Figure 13-9. The signal at each ear is divided into frequency bands. The left and right ear signals in each band are cross-correlated, and the cross-correlation is combined with the estimated signal power at each ear to form a gain function. The gain ranges from 1, when the left-ear and right-ear signals in the frequency band are completely correlated, to 0 if they are completely uncorrelated.

The binaural correlation algorithms in the literature are typically derived in the frequency domain. Those descriptions, however, require mathematics (functions of a complex variable) that lie beyond the knowledge assumed for this book. The signal processing will be described here in the time domain; the interested reader is referred to

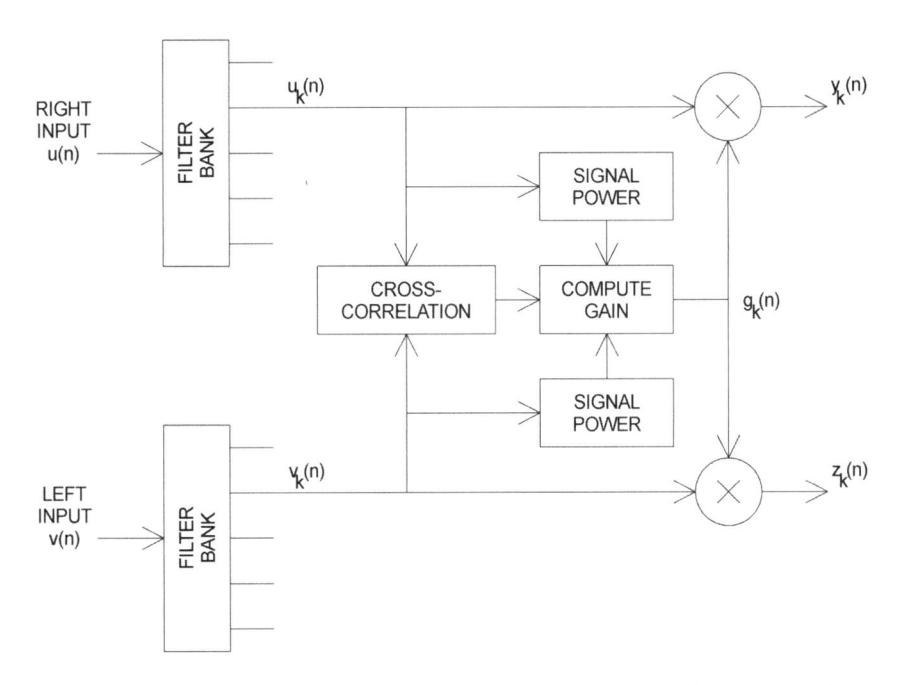

Figure 13-9. Block diagram of a binaural cross-correlation system for adjusting the gain at the right and left ears.

the cited papers for the more complete descriptions of the frequency-domain processing.

Let the right input signal be $u(n)$, and the left signal be $v(n)$. Each signal consists of sound from the desired source in front of the listener, combined with independent noise at each ear. The right-ear signal can be written as $u(n) = s(n) + p(n)$, where $s(n)$ is the signal from the desired source and $p(n)$ is the interference. Similarly, the left-ear signal is $v(n) = s(n) + q(n)$, where $s(n)$ is the same desired source and $q(n)$ is an independent source of interference. We will assume that the interference is uncorrelated with the desired signal, and that the two interference signals are uncorrelated with each other. These assumptions can be written as:

$$\langle s(n)p(n) \rangle = 0$$
$$\langle s(n)q(n) \rangle = 0 \quad \text{Equation (13.1)}$$
$$\langle p(n)q(n) \rangle = 0$$

where the angle brackets denote the signal average. The average is generally implemented as a low-pass filter, and the lack of correlation means that the average of the various signal products within the angle brackets is 0.

Assume that there are K frequency bands in the filter bank, numbered from 1 to K. The outputs for frequency band k are denoted by $u_k(n)$ and $v_k(n)$ for the left and right ears, respectively. The signal power in band k for the right ear is given by:

$$\langle u_k^2(n) \rangle = \langle [s_k(n) + p_k(n)]^2 \rangle = \langle s_k^2(n) + 2s_k(n)p_k(n) + p_k^2(n) \rangle$$

Equation (13.2)

Because the desired signal and the interference are uncorrelated, the cross-product $s_k(n)p_k(n)$ within the bracket averages out to zero and the signal power becomes:

$$\langle u_k^2(n) \rangle = \langle s_k^2(n) \rangle + \langle p_k^2(n) \rangle \quad \text{Equation (13.3)}$$

Similarly, the signal power in band k for the left ear is:

$$\langle v_k^2(n) \rangle = \langle s_k^2(n) \rangle + \langle q_k^2(n) \rangle \quad \text{Equation (13.4)}$$

The cross-correlation between the right and left ears is:

$$\langle u_k(n)v_k(n) \rangle = \langle [s_k(n) + p_k(n)][s_k(n) + q_k(n)] \rangle$$
$$= \langle s_k^2(n) + s_k(n)p_k(n) + s_k(n)q_k(n) + p_k(n)q_k(n) \rangle$$

Equation (13.5)

All of the terms except the first in this equation average out to zero because of the assumptions that the desired signal and interference are uncorrelated and that the interference at the two ears is also uncorrelated. The average interaural cross-correlation then becomes:

$$\langle u_k(n)v_k(n)\rangle = \langle s_k^2(n)\rangle \quad \text{Equation (13.6)}$$

The interaural cross-correlation thus returns the average power of the desired signal.

If the desired source of sound is not directly in front of the listener, it will arrive at one ear before the other. Compensation for the difference in arrival times at the two ears can be provided by delaying the signal that arrives first so that it is temporally aligned with the signal that arrives later at the other ear. The cross-correlations and power calculations would then proceed as outlined above. The frequency-domain implementations of the binaural signal processing used in the literature are more general in that they can automatically provide compensation for the interaural time delays associated with an off-axis desired source of sound.

BINAURAL WIENER FILTER

One of the earliest systems for binaural noise suppression was proposed by Allen et al. (1977). This system starts with the block diagram of Figure 13-9. The cross-correlation between the right- and left-ear signals is computed along with the power in the signals at each ear. A gain value is then computed using these values, and the same gain $g_k(n)$ is applied to the signal in each frequency band to produce the right and left outputs $y_k(n)$ and $z_k(n)$.

Allen et al. (1977) proposed two procedures for adjusting the gain. For the first approach, the gain is given by:

$$g_k(n) = \frac{\langle u_k(n)v_k(n)\rangle}{\frac{1}{2}\left[\langle u_k^2(n)\rangle + \langle v_k^2(n)\rangle\right]} \quad \text{Equation (13.7)}$$

after the signals $u_k(n)$ and $v_k(n)$ have been aligned to compensate for the difference in arrival times at the two ears. The desired signal and interference correlation assumptions mean that the numerator of Eq. (13.7) can be replaced by Eq (13.6), and the terms in the denominator can be replaced by Eqs. (13.3) and (13.4). Making these substitutions results in:

$$g_k(n) = \frac{\langle s_k^2(n) \rangle}{\langle s_k^2(n) \rangle + \frac{1}{2}\left[\langle p_k^2(n) \rangle + \langle q_k^2(n) \rangle\right]} \quad \text{Equation (13.8)}$$

The numerator is the desired signal power, whereas the denominator is the sum of the desired signal power plus the average of the interference power at each ear. A related approach (Lindemann, 1995, 1996; Lindemann & Melanson, 1997) does not compensate for the difference in arrival times at the two ears, with the result that off-axis sounds are suppressed relative to those arriving from directly in front.

Comparing Eq. (13.8) with Eq. (10.6) from Chapter 10 shows that Eq. (13.8) is a Wiener filter. The processing given by Eq. (13.7) therefore minimizes the mean-squared error between the original desired signal and processed output at the ears. The signal power in the numerator of the Wiener filter in the binaural case is formed by computing the interaural cross-correlation of the signals at the two ears, whereas the signal plus noise power in the denominator is the average of the power at each ear. If the interference power is low, that is the listener is in a good SNR, the denominator will be dominated by the desired signal power and the gain will approach 1. As the level of the interference increases the denominator grows along with the interference whereas the numerator remains constant. Thus as the SNR gets worse the gain decreases. In the limit of no desired signal the numerator of Eq. (13.8) becomes 0 and the gain is set to 0 as well.

The second approach proposed by Allen et al. (1977) computes the gain as:

$$g_k(n) = \frac{\langle u_k(n) v_k(n) \rangle}{\left[\langle u_k^2(n) \rangle \langle v_k^2(n) \rangle\right]^{1/2}} \quad \text{Equation (13.9)}$$

This alternative formulation is the coherence function between the signals at the two ears. If just the desired signal from the front is present the signals at the two ears are identical, yielding $u_k(n)v_k(n) = u_k^2(n) = v_k^2(n)$. For this situation the gain given by Eq. (13.9) is exactly 1. If only interference is present the cross-correlation in the numerator of Eq. (13.9) is 0 and the gain is also 0. Thus, Eq. (13.9) provides an alternative formulation that, like Eq. (13.7), varies smoothly from a gain of 1 in a frequency band that contains just the desired signal to a gain of 0 when the band contains only interference.

The binaural signal processing of Allen et al. (1977) was proposed as a dereverberation technique to improve speech intelligibility in rooms. However, a test of the Wiener filter approach given by *Eq. (13.7)* showed no improvement in speech intelligibility for normal-hearing or hearing-impaired listeners for speech recorded in a reverberant room (Bloom, 1980), and a test of the coherence approach given by *Eq. (13.9)* using normal-hearing listeners also showed no improvement in intelligibility under conditions of reverberation (Bloom & Cain, 1982). On the other hand, a test using hearing-impaired listeners reported by Lindemann (1995) shows an improvement in intelligibility for the binaural processing in comparison with the subjects' own (monaural) hearing aids for sentences in diffuse multitalker babble, and Schweitzer et al. (1996) found a reduction in the perceived difficulty of listening for the hearing-impaired subjects under the same conditions. These results suggest that binaural noise suppression, like so many other hearing-aid algorithms, does not improve speech intelligibility but may reduce listening effort.

BINAURAL SIGNAL DIFFERENCE

The binaural Wiener filter measures the degree of similarity between the signals at the two ears. It is also possible to design a binaural algorithm based on measuring the differences in the two signals (Kates, 2004b). The normalized signal difference is given by:

$$d_k(n) = \frac{\langle [u_k(n) - v_k(n)]^2 \rangle}{\langle u_k^2(n) \rangle + \langle v_k^2(n) \rangle} \quad \text{Equation (13.10)}$$

Taking the difference removes the desired signal from the numerator of *Eq. (13.10)*, leaving only the interference. The denominator of *Eq. (13.10)* is the same as for *Eq. (13.7)*, and gives the signal power at the two ears. In terms of the signal and interference components, *Eq. (13.10)* can be rewritten as:

$$d_k(n) = \frac{\frac{1}{2}\left[\langle p_k^2(n) \rangle + \langle q_k^2(n) \rangle\right]}{\langle s_k^2(n) \rangle + \frac{1}{2}\left[\langle p_k^2(n) \rangle + \langle q_k^2(n) \rangle\right]} \quad \text{Equation (13.11)}$$

424 Digital Hearing Aids

The normalized signal difference thus yields the noise/(signal+noise), as opposed to the Wiener filter which gives the signal/(signal+noise).

The processing approach proposed by Kates (2004b) is designed to minimize the noise in the processed signal. A trivial solution to this problem is to set the gain in each frequency band to zero: no output means that there is no noise. Of course, there will be no signal either, which is not very useful, so to prevent this degenerate solution the problem was restated. The problem becomes: Minimize the interference power in the processed signal, subject to the constraint that the sum of the gains across the frequency bands equals the number of bands. Stated mathematically, the constraint is that:

$$\sum_{k=1}^{K} g_k(n) = K \quad \text{Equation (13.12)}$$

The constraint means that if the gain is reduced in one frequency band because it contains a large amount of interference, the gain must be increased in some other band or bands that contain more of the desired signal. The result of the constraint is that the processed signal has about the same overall intensity as the original unprocessed signal, but the emphasis has been shifted to those frequency bands that contain a preponderance of the signal from the desired source. Additional processing can be applied to reduce the overall gain if no frequency band appears to contain a preponderance of signal power.

The solution for the gains is given by:

$$g_k(n) = \frac{\dfrac{1}{d_k(n)}}{\dfrac{1}{K} \sum_{k=1}^{K} \dfrac{1}{d_k}(n)} \quad \text{Equation (13.13)}$$

This solution can be compared to the Wiener filter solution. Let $w_k(n)$ be the gains for the Wiener filter given by Eq. (13.7). The normalized signal difference can then be written as $d_k(n) = 1 - w_k(n)$. The gains given by Eq. (13.13) are proportional to the inverse of $d_k(n)$, giving

$$g_k(n) \propto \frac{1}{1-w_k(n)} \quad \text{Equation (13.14)}$$

The Wiener filter of Eq. (13.7) creates broad peaks around those frequency bands that contain the desired signal, whereas the difference solution of Eq. (13.14) creates broad valleys for those frequency regions that contain mostly interference.

The result of Eq. (13.14) is that the frequency regions having high signal gain are narrower than for the Wiener filter, providing a greater degree of noise and interference suppression. The power spectrum for a segment of speech is plotted in Figure 13-10A. The source of the speech is in front of the simulated head. The interference is stationary speech-shaped noise in a simulated diffuse sound field at a SNR of 5 dB. The gains computed for the Wiener filter of Eq. (13.7) are plotted as a function of frequency in Figure 13-10B along with the gains computed using Eq. (13.13) for the same speech segment. Both filters set the gain high in those frequency bands where the speech dominates and low in those bands where the noise dominates. However, the approach proposed by Kates (2004b) has narrower peaks and broader valleys in the gain function than the Wiener filter.

BINAURAL SPECTRAL SUBTRACTION

The spectral subtraction algorithms discussed in Chapter 10 can also be implemented binaurally. The objective of the binaural implementation is to use the interaural cross-correlation to improve the noise estimates at each ear. A block diagram of one such system (Dörbecker & Ernst, 1996) is presented in Figure 13-11. One procedure for estimating the level of the interference (Dörbecker & Ernst, 1996), assuming that it is the same at each ear, is to use:

$$\langle p_k^2(n) \rangle = \langle q_k^2(n) \rangle \approx \left[\langle u_k^2(n) \rangle \langle v_k^2(n) \rangle \right]^{1/2} - \langle u_k(n)v_k(n) \rangle$$

Equation (13.15)

The first term in the right-hand side of Eq. (13.15) gives the combined signal plus interference powers, whereas the second term gives the signal power alone. The difference then yields the estimated power in the

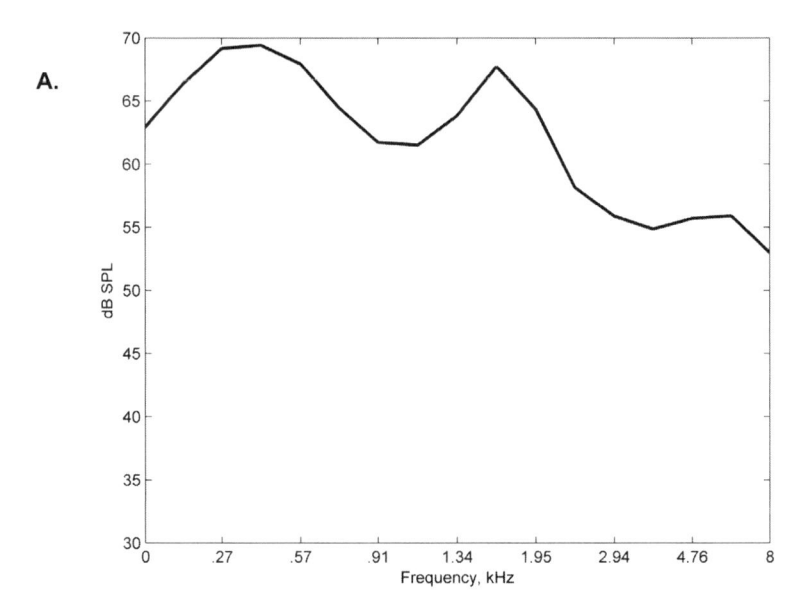

Figure 13-10. A. Spectrum for a segment of speech in diffuse speech-shaped noise at a SNR of 5 dB; and **B.** binaural gains for the segment computed using the Wiener filter and the approach of Kates (2004b).

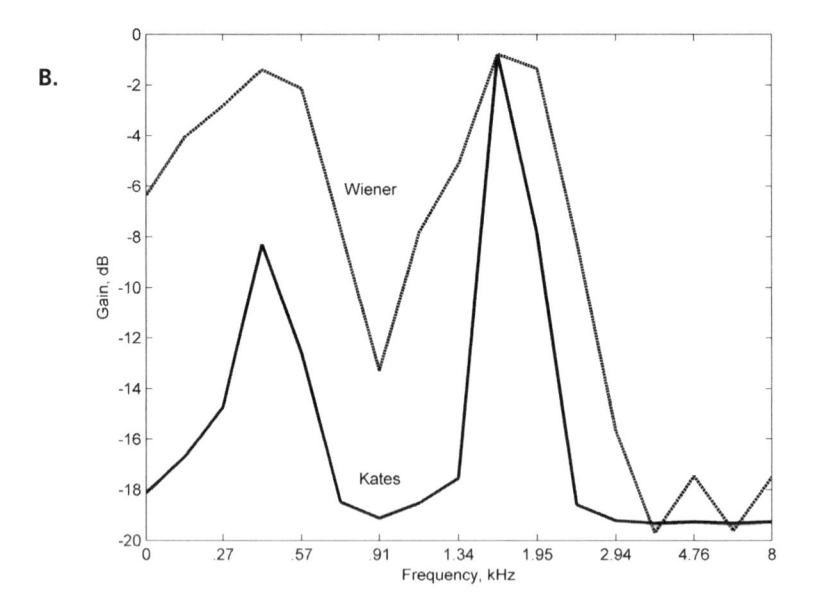

interference. A second approach is to use separate estimates of the interference power at each ear (Vary et al., 1998):

$$\langle p_k^2(n) \rangle = \langle u_k^2(n) \rangle - \langle u_k(n) v_k(n) \rangle$$
$$\langle q_k^2(n) \rangle = \langle v_k^2(n) \rangle - \langle u_k(n) v_k(n) \rangle$$

Equation (13.16)

The noise estimates using this second approach may differ at the two ears.

Given the desired signal and interference power estimates at each ear, the spectral subtraction algorithm then operates independently in the two hearing aids. As a result of the independent operation, the spectral subtraction gains at the two ears will be different. An alternative would be to average the desired signal levels and the interference levels across the two ears and to compute the spectral subtraction gain using the averaged signal powers. In this case the spectral subtraction gains would be identical at the two ears, which might of benefit in preserving interaural level difference (ILD) cues used in localization. A further advantage of averaging the desired signal and interference powers is that the averages will have lower variances than the signals at either ear alone, and the errors in estimating the signal power levels and the fluctuations in the spectral subtraction gains will be reduced.

Hamacher (2002) measured the amount of noise reduction provided by binaural spectral subtraction for a desired signal source in front of a dummy head in a crowded cafeteria. BTE hearing aids were mounted over the two ears of the dummy head. The spectral subtraction was operated in a binaural mode using the noise estimation of *Eq. (13.16)*, and was also operated independently at the two ears. The spectral subtraction algorithms were compared to a directional microphone at each ear. The measured amounts of noise suppression, averaged across the two ears, indicate that the binaural spectral subtraction processing is more effective than the independent monaural spectral subtraction. However, the directional microphones were found to be more effective than either spectral subtraction approach in suppressing the interference, and caused less distortion in the processed speech.

DIRECTIONAL CUES

Localization refers to the ability of a human observer to determine the direction from which sound arrives. The directional cues used for localization are the interaural phase or timing difference (ITD) between the

428 Digital Hearing Aids

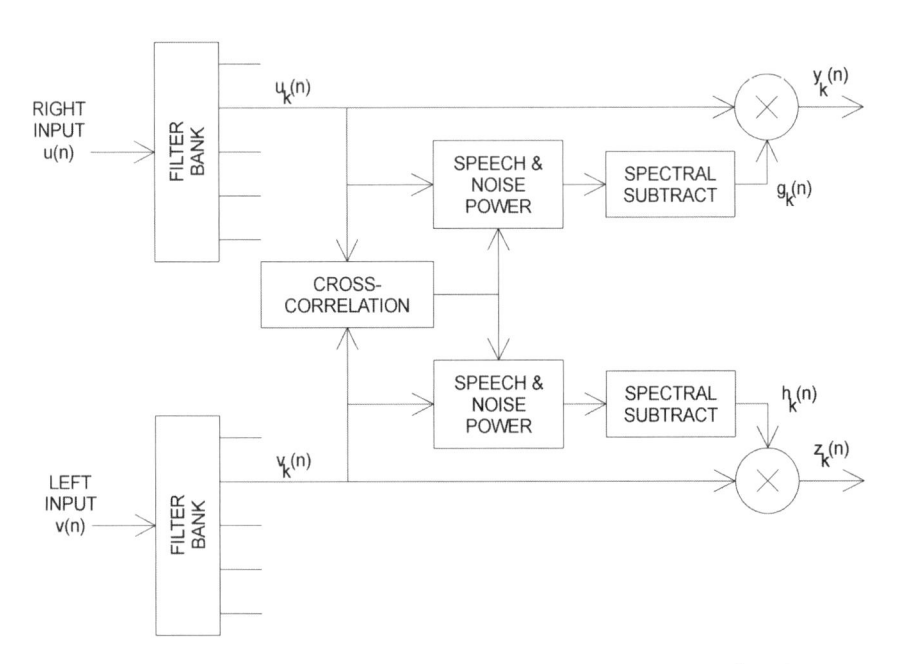

Figure 13-11. Block diagram of a binaural spectral subtraction system for adjusting the gain at the right and left ears.

signals arriving at the two ears at low frequencies, and the interaural level difference (ILD) at high frequencies (Moore, 2003). One approach to binaural noise suppression is to design digital systems that model the assumed human binaural processing. If the directional hearing cues indicate that the source of sound is in front of the listener, the gain in the frequency band is set close to 1. If the directional cues indicate that the source is located in some other direction or is diffuse, the gain in the frequency band is reduced.

An example of system that uses binaural directional cues (Kollmeier et al., 1993) is shown in Figure 13-12. The processing is performed in the frequency domain using the FFT of the signals at each ear. The autocorrelation of the two signals is used to estimate the signal power, and the cross-correlation between them is also computed. The power and cross-correlation values are used to compute the interaural coherence function (the frequency-domain version of Eq. (13.9)), the phase difference between the signals at the two ears, and the interaural level difference. The coherence, phase, and level values are then combined to produce the gain in each FFT bin. A source directly in front of the listener will have a high interaural coherence, zero degree phase difference between the left and right signals, and zero-dB level difference. This combination of signal characteristics will lead to a gain near 1 in the frequency band. A weighted combination of the three signal characteristics is used to compute a gain reduction for conditions, such as reduced coherence, increased interaural phase difference, or increased level difference, that are indicative of interference rather than the desired center-front source. Further developments of this processing strategy include probabilistic weighting of the signal characteristics (Nix & Hohmann, 2001) and weights that vary depending on the amount of interaural correlation (Hohmann et al., 2002; Wittkop & Hohmann, 2003).

Tests of an early (Kollmeier et al., 1993) version of the binaural algorithm using hearing-impaired listeners showed no benefit in intelligibility, but did indicate a preference for the sound quality of the processed stimuli when listening to sounds produced in a reverberant room. The speech was reproduced using a loudspeaker 1.5 m in front of a dummy head and the interference was noise reproduced using a single loudspeaker located 30 degrees to the left. Tests of later versions of the processing approach (Hohmann et al., 2002; Wittkop & Hohmann, 2003) using hearing-impaired listeners show statistically significant improvements in the speech reception threshold (SRT) for the processed speech in comparison with linear binaural amplification for both a single source of interference and diffuse interference for subjects tested using loudspeakers in an audiometric booth. The average improvement in SRT was about 3 dB for the diffuse noise test condition. Quality judgments for the processing under similar test conditions (Wittkop & Hohmann, 2003) show a preference for the system with the variable weights over the version of the processing that used fixed weights or the linear binaural amplification.

LOCALIZATION MODEL

Another approach is to compare the signals at the two ears by subtracting one signal from the other. Two signals that are similar will cancel, leading to a low output when the difference is taken. On the other hand, the power for two dissimilar (uncorrelated) signals will sum when one is subtracted from the other, leading to a high output. The direction of a source of sound can thus be determined by adjusting the delay and relative amplitude between the right and left ear signals so as to produce

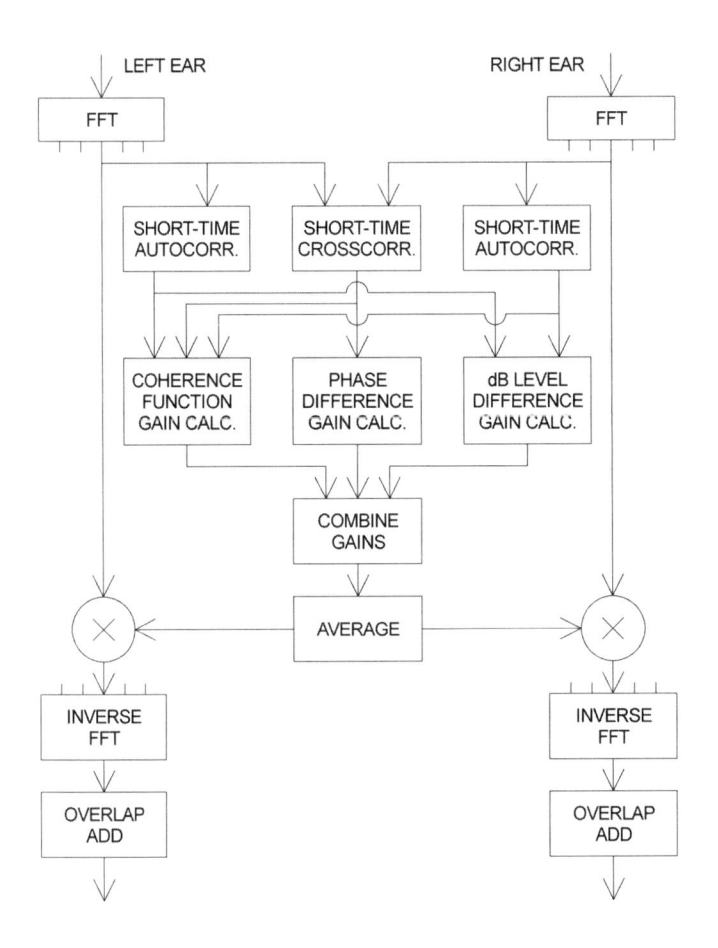

Figure 13-12. Block diagram of a binaural spatial enhancement (after Kollmeier et al., 1993).

the best degree of cancellation (Durlach, 1963; Jeffress, 1948). A system that performs this operation is shown in Figure 13-13. The right- and left-ear signals in each frequency band are compared through a cascade of delay stages. The gains are adjusted at each stage to produce the greatest possible amount of signal cancellation.

If the signal originates at the right ear, for example, the left-ear signal will need to be adjusted for the head shadow attenuation as a function of frequency. The signal arrives at the left ear later than at the right, so the right-ear signal will need to be delayed to compensate for the ITD. Thus, the maximum cancellation will occur at the end of the right-ear delay line, which is also the beginning of the left-ear delay line, and the left-ear signal will require additional amplification to give the best match to the delayed right-ear signal and the best cancellation. If the source of sound is in front of the listener, equal delays for the signals from the right and left ears will produce the best cancellation in the middle of the delay lines. The location of the delay tap at which the best cancellation occurs thus is an accurate indicator of the azimuth of the sound source.

The locations of the best cancellation can be used to indicate the azimuths of multiple sources of interference. Liu et al. (2001) and Feng et al. (2001) have designed a system in which the locations of multiple talkers can be identified by finding the best signal cancellation for each talker during the pauses in the speech from the other talkers. The cancellation delays and relative gains are then used to subtract the interfer-

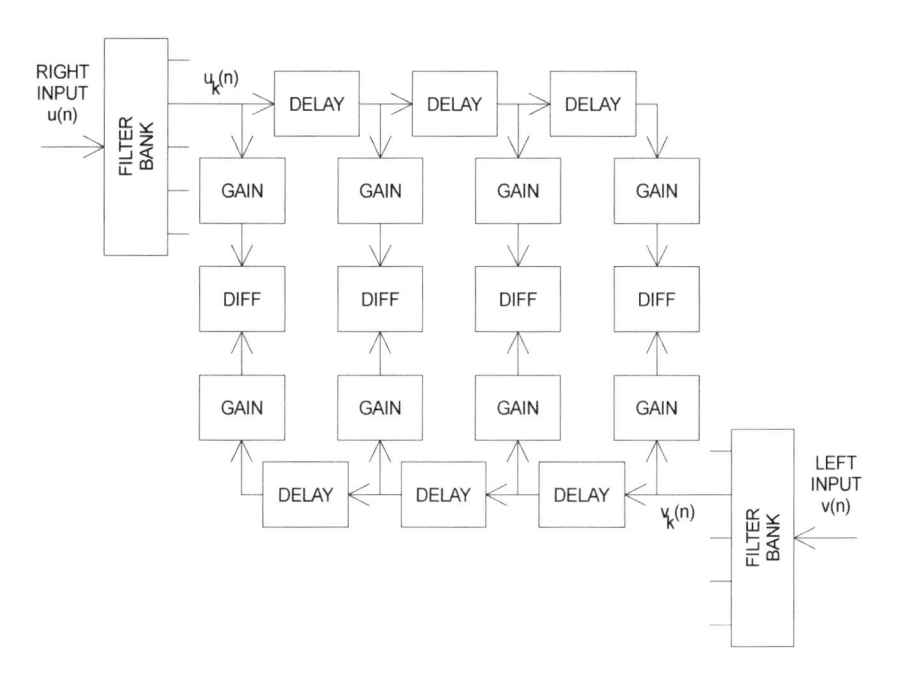

Figure 13-13. Signal-processing model showing the equalization-cancellation model of binaural interaction.

ence signal from the speech of the desired talker. The processing gives improvements in SNR of about 8 dB for four competing talkers in an anechoic chamber, and an improvement in SNR of about 6 dB in a room having a reverberation time of 400 msec.

Dichotic Band Splitting

There is ample evidence that the auditory filters are broader in impaired ears than in normal ears (see Chapter 11, Spectral Contrast Enhancement). The broader filters reduce the frequency resolution in the impaired ear, and can also modify the temporal responses and the envelopes of the filter outputs in comparison with those of the filters in a normal ear. The reduced frequency resolution means that the spectrum in the impaired ear is smeared relative to that in the normal ear and the spectral contrast is reduced. Upward spread of masking is also greater in the impaired ear, leading to reduced internal SNRs as the speech in a given frequency band is masked to a greater degree by the signals found in the lower frequency bands.

One way to reduce the upward spread of masking in the impaired ear is to move the auditory filter outputs further apart in frequency. For example, if every other frequency band were presented to the impaired ear, then the spread of masking effects would be reduced due to the increased separation between the bands; the signal in a given band would no longer be subject to masking from the signals in the two adjacent bands. Of course, reproducing only every other frequency band removes half of the spectrum, which may not be desirable. A way around this problem is to split the speech signal into auditory frequency bands using a filter bank, and then present the even-numbered bands to one ear and the odd-numbered bands to the other ear (Lunner et al., 1993). The band-splitting is diagrammed in Figure 13-14. The interleaved frequency bands, despite being presented dichotically, are perceptually integrated in the auditory cortex to form a single speech stream (Chaudari & Pandey, 1998).

Lunner et al. (1993) used a filter bank having eight bands, and presented the odd-numbered bands to one ear and the even-numbered bands to the other. Compared to diotic listening in which the same full-band signal was presented to both ears, the dichotic even-odd condition improved the SRT by an average of 2 dB for the three hearing-im-

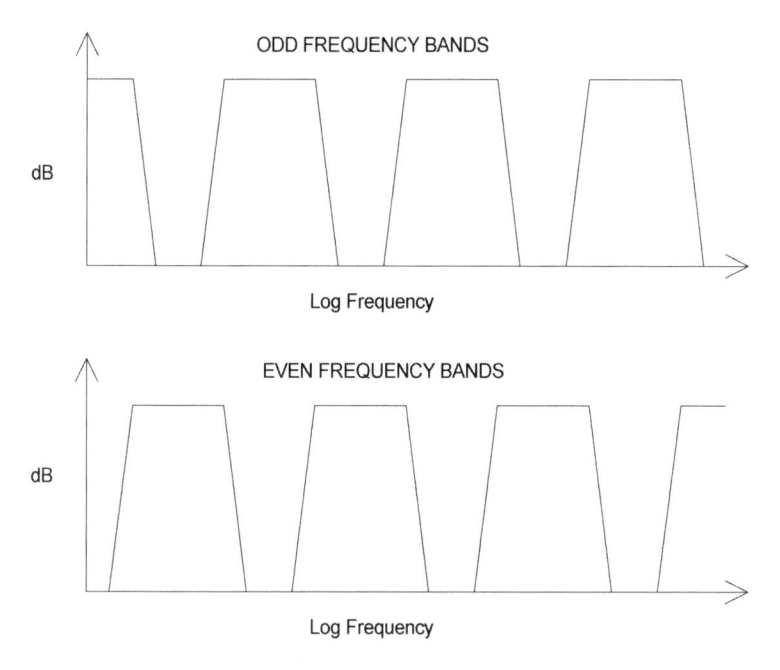

Figure 13-14. Filter structure for splitting the speech signal into alternating bands presented to each ear.

paired listeners used in the experiments. NAL-R frequency equalization was provided to compensate for the hearing loss. It made no difference whether the even-numbered bands were sent to the right ear and the odd-numbered bands to the left or if the opposite arrangement was used. Chaudhari and Pandey (1998) used a 17-band filter bank, with the band spacing approximating auditory critical bands, and tested normal-hearing listeners. They found no benefit for the dichotic even-odd presentation for isolated syllables in quiet, but found improvements in overall intelligibility and in the transmission of manner, place, and voicing speech features at the tested SNRs ranging from 6 to −3 dB for syllables in white Gaussian noise. Cheeran and Pandey (2004) tested a similar system using hearing-impaired listeners. They used phonetically balanced lists of words in quiet as the stimuli, and found an overall improvement of 31% in the number of words identified correctly for the dichotic even-odd presentation as compared to diotic full-band presentation at the two ears.

The experiments to date have compared dichotic even-odd band presentation to diotic full-band presentation of the stimuli. However, the dichotic presentation removes the binaural cues that may be used to separate speech from noise in the real world as a monaural signal is processed via the band splitting to produce the inputs to the two ears. An experiment that needs to be done is to evaluate the band-splitting approach for binaural listening. The reference condition would be full-band binaural presentation of the test stimuli in a room, with the full-band right ear signal presented to the right ear and the full-band left ear signal presented to the left ear of the listener. The test condition would then be to present the odd-numbered frequency bands of the right ear signal to the right ear and the even-numbered bands of the left ear signal to the left ear (or vice versa). The effects of the binaural band-splitting on speech intelligibility, sound quality, and localization accuracy would need to be determined for hearing-impaired listeners. Note that the band splitting will not necessarily destroy localization as there will still be overlap along the filter band edges in the two ears.

Concluding Remarks

A limiting factor in binaural processing is the data link between the hearing aids. The technology available today requires at least as much power to transmit the signals between the hearing aids as is needed for the signal processing already built into each monaural device. Various forms of data coding, such as MP3, can be applied to the signals before transmission to reduce the data rate, but increased data compression often comes at the expense of increased transmission latency. Thus, there are a large number of engineering tradeoffs that need to be considered in designing a binaural transmission link, including the data rates needed to implement a given algorithm, the transmission latency that can be tolerated, and the acceptable decrease in battery life in the hearing aid.

A compromise is to transmit processing parameters rather than the raw signals from one hearing aid to the other. The signal processing in the two hearing aids can then be synchronized rather then operating completely independently from each other. Synchronization is intuitively appealing, but the success of many years of conventional binaural fittings suggests that it may not be necessary. The benefits of interaural synchronization may be small, as was shown in the section on binaural compression.

The binaural signal processing considered in this chapter encompasses a number of different algorithms. Two procedures for binaural compression were discussed, one based on binaural loudness summation and the other based on modeling the effects of the efferent nerve fibers in the cochlea. Binaural noise suppression was introduced 30 years ago with the binaural Wiener filter, but no improvement in speech intelligibility has been demonstrated for this approach. More complex algorithms that incorporate aspects of auditory localization, however, have shown some improvement in intelligibility and in perceived sound quality. Dichotic band-splitting has also shown improvement in intelligibility under laboratory conditions, but the tests to date are incomplete and better binaural control and test conditions are needed before this approach can be recommended in a binaural fitting.

References

Allen, J. B., Berkley, D. A., & Blauert, J. (1977). Multimicrophone signal-processing technique to remove room reverberation from speech signals. *Journal of the Acoustical Society of America, 62,* 912–915.

Arsenault, M. D., & Punch, J. L. (1999). Nonsense-syllable recognition in noise using monaural and binaural listening strategies. *Journal of the Acoustical Society of America, 105,* 1821–1830.

Balfour, P. B., & Hawkins, D. B. (1992). A comparison of sound quality judgments for monaural and binaural hearing aid processed stimuli. *Ear and Hearing, 13,* 331–339.

Berlin, C. I., Hood, L. J., Hurley, A. E., Wen, H., & Kemp, D. T. (1995). Binaural noise suppresses linear click-evoked otoacoustic emissions more than ipsilateral or contralateral noise. *Hearing Research, 87,* 96–103.

Berlin, C. I., Hood, L. J., Wen, H., Szabo, P., Cecola, R. P., Rigby, P., & Jackson, D. F. (1993). Contralateral suppression of non-linear click-evoked otoacoustic emissions. *Hearing Research, 71,* 1–11.

Bloom, P. J. (1980). Evaluation of a dereverberation process by normal and impaired listeners. *Proceedings of the IEEE International Conference on Acoustics, Speech and Signal Processing* (pp. 500–503); Denver, April 9–11, 1980.

Bloom, P. J., & Cain, G. D. (1982). Evaluation of two-input dereverberation techniques. *Proceedings of the IEEE International Conference on Acoustics, Speech, and Signal Processing* (pp. 164–167); Paris, May 3–5, 1982.

Bronkhorst, A. (2000). The cocktail party phenomenon: A Review of research on speech intelligibility in multiple-talker conditions. *Acustica, 86*, 117–128.

Bronkhorst, A. W., & Plomp, R. (1988). The effect of head-induced interaural time and level differences on speech intelligibility in noise. *Journal of the Acoustical Society of America, 83*, 1508–1516.

Bronkhorst, A. W., & Plomp, R. (1989). Binaural speech intelligibility in noise for hearing-impaired listeners. *Journal of the Acoustical Society of America, 86*, 1374–1383.

Bronkhorst, A.W., & Plomp, R. (1992). Effect of multiple speechlike maskers on binaural speech recognition in normal and impaired hearing. *Journal of the Acoustical Society of America, 92*, 3132–3139.

Brown, C. P. (1996). *Modeling the elevation characteristics of the head-related impulse response.* Masters Thesis, Department of Electrical Engineering, San Diego State University.

Brown, C. P., & Duda, R.O. (1998). A structural model for binaural sound synthesis. *IEEE Transactions on Speech and Audio Processing, 6*, 476–488.

Carhart, R. (1965). Monaural and binaural discrimination against competing sentences. *International Journal of Audiology, 1*, 5–10.

Chaudhari, D. S., & Pandey, P.C. (1998). Dichotic presentation of speech signal with critical band filtering for improving speech perception. *Proceedings of the International Conference on Acoustics, Speech, and Signal Processing* (paper AE3.1), Seattle, May 12–15, 2004.

Cheeran, A. N., & Pandey, P. C. (2004). Speech processing for hearing aids for moderate bilateral sensorineural hearing loss. *Proceedings of the International Conference on Acoustics, Speech, and Signal Processing, IV* (pp. 17–20), Montreal, May 17–21, 2004.

Cherry, E. C. (1953). Some experiments on the recognition of speech with one and two ears. *Journal of the Acoustical Society of America, 25*, 975–979.

Chéry-Croze, S., Moulin, A., & Collet, L. (1993). Effect of contralateral sound stimulation on the distortion product $2f_1$-f_2 in humans: Evidence of a frequency specificity. *Hearing Research, 68*, 53–58.

Dirks, D. D., & Wilson, R. A. (1969a). The effect of spatially separated sound sources on speech intelligibility. *Journal of Speech and Hearing Research, 12*, 5–38.

Dirks, D. D., & Wilson, R. A. (1969b). Binaural hearing of speech for aided and unaided conditions. *Journal of Speech and Hearing Research, 12*, 650–664.

Dörbecker, M., & Ernst, S. (1996). Combination of two-channel spectral subtraction and adaptive Wiener post filtering for noise reduction and dereverberation. *Proceedings of EUSIPCO* (pp. 995–998); Trieste, Sept. 1996,.

Durlach, N. I. (1963). Equalization and cancellation theory of binaural masking-level differences. *Journal of the Acoustical Society of America, 35*, 1206–1218.

Ebata, M. (2003). Spatial unmasking and attention related to the cocktail party problem. *Acoustic Science and Technology, 24*, 208–219.

Feng, A. S., Lansing, C. R., Liu, C., O'Brien, W., & Wheeler, B. C. (2001). *Binaural signal processing system and method*. U.S. Patent 6 222 927, issued April 24, 2001.

Gennum Corp. (2006). *Digital wireless: Falcon™*. Specification Sheet available on-line at http://www.gennum.com/audio/hip/wireless/falcon/index.htm

Hamacher, V. (2002). Comparison of advanced monaural and binaural noise reduction algorithms for hearing aids. *Proceedings of the International Conference on Acoustics, Speech, and Signal Processing* (pp. 4008–4011), Orlando, FL, May 13–17, 2002.

Hawkins, D. B., Prosek, R. A., Walden, B. E., & Montgomery, A. A. (1987). Binaural loudness summation in the hearing impaired. *Journal of Speech, Language, and Hearing Research, 30*, 37–43.

Hawley, M. L., Litovsky, R. Y., & Culling, J. F. (2004). The benefit of binaural hearing in a cocktail party: Effect of location and type of interferer. *Journal of the Acoustical Society of America, 115*, 833–843.

Haykin, S., & Chen, Z. (2005). The cocktail party problem. *Neural Computers, 17*, 1875–1902.

Hohmann, V., Nix, J., Grimm, G., & Wittkop, T. (2002). Binaural noise reduction for hearing aids. *Proceedings of the IEEE International Conference on Acoustics, Speech, and Signal Processing* (pp. IV:4000–4003), Orlando, May 13–17, 2002.

Hood, L. J., Berlin, C. I., Hurley, A., Cecola, R. P., & Bell, B. (1996). Contralateral suppression of transient-evoked otoacoustic emissions in humans: Intensity effects. *Hearing Research, 101*, 113–118.

Jeffress, L. A. (1948). A place theory of sound localization. *Journal of Comparative Physiology and Psychology, 41*, 35–39.

Kates, J. M. (2004a). *Binaural compression system*. U.S. Patent Application 20040190734 A1, Published Sept. 30, 2004.

Kates, J. M. (2004b). *Binaural signal enhancement system*. U.S. Patent Application 20040196994 A1, Published Oct. 7, 2004.

Kates, J. M., & Arehart, K. H. (2005). Multi-channel dynamic range compression using digital frequency warping. *EURASIP Journal of Applied Signal Processing, 18*, 3003–3014.

Kollmeier, B., Gabriel, B., Nix, J., Hohmann, V., Wittkop, T., & Otten, J. (2002). *Clinical test of binaural dynamic compression schemes with hearing-impaired subjects*. Final Report, Project 200110037, Hörzentrum Oldenburg GmbH.

Kollmeier, B., Peissig, J., & Hohmann, V. (1993). Real-time multiband dynamic range compression and noise reduction for binaural hearing aids. *Journal of Rehabilitation Research and Development, 30*, 82–94.

Kuhn, G. F. (1977). Model for the interaural time differences in the azimuthal plane. *Journal of the Acoustical Society of America, 62*, 157–167.

Levitt, H., & Rabiner, L.R. (1967a). Binaural release from masking for speech and gain in intelligibility. *Journal of the Acoustical Society of America, 42*, 601–608.

Levitt, H., & Rabiner, L. R. (1967b). Predicting binaural gain in intelligibility and release from masking for speech. *Journal of the Acoustical Society of America, 42*, 820–829.

Liberman, M. C., & Kujawa, S. G. (1999). The olivocochlear system and protection from acoustic injury: Acute and chronic effects. In C. Berlin (Ed.), *The efferent auditory system: Basic science and clinical applications*. San Diego, CA: Singular Publishing Group.

Lindemann, E. (1995). Two microphone nonlinear frequency domain beamformer for hearing aid noise reduction. *Proceedings of the 1995 Workshop on Applications of Signal Processing to Audio and Acoustics*, Mohonk Mountain House, New Paltz, NY.

Lindemann, E. (1996). *Dynamic intensity beamforming system for noise reduction in a binaural hearing aid*. U.S. Patent No. 5 511 128, issued April 23, 1996.

Lindemann, E., & Melanson, J. (1997). *Noise reduction system for binaural hearing aid*. U.S. Patent No. 5 651 071, issued July 22, 1997.

Liu, C., Wheeler, B. C., O'Brien, W. D., Lansing, C. R., Bilger, R. C., Jones, D. L., & Feng, A. S. (2001). A two-microphone dual delay-line approach for extraction of a speech sound in the presence of multiple interferers. *Journal of the Acoustical Society of America, 110*, 3218–3231.

Lunner, T., Arlinger, S., & Hellgren, J. (1993). 8-channel digital filter bank for hearing aid use: Preliminary results in monaural, diotic, and dichotic modes. *Scandinavian Audiology* (Suppl. 38), 75–81.

Maison, S., Micheyl, C., & Collet, L. (1998). Contralateral frequency-modulated tones suppress transient-evoked otoacoustic emissions in humans. *Hearing Research, 117*, 114–118.

Markides, A. (1977). *Binaural hearing aids* (pp. 31–86). New York: Academic Press.

McKenzie, A. R., & Rice, C. G. (1990). Binaural hearing aids for high-frequency hearing loss. *British Journal of Audiology, 24*, 329–334.

Moore, B. C. J. (2003). Space perception. In *An introduction to the psychology of hearing* (5th ed., pp. 233–268). New York: Academic Press.

Nix, J., & Hohmann, V. (2001). Enhancing sound sources by use of binaural spatial cues. *Proceedings of the Eurospeech 2001 Workshop on Consistent and Reliable Acoustical Cues* (CRAC) (pp. 1–4); Aalborg, Sept 3–7, 2001.

van de Par, S., & Kohlrausch, A. (1999). Dependence of binaural masking level differences on center frequency, masker bandwidth, and interaural parameters. *Journal of the Acoustical Society of America, 106*, 1940–1947.

Pickles, J. O. (1988). The centrifugal pathways. *An Introduction to the physiology of hearing* (2nd ed., pp. 235–255). New York: Academic Press.

Puel, J.-L., & Rebillard, G. (1990). Effect of contralateral sound stimulation on the distortion product $2F_1$-F_2: Evidence that the medial efferent system is involved. *Journal of the Acoustical Society of America, 87*, 1630–1635.

Rafaely, B. (2000). Spatial-temporal correlation of a diffuse sound field. *Journal of the Acoustical Society of America, 107*, 3254–3258.

Schweitzer, C., Terry, M., & Grim, M. (1996). Three experimental measures of a digital beamforming signal processing algorithm. *Journal of the American Academy of Audiology, 7*, 230–239.

Shaw, E. A. G. (1974). Transformation of sound pressure level from the free field to the eardrum in the horizontal plane. *Journal of the Acoustical Society of America, 56*, 1848–1861.

Shaw, E. A. G., & Vaillancourt, M. M. (1985). Transformation of sound pressure level from the free field to the eardrum presented in numerical form. *Journal of the Acoustical Society of America, 78*, 1120–1123.

Sridhar, T. S., Liberman, M. C., Brown, M. C., & Sewell, W. F. (1995). A novel cholinergic 'slow effect' of efferent stimulation on cochlear potentials in the guinea pig. *Journal of Neuroscience, 15*, 3667–3678.

Vary, P., Heute, U., & Hess, W. (1998). *Digitale Sprachsignalverarbeitung*, Stuttgart: Teubner-Verlag.

Wittkop, T., & Hohmann, V. (2003). Strategy-selective noise reduction for binaural digital hearing aids. *Speech Communication, 39*, 111–138.

Zwicker, E., & Zwicker, U. T. (1991). Dependence of binaural loudness summation on interaural level differences, spectral distribution, and temporal distribution. *Journal of the Acoustical Society of America, 89*, 756–764.

Index

A

Adaptive multimicrophone arrays, 129–133. *See also main entry* Multimicrophone arrays
Aliasing
  distortion, 46
  temporal, 46–47
Analog to digital aids. *See main entry* Digital from analog
Analog-to-digital converter, 10–11
Anatomy, head and ear, 55
Auricle of ear, 55–56, 58, 59

B

Batteries, 14–15
Bayes classifiers, 379–381
Binaural signal processing. *See also main entry* Signal processing
  afferent neural fibers, 409
  auditory efferents, 409–410
  BILD (binaural intelligibility level difference), 403
  BMLD (binaural masking level difference), 403
  COCB (crossed olivo-cochlear bundle), 409–411, 412, 413, 414, 415, 416
  "cocktail party" problem, 402–404
  compression, binaural,
    auditory efferent use, 410–416
    efferent use, 410 416
    loudness summation use, 406–409
    using loudness summation, 406–409
  dichotic band splitting, 432–434

directional cues, 427–429
efferents, 409–410
IID (interaural intensity difference), 404
ILD (interaural level difference), 402, 427, 428
interaural cross correlation, 418–421
localization model, 429–432
loudness summation, 406, 415
MP3, 405, 434
noise suppression, 416–432 (*See also* Noise suppression, single-microphone)
OAE (otoacoustic emissions), 409
overview, 401–402, 434–435
signal difference, 423–425
signal transmission, 404–406
spectral subtraction, 425–427 (*See also main entry* Spectral subtraction)
TEOAE (transient-evoked otoacoustic emissions), 409
transmission latency, 434
Wiener filter, binaural, 421–423
wireless link, 404–405
Block processing, 40–42
Body-worn aids, 4
Brownian motion, 76
BTE (behind-the-ear) aids, 3
  acoustic resonation, 54
  A/D (analog-to-digital) converter, 53
  D/A (digital-to-analog) converter, 53
  feedback loop, 52, 54
  microphone location and head, 94–96
  microphone separation, 90

442 Index

open fitting, 4, 69–70
open fitting type, 4
overview, 4
receiver, 54
tubing, 54
venting, 52–54
and wind noise,
    airflow/turbulence, 152–155
    reduction, 165
    sound pressure, 155–157

C
CIC (completely in-the-canal) aids
    overview, 2–3
    and wind noise,
        airflow/turbulence, 150, 152
        sound pressure, 157–158
Clock, digital system, 7, 8, 13–14
Clock jitter, 14
"Cocktail party" problem, 402–404
Current drain from digital
        circuit, 7, 9, 12

D
DFT (discrete Fourier transform), 30–32
Digital circuit components, 10–14
Digital from analog aids, 4–6
    circuit complexity, 6–7
    digital complexity drain, 7–8
    Moore's law, 6–7
    overview, 4–6, 15–16
    power consumption, 8–10
    Project Phoenix, 8
Digital system concerns, 42–49
Directional microphones
    benefit, real world, 105–108
    construction, 76–78
    directional response patterns, 83–85
    DI values, 100
    frequency response, 85–93
    on head, 93–102
    illustrated, 78, 79
    and listening environment
        intelligibility, 104–105
    magnitude frequency response,
        85–90

    microphone mismatch, 85, 86, 90–91
    microphone noise, 93
    versus omnidirectional, 107–108
    overview, 75, 108–109
    PHAB (Profile of Hearing Aid
        Benefit), 106–107
    ports, 77–78
    reflections (late/early), 105–106
    spacing and time delay, 83–84
    spatial signal processing, 78–82
    vent interaction, 91–92
    wind noise reduction, 163–164
Distortion
    linear, 29
    nonlinear, 29–30
DSP (digital signal processors)
    overview, 7, 11–12
Dynamic-range compression
    algorithm design concerns, 224–226
    all-pass filters, 226, 247–254, 257, 258
    attack time, 233, 234, 235,
        236, 237, 240
    binaural, 225, 248–249
    and feedback, 229, 231
    feed-forward, 230, 232
    and FFT (fast Fourier transform),
        222, 242–247, 249–258
    frequency-domain compression,
        ideal FFT system, 242–243
        practical FFT system, 244–245
        side-branch, 246–247
    and frequency resolution, 224
    frequency warping,
        digital, 247–249
        system delay comparison, 255–258
        warped compressor
            system, 249–255
    multichannel compression,
        swept frequency response, 240–241
        temporal response, 236–239
    overshoot, 236, 237, 247
    overview, 221–222, 258–259
    peak detection, 227, 232–
        236, 237, 247
    and processing delay, 224–226
    recruitment, 221, 222

Index   **443**

release time, 223, 233, 234,
   235, 236, 237, 240, 242
single-channel compression,
   envelope detection, 231–236
   input/output rules, 227–229
   volume control, 229–231
syllabic, 222, 234, 235

E
Ear/head
   acoustic environment
      modification, 60–61
   ear canal and aid, 55
   hearing aid transfer function
      blocking (*See also* main
      entry Occlusion effect)
   helix, 55–56
   HRTF (head-related transfer
      function), 57–60
   and microphones, 59
   resonance, 55
   tragus, 55–56
Electroacoustic system
   hearing aid system, 52–54 (*See
      also* BTE (behind-the-ear)
      aids *main entry;* ITE (in-
      the-ear) aids *main entry*)
   overview, 51
Ephraim-Malah algorithm,
   307–309, 312–313
EPROM (erasable programmable
   read-only memory), 13
Equations
   adaptive gain multimicrophone
      array, 116
   adaptive gain update
      multimicrophone array, 118
   air in vent acoustic mass, 63
   amplitude modulation, 28–29
   autocorrelation, 22
   Bayes classifiers, 380
   binaural signal difference, 423–425
   binaural spectral subtraction, 425,
      427
   broadband envelope correlation
      lag/peak level, 393–394

centroids, sound classification,
   392–393
compliance (in ear canal), 63
compliance (tympanum), 63
compression cascade, spectral
   contrast modification, 346
compression gain filter (dynamic-
   range compression), 250–251
for convolution, 20–21
cross-correlations, 23
current drain from digital circuit, 7
DFT (discrete Fourier
   transform), 31–32
digital all-pass filter (dynamic-
   range compression), 248
digital frequency, 18
directional microphone low-frequency
   magnitude response, 82
directional microphone output, 80
ear canal residual air, 63
envelope valley filters, 280
feedback, 25–26
feedback, system, 177–179
feedback cancellation
   adaptation, 192–193
feedback-cancellation filter, 188–189
filtered-X algorithm, 199–201
FIR filter, 37
four-band envelope correlation
   lag/peak level, 394–395
front/rear microphone time delay, 79
IIR (infinite-impulse) filter, 34
interaural cross correlation, 419–421
linear model (feedback), 215
magnitude spectral subtraction, 304
masking, excess upward
   spread, 340–341
mean-squared signal power, 389
mel cepstrum coefficients, 390
microphone output, 79–80
microphone spacing, 83, 86–88
microphones time delay, 79–81
multiple-sample unit impulse
   sequences, 20–21
naïve Bayes classifiers, 381
neural network hidden layer, 375

444 Index

noise magnitude (spectral subtraction), 297
noise update (spectral subtraction), 296
nonlinear distortion, 215
omnidirectional microphone output, 80
omnidirectional microphone pattern/cosine sum, 84
peak detector output (single-channel compression), 232–233
power consumption, digital circuit, 7
power spectral subtraction, 303
power spectrum entropy, 393
Q (quality) of resonance, 64
quantization noise, 44–45
raising spectrum to a power, spectral contrast modification, 331–332
resonance frequency, 64
sharpening filter, spectral contrast modification, 335
signal envelope standard deviation, 389
simple spectral-enhancement filter, spectral contrast modification, 336
sinusoid sequence, 18
SNR, a posteriori/a priori (spectral subtraction), 308
spectral contrast modification, 331–332, 336, 340–341, 346
spectral subtraction, 297, 303–304, 306, 425, 427
spectral subtraction, binaural, 297, 425, 427
spectral subtraction, Ephraim-Malah algorithm, 308
spectral subtraction, general, 304
spectral subtraction, intelligibility compromise, 311
suppression gain (spectral subtraction), 306
transfer function, 24–25
U_{50} (room speech intelligibility), 104–105
unit impulse sequence, 18

valley detector output, 293–294
Wiener filters, 300–301, 303, 421–422
wind noise spatial correlation, 160–162
ZCR (zero crossing rate), 391–392

F
Feedback
acoustic, 175, 177, 179, 180, 183, 184, 206
cancellation (*See* Feedback cancellation)
mechanical, 175, 177
overview, 216
signal processing overview, 25–27
system equations, 177–179
system overview, 176–184
system response, 179–184
and venting feedback loop, 52, 54
Feedback cancellation
adaptive notch filter, 202
clamp constraint, 192, 195–196
constrained adaptation, 191–198
cost function constraint, 195–196, 197
and delay, 199
equations, system, 188–200
filtered-X algorithm, 199–203
frequency-domain adaptation, 203–205
gain-reduction solutions, 185–188, 197
interrupted adaptation, 197, 199
LMS adaptation, 190–191
nonlinear distortion, 215–216
overview, 175–176, 216–217
processing limitations, 205–216
and room reflections, 206–215
FFT (fast Fourier transform), 30, 40, 41, 43
and dynamic-range compression, 222, 242–247, 249–258
Filter banks
and filter definitions, 32–33
FIR filers, 37–40, 43
frequency analysis, 32
frequency resolution, 40

group delay, 40
IIR (infinite-impulse) filters,
    34–37, 38, 43
nonrecursive filters, 37–40
and nonrecursive filters, 37–40
Nyquist theorem, 40
recursive filters, 34–37
Wiener filters, 300–302,
    303, 312, 421–423
Filters
  auditory filters in damaged cochlea,
      320–328 (See also Spectral
      contrast enhancement)
  Butterworth, 34–35
  FIR filers, 37–40, 43
  frequency analysis, 40, 41
  high-pass, 32–33
  IIR (infinite-impulse) filter,
      34–37, 38, 43
  linear phase, 37, 38
  low-pass, 32–33
  nonrecursive, 37–40
  recursive filters, 34–37
  tapped delay line, 37
Fourier transform, 32, 40, 42,
    46–47. See also DFT (discrete
    Fourier transform); FFT
    (fast Fourier transform)
  inverse, 31–32

H
Head/ear
  acoustic environment
      modification, 60–61
  ear canal and aid, 55
  hearing aid transfer function
      blocking (See also main
      entry Occlusion effect)
  helix, 55–56
  HRTF (head-related transfer
      function), 57–60
  and microphones, 59
  tragus, 55–56
Hirsch-Ehrlicher algorithm, 300
HMMs (hidden Markov
    models), 377–379

HRTF (head-related transfer
    function), 57–60

I
ITC (in-the-canal) aids
  overview, 2–3
  wind noise,
      sound pressure, 157–158
ITE (in-the-ear) aids
  A/D (analog-to-digital) converter, 53
  cross section, 52
  D/A (digital-to-analog) converter, 53
  feedback loop, 52, 54
  hearing aid transfer function
      blocking, 59–60
  microphone separation, 90
  overview, 3
  receiver, 54
  tubing, 54
  vented, 64–65, 66
  venting, 52–54
  and wind noise, 152
      airflow/turbulence, 150

M
Memory (digital processing), 12–13
Microphones
  and AI (articulation index), 102
  arrays overview, 113–114 (See main
      entry Multimicrophone arrays)
  cardioid directional pattern, 84–85,
      88, 90–93, 93, 97–100, 108
  cosine directional pattern, 84, 100
  DI (directivity index), 99–101, 102
  dipole (figure-eight) directional
      pattern, 86, 90, 98
  directional, 75–109 (See
      main entry Directional
      microphones for details)
  directional response patterns,
      83–84, 86–88
  and ear/head, 59
  FBR (front-to-back ratio), 98–99 (See
      also SNR (signal-to-noise) ratio)
  figure-eight (dipole) directional
      pattern, 86, 90, 98

frequency response, 61–62
on head, 93–102
and head/ear, 59
hypercardioid directional pattern, 84, 86, 98, 100, 102
noise of, 93
omnidirectional, 76–77
performance indexes, 98
PHAB (Profile of Hearing Aid Benefit), 106–107
reflections (late/early), 105–106
and reverberation, 102–105 (*See also main entry* Reverberation)
and rooms, 102–105
and SII (speech intelligibility index), 102
single-microphone noise suppression, 263–287 (*See also main entry* Noise suppression, single-microphone)
UI (unidirectional index), 101–102
Moore's law, 6–7
Multimicrophone arrays
adaptive arrays, 129–133
beamwidth, 124, 126–127
benefits of, 139–142
broadside, 124–127, 134, 136–137, 141
delay-and-sum beam-forming, 123–129
endfire, 124, 125, 126–128, 129, 131–132, 134–136, 140, 142
and frequency domain, 131, 132, 139, 141, 142
Griffiths-Jim adaptive array, 136–137, 139
and main lobes, 124, 126, 128, 129, 134, 136, 137
scaled projection algorithm, 131
and sidelobes, 127, 128, 129, 133, 134
and SRT (speech reception threshold), 139–141
superdirective arrays, 133–136
two-microphone arrays, adaptive delay, 114–115
adaptive filter, 118–123
adaptive gain, 116–118
widely spaced arrays, 136–139

N
NiMH batteries, 14–15
Noise
background, 263 (*See also* Noise suppression, single-microphone)
estimation of, 293–300 (*See also* Spectral subtraction)
musical, 302, 305, 306, 307, 308, 309, 310, 315
quantization noise, 43–45
and reverberation, 104–105
speech/noise signals, 264–265
suppression, single microphone, 263–287 (*See also main entry* Noise suppression, single microphones)
suppression, single-microphone, 263–287
suppression, spectral subtraction, 291–315 (*See also main entry* Spectral subtraction)
wind noise, 147–172 (*See also main entry* Wind noise *for details*)
Noise suppression, single-microphone, 292. *See also* binaural noise suppression *under* Binaural signal processing; Spectral subtraction; Wind noise
adaptive high-pass filters, 275–276
adaptive low-pass filters, 276–277
bandwidth reduction, 274–278
envelope valley filters, 278–286
envelope valley tracking, 272–274
Gaussian noise, 266–269
low-level expansion, 270–272
noise suppression algorithms, 264–269, 281–283
overview, 263–264, 286–287
RASTA algorithm, 281–283
spectrogram analysis, 269
speech envelope, 264–268

Index 447

speech *versus* noise
  perception, 265–270
"Zeta Noise Blocker," 277–278
Nyquist frequency, 46
Nyquist theorem, 40

O
OAE (otoacoustic emissions), 409
Occlusion effect, 70
Open fitting BTE aids, 4
  overview, 4
  and venting, 69–70

P
PHAB (Profile of Hearing Aid
  Benefit), 106–107
Pinna of ear, 55–56, 58, 59
Project Phoenix, 8

R
RAM (random access memory), 13
Receivers
  frequency response, 62
Reverberation
  critical distance, 103
  and noise, 104–105
  reflections, early, 103–104
  reflections (late/early), 105–106
ROM (read-only memory), 13
Rooms
  and microphones, 102–105
  reflection and feedback, 206–215

S
Signal processing. *See also main entry*
    Binaural signal processing
  and algorithm complexity, 47–48
  and algorithm interaction, 48–49
  and aliasing distortion, 46
  amplitude modulation, 28–29
  autocorrelation, 22
  block processing, 40–42
  cascade transfer function, 24–25
  convolution, 19–22, 23
  correlation, 22–24
  cross-correlation, 22, 23

DFT (discrete Fourier
  transform), 30–32
digital system concerns, 42–49
distortion, 29–30, 46
feedback, 25–27
FFT (fast Fourier transform),
  30, 40, 41, 43
filter banks, 32–40 (*See also main
  entry* Filter banks; Filters)
filter impulse response, 19–20
Fourier transform, 32, 40, 42, 46–47
frequency analysis, 30, 32, 40, 41
frequency resolution, 40
group delay, 27–28
and integer arithmetic, 42–43
inverse Fourier transform, 31–32
linear distortion, 29
linear phase, 28, 37
linear shift invariance, 18, 19
linear time invariance, 18–19
MATLAB software, 32
minimum-phase system, 27–28
nonlinear distortion, 29–30
Nyquist frequency, 46
Nyquist theorem, 40
overlap-add technique, 41–42
parallel transfer function, 25
power of 2 FFT segment length, 32
and quantization noise, 43–45
and saturation, 43
segment length, FFT, 32
series transfer function, 25, 27
signal/system properties, 17–30
tapped delay line filtering, 37
and temporal aliasing, 46–47
transfer functions, 24–25, 26
and underflow, 43
unit impulse sequence, 18
zero/transfer function, 27
SII (speech intelligibility index), 102
SNR (signal-to-noise) ratio
  and adaptive two-microphone
    system, 114–115
  and microphones, 75, 102
Sound classification
  Bayes classifiers, 379–381

Bayes classifiers, naïve, 381
broadband envelope correlation
  lag/peak level, 393–394
centroids, 392–393
classifier algorithms, 367–382
classifier personalization, 381–382
classifier training, 368–369
classifier types, 369–370
clustering, 370–371
delta cepstrum coefficients, 390
distance metric, clustering, 370
examples of, 382–387
feature numbers, 383–385
feature selection, 361–362, 364–367
four-band envelope correlation
  lag/peak level, 394–395
generalization, 372, 374
HMMs (hidden Markov
  models), 377–379
isolated signals *versus*
  mixtures, 385–387
k-means clustering, 370
learning, supervised, 368, 372
learning, unsupervised, 369
linear discriminant, 371–372
mean-squared signal power, 389
mel cepstrum coefficients, 390, 391
mixtures *versus* isolated
  signals, 385–387
mutual information, 361–367
neural network, 374–376
  activation function, 374–375, 375
  overfitting, 376
overview, 355–356, 387–388
power spectrum entropy, 393
rationale for, 357–358
RVM (relevance vector machine), 375
saturation, 374, 375
signal envelope standard
  deviation, 389
signal features, 359–361, 388–395
SVM (support vector
  machine), 372–374
ZCR (zero crossing rate), 391–392
Spectral contrast enhancement
  and cochlea, damaged,
    neural firing patterns, 321–324
    perceptual measurements, 324–328
    physiologic measurements, 320–324
    processing strategies, 328
    tuning curves, 320–321
  with compression, 345–348
  excitation spread, 335
  f2/f1 ratio, 321–322, 323, 324,
    328, 341–342, 349–350
  formant transition, 339, 343
  and inner hair cell loss, 321, 323
  masking, excess upward
    spread, 340–341
  neural firing patterns, 321–324
  and outer hair cell loss, 321, 325
  overview, 319–320, 348–350
  principal components, speech
    intelligibility, 327
  processing comparison, 342–345
  processing interactions, 345
  raising spectrum to a power, 331–334
  sinusoidal modeling, 320, 329
  spectral contrast modification, 331–339
  spectral filtering, 334–339
  spectral valley suppression, 328–331
  suppression, spectral valley, 328–331
  tip-to-tail ratio, 320, 328, 342, 349
Spectral subtraction. *See also*
  spectural subtraction *under*
  Binaural signal processing
  algorithm effectiveness, 312–314
  attenuation floor, 305
  auditory masking, 309–311
  classical approaches, 302–304
  Ephraim-Malah algorithm,
    307–309, 312–313
  Gaussian distribution, 300, 308
  general equation, 304–306
  Hirsch-Ehrlicher algorithm, 300
  and histograms, 298–300
  and minima statistics, 294–298
  musical noise, 302, 305, 306,
    307, 308, 309, 310, 315
  noise estimation, 293–300
  nonlinear expansion, 306–307
  oversubtraction, 305, 314

overview, 291–293, 314–315
process, 302–311
SNR, a posteriori/a priori, 308
speech distortion, 311
VAD (voice activity detector), 293
valley detection, 293–294
Wiener filters, 300–302, 303, 305, 312
Speech perception, 264–270, 291–292. *See also* Noise suppression, single-microphone; Spectral subtraction
SRT (speech reception threshold) multimicrophone arrays, 139–141

T
Telephone handsets, 60–61
TEOAE (transient-evoked otoacoustic emissions), 409
Types of hearing aids
  body-worn aids, 4 (*See also* Body-worn aids *main entry*)
  BTE aids, 3, 4
  canal aids, 2–3 (*See also* CIC (completely in-the-canal) aids; ITC (in-the-canal) aids)
  ITE aids, 3 (*See also* ITE (in-the-ear) *main entry*)
  open fitting BTE aids, 4, 69–70
  overview, 1–2

V
Vent acoustics
  acoustic elements, 63–65
  feedback/system response, 179–180
  overview, 52–54, 62
  residual ear canal volume, 67–69
  and vent size, 65–67
Vents
  and directional microphones, 91–92

W
Wiener filters, 300–302, 303, 312, 421–423
Wind noise
  hearing aid measurement of,
    airflow and turbulence, 150–155
    sound pressure, 155–158
  laminar flow, 2, 3, 4
  overview, 147–148, 171–172
  reduction,
    adaptive arrays, 169–171
    correlation algorithms, 166–169
    directional microphones, 163–164
    spectrum algorithms, 165–166
    wind screens, 164–165
  signal characteristics, 158–163
  spatial correlation of, 160–163
  spectrum of, 158–159
  temporal fluctuations of, 160
  and turbulence, 148–149

Z
Zinc-air batteries, 14–15

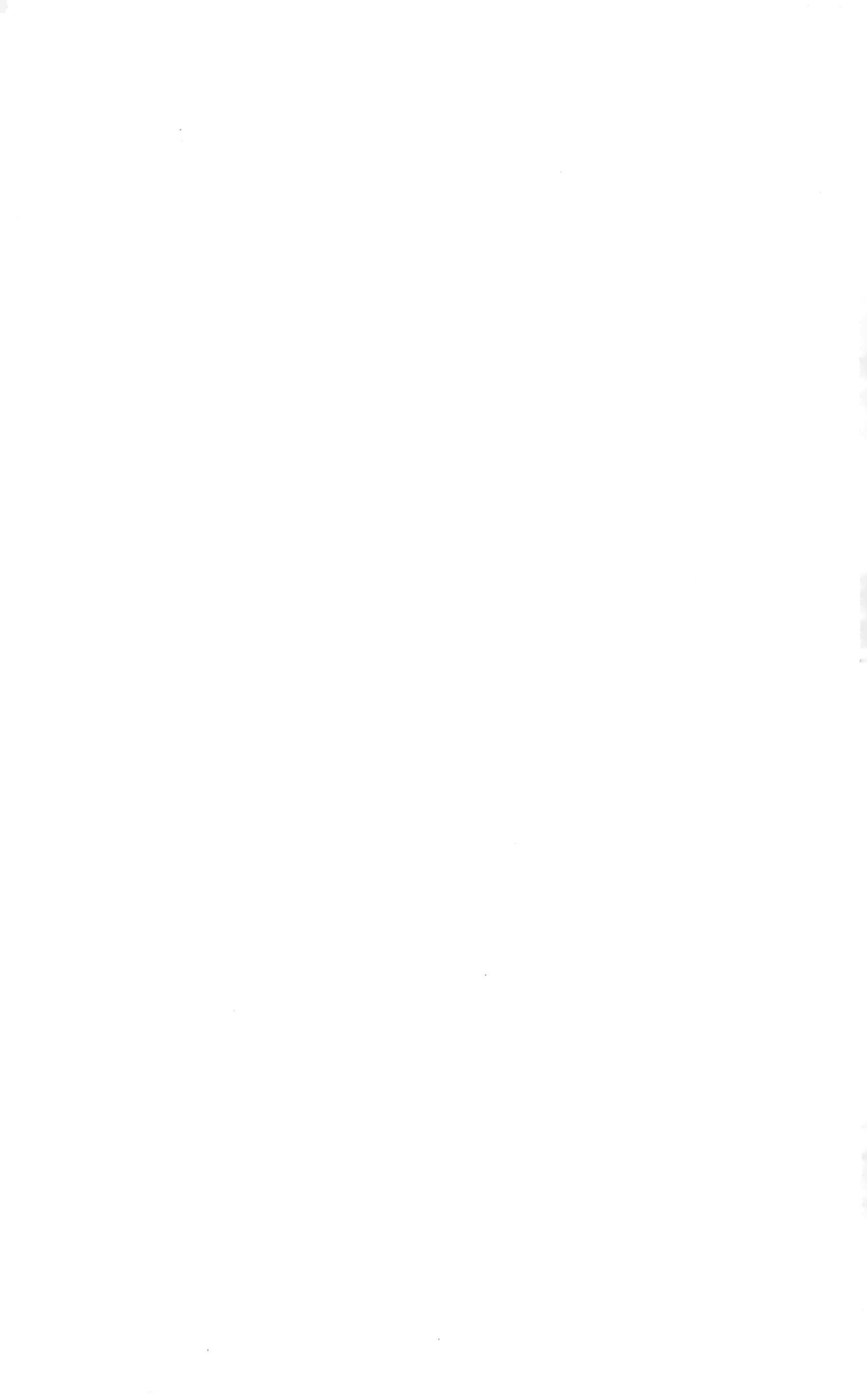